STUDENT WORKBOOK
FOR
UNDERSTANDING
MEDICAL-SURGICAL NURSING

STUDENT WORKBOOK FOR UNDERSTANDING MEDICAL-SURGICAL NURSING

PAULA D. HOPPER, MSN, RN

Associate Professor of Nursing

Jackson Community College

Case Manager on Call

W.A. Foote Memorial Hospital

Jackson, Michigan

LINDA S. WILLIAMS, MSN, RNC

Professor of Nursing

Jackson Community College

Registered Nurse

W.A. Foote Memorial Hospital

Jackson, Michigan

F.A. DAVIS COMPANY / Philadelphia

F. A. Davis Company
1915 Arch Street
Philadelphia, PA 19103
www.fadavis.com

Printed in the United States of America

Last digit indicates print number: 10 9 8 7 6 5 4

Acquisitions Editor: Lisa B. Deitch
Developmental Editors: Melanie J. Freely, Catherine Harold
Cover Designer: Louis Forgione

As new scientific information becomes available through basic and clinical research, recommended treatments and drug therapies undergo changes. The author(s) and publisher have done everything possible to make this book accurate, up to date, and in accord with accepted standards at the time of publication. The authors, editors, and publisher are not responsible for errors or omissions or for consequences from application of the book, and make no warranty, expressed or implied, in regard to the contents of the book. Any practice described in this book should be applied by the reader in accordance with professional standards of care used in regard to the unique circumstances that may apply in each situation. The reader is advised always to check product information (package inserts) for changes and new information regarding dose and contraindications before administering any drug. Caution is especially urged when using new or infrequently ordered drugs.

Preface

▶ NOTE TO THE STUDENT:

The study guide for Understanding Medical-Surgical Nursing has been written and edited by the authors to accompany the second edition of Understanding Medical-Surgical Nursing. Many of the exercises included have been used by our own licensed practical nurse/licensed vocational nurse (LPN/LVN) students. We have included exercises that will help you develop your critical thinking abilities. We feel this is an important part of understanding the material and will also help you as you prepare for the NCLEX-PN. We hope you find the materials included helpful in increasing your understanding and critical thinking abilities.

The major themes in the study guide include:

1. Chapter Checklist for Learning Success
2. Chapter vocabulary practice
3. Anatomy and physiology review
4. Chapter content-focused exercises
5. Critical Thinking practice
6. NCLEX-PN style questions with answers and rationale

The study guide is organized by chapters that correspond to textbook chapters. The information reinforced in the study guide exercises is found in the textbook. Answers are provided for all exercises.

▶ SUGGESTIONS FOR USING THE STUDY GUIDE:

Chapter Checklists for Learning Success are included at the beginning of each unit. You can use these checklists to track your study of the major topics.

A good foundation for understanding the information in the textbook is being comfortable with the medical vocabulary being used. Completing the vocabulary review will assist you in building this foundation.

Basic matching, true/false, word scrambles, and other exercises are included for all chapters to allow you to practice understanding medical-surgical nursing information in a fun way. These exercises are most helpful for developing knowledge and recall of material.

Critical Thinking exercises have been included for most chapters. We feel strongly that you must learn to think critically, rather than just memorize facts. The answers we give are just some of the possibilities. You will come up with additional answers of your own as your knowledge base expands.

NCLEX-PN style questions have been provided to give you practice in applying the knowledge you have gained. Rationale for why an answer is correct or incorrect has been included to strengthen your critical thinking abilities for test taking.

We hope you find this study guide useful. Happy studying!

PAULA HOPPER LINDA WILLIAMS

Contents

UNIT ONE

UNDERSTANDING HEALTH CARE ISSUES

CHECKLIST FOR LEARNING SUCCESS

Critical Thinking	Legal Ethical	Cultural Influences	Alternative/Complementary
☐ Problem solving	☐ Ethical obligations and nursing	☐ Terminology	☐ Terminology
☐ Role of the licensed practical nurse/licensed vocational nurse (LPN/LVN)	☐ Nursing Code of Ethics	☐ Communication styles	☐ Allopathy
	☐ Virtues	☐ Family organization	☐ Ayurveda
	☐ Rights	☐ Nutrition	☐ Chinese medicine
☐ Nursing process	☐ Building blocks of ethics	☐ Death & dying	☐ Chiropractic
☐ Data collection	☐ Ethical principles	☐ Health beliefs	☐ Homeopathy
☐ Documentation of data	☐ Ethical theories	☐ Health practitioners	☐ Naturopathy
☐ Nursing diagnosis	☐ Ethical decision-making	☐ Cultural groups	☐ Native-American medicine
☐ Plan of care	☐ Regulation of the practice of nursing		☐ Osteopathy
☐ Implementation	☐ Nursing liability and the law		☐ Herb use
☐ Evaluation	☐ Criminal and civil law		☐ Safety/effectiveness
			☐ Role of LPN/LVN

1
CRITICAL THINKING AND THE NURSING PROCESS

► VOCABULARY
Define the following terms and use them in sentences.

Auscultation _____

    Definition: _____

    Sentence: _____

Assessment _____

    Definition: _____

    Sentence: _____

Critical thinking_____

    Definition: _____

    Sentence: _____

Inspection _____

    Definition: _____

    Sentence: _____

Objective data _____

    Definition: _____

    Sentence: _____

Palpation _____

    Definition: _____

    Sentence: _____

Percussion _____

    Definition: _____

    Sentence: _____

Subjective data

    Definition: _____

    Sentence: _____

▶ SUBJECTIVE AND OBJECTIVE DATA

Identify the following data as subjective (symptom) or objective (sign).

1. Pain _____

2. Dyspnea _____

3. Edema _____

4. Capillary refill 2 seconds _____

5. Nausea _____

6. Vomiting _____

7. Dizziness_____

8. Cyanosis _____

9. Numbness _____

10. Indigestion _____

11. Pale _____

12. Serum potassium 3.6 mEq/L _____

13. Palpitations _____

14. Blood pressure 130/82 _____

15. White blood cell count 7000/mm^3 _____

▶ INSPECTION, PERCUSSION, PALPATION, AUSCULTATION

Identify the appropriate technique to assess the following.

1. _____ Bowel sounds

2. _____ Pitting edema

3. _____ Radial pulse

4. _____ Capillary refill

5. _____ Mucous membranes

6. _____ Bladder distention

7. _____ Apical pulse

8. _____ Cyanosis

9. _____ Subcutaneous crepitation

10. _____ Liver size

A. Inspection
B. Percussion
C. Palpation
D. Auscultation

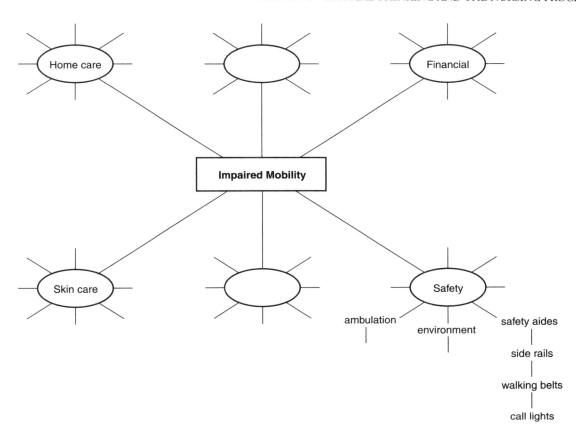

▶ CRITICAL THINKING

Make a cognitive map for a patient with impaired mobility related to multiple sclerosis. A cognitive map helps the nurse visualize the patient's needs. Think of possible needs categories of this patient and then complete possible patient needs in each category. See the example to get started.

R E V I E W   Q U E S T I O N S

Choose the best answer.

1. Which one of the following is a nursing diagnosis?
   A. Peptic ulcer
   B. Pneumonia
   C. Ineffective airway clearance
   D. Myocardial infarction

2. Which one of the following is a medical diagnosis?
   A. Hiatal hernia
   B. Impaired mobility
   C. Powerlessness
   D. Anxiety

3. During physical assessment of the abdomen the inspection, palpation, percussion, auscultation (IPPA) format order is changed to IAPP. Which of the following is the reason for this format order change?
   A. Inspection of abdomen can alter auscultation findings.
   B. Palpation of abdomen can alter auscultation findings.
   C. Auscultation can alter palpation findings of abdomen.
   D. Auscultation can alter inspection findings of abdomen.

4. The LPN/LVN is admitting a patient with diabetes. Which of the following steps in the nursing process should the nurse perform first?
   A. Implement
   B. Evaluate
   C. Collect data
   D. Set goals

5. Which of the following defines *critical thinking*?
   A. Goal-focused directed thinking
   B. Used to resolve critical situations
   C. Negative feedback about a situation
   D. Used to resolve life-threatening situations

6. The LPN/LVN is reviewing the nursing care plan of a patient with a fractured ankle. Which of the following steps in the nursing process does the nurse use to determine the effectiveness of the plan of care?
   A. Assessment
   B. Diagnosis
   C. Goal setting
   D. Evaluation

7. Which of the following is a role of the LPN/LVN in using the nursing process?
   A. Collect data
   B. Formulate nursing diagnoses
   C. Determine outcomes
   D. Plan interventions

8. The LPN/LVN is documenting patient data. Which of the following should the nurse document under objective data?
   A. No nausea
   B. Shortness of breath
   C. Strong bilateral grasps
   D. Midsternal chest pain

9. A patient is admitted with chest pain, which has been resolved. The patient states, "I hope I can live a normal life." According to Maslow's hierarchy of needs, at which of the following levels does this statement indicate the patient to be?
   A. Physiological needs
   B. Safety and security
   C. Love and belonging
   D. Self-esteem

10. A patient has a nursing diagnosis of impaired swallowing related to muscle weakness as evidenced by drooling, coughing, and choking. Which of the following outcomes is appropriate for this patient's nursing diagnosis?
    A. Improved airway clearance within 8 hours as evidenced by clear lung sounds and productive cough
    B. Baseline body weight maintained as evidenced by no weight loss
    C. Improved airway clearance within 8 hours as evidenced by reduced secretions
    D. Improved swallowing within 48 hours as evidenced by no drooling, coughing, or choking

2
ETHICAL AND LEGAL ISSUES FOR NURSES

▶ VOCABULARY
Match the following legal terms and definitions.

1. _____ Assault

2. _____ Battery

3. _____ Defamation

4. _____ False imprisonment

5. _____ Outrage

6. _____ Invasion of privacy and wrongful disclosure of confidential information

A. Unlawful touching of another

B. Unlawful conduct that places another in the immediate fear of an unlawful touching or battery; the real threat of bodily harm

C. Unlawful restriction of a person's freedom

D. Extreme and outrageous conduct by a defendant relating to the care of the patient or the body of a deceased individual

E. Wrongful injury to another's reputation or standing in a community; may be written (libel) or spoken (slander)

F. Liability when a patient's privacy is invaded physically or if records are released without authority

▶ ETHICAL AND LEGAL PRINCIPLES

1. Nurses must be _____-licensed to practice to _____ the public and maintain the _____ of health care services.

2. A _____ approach to patient care is necessary in a professional role.

3. Nursing care uses the following principles: ensuring _____ and respect, _____ confidentiality, including the patient and _____ in care explanations and decisions, respecting the patient's _____ to make care choices, and maintaining a professional relationship with the patient.

▶ VALUES CLARIFICATION
Complete the following sentences.

1. The one thing I have always wanted to do is _____.

2. If I inherited 5 million dollars, I would _____.

3. As president of the United States, I would _____.

4. If I died today, I would like my obituary to say _____.

5. If I could control the world and its destiny, I would _____.

Complete this list of things people value with items you believe should be included, then rank the value you believe each item has, with 1 being the highest value.

_____ Family   _____ Professionalism

_____ Career   ___ _____

_____ Religion   ___ _____

_____ Honor   ___ _____

_____ Material possessions   ___ _____

_____ Health   ___ _____

_____ Recreation   ___ _____

What have you learned about yourself by doing this exercise? What do the rankings signify? Can you identify yourself as more utilitarian, or more deontological? (There are no answers to this section because this is an exercise requiring personal responses.)

► CRITICAL THINKING

Read the following case study and answer the questions.

Mrs. Reo, a 5'3", 105-lb, 86-year-old retired cleaning lady, was admitted to a general medical-surgical unit in a small rural hospital. She had been diagnosed 3 months previously as having metastatic cancer that had spread from her liver to her lungs and bone marrow. She received chemotherapy and radiation therapy for several weeks, but the treatment was not effective. She was admitted to the hospital because she became too weak to walk or care for herself at home. The cancer returned, and the large doses of oral narcotic medications taken at home were having little effect on her pain while increasing her confusion and weakness.

Her oncologist decided that further chemotherapy or radiation therapy would not be effective, and she ordered Mrs. Reo to be kept comfortable with medications. A continuous morphine intravenous drip was started to help control the pain. Even with this medication, Mrs. Reo cried out in pain, particularly when morning care was given, and begged the nurses not to move her. Because she was severely underweight, the skin over her bony prominences quickly became reddened and showed the beginning signs of breakdown.

The hospital standards of care for immobile patients require that they be turned from side to side at least every 2 hours. Mrs. Reo yelled so loudly when she was turned that the nursing staff wondered if they were helping or hurting her.

To help decide what should be done, a patient care conference was called by the nurses who gave care to Mrs. Reo. The head nurse of the unit stated very clearly that the hospital standards of care required that she be turned at least every 2 hours to prevent skin breakdown, infections, and perhaps sepsis. In her already weakened condition, an infection or sepsis would most likely be fatal. Betsy, who had been a licensed practical nurse for some 15 years, disagreed with the head nurse. Her feeling was that causing this obviously terminal patient so much pain by turning her was cruel and violated her dignity as a human being. She stated that she could not stand to hear Mrs. Reo yell anymore and refused to take care of her until some other decision was made about her nursing care. Sally, a new graduate nurse, felt that the patient should have some say in her own care and that perhaps some type of compromise could be reached about turning her, perhaps turning her less frequently. Monica, a registered nurse who had worked on the unit for 2 years, felt that the physician should make the decision about turning this patient, and then the nurses should follow the order. This last suggestion was met with strong negative comments by the other nurses present. They felt that patient comfort and turning were nursing measures.

1. What are the important ethical principles in this dilemma? _____

_____

2. How does the Code of Ethics apply to this situation? _____

_____

3. What are the legal issues? _____

4. Are there ever any situations when a nurse might legally and ethically violate a standard of care? _____

_____

5. What are some other possible solutions to this dilemma? What types of consequences might they have? _____

_____

(There are no right answers to this section because this is an ethical exercise that has many choices to be considered for the best outcome for the patient. Discuss your options with classmates.)

Choose the best answer.

1. Which of the following do governments create to regulate citizen behaviors?
   A. Ethos
   B. Laws
   C. Liability limitation
   D. Contracts

2. One nurses' code of ethics states, "The nurse safeguards the patient's right to privacy by judiciously protecting information of a confidential nature." This statement is based on which of the following principles?
   A. The right to privacy is an inalienable right of all persons.
   B. The nurse-patient relationship is based on trust.
   C. A breach of confidentiality may expose the nurse to liability.
   D. Nurses know what is best for patients' health care.

3. The ethical principle that the primary goal of health care and nursing is to do good for others is called which of the following?
   A. Autonomy
   B. Fidelity
   C. Beneficence
   D. Veracity

4. The ethical principle of nonmaleficence is defined as which of the following?
   A. Health care workers avoiding harm to patients
   B. Telling the truth to patients in all matters
   C. Being faithful to commitments made to patients
   D. The right of self-determination of patients

5. Which of the following is the term used to describe an ethical situation that arises in which there is a choice between two equally unfavorable alternatives?
   A. A tort
   B. Ethical antagonism
   C. Contraindication
   D. Ethical dilemma

6. Which of the following is the first step in the ethical decision-making process?
   A. Analyze the alternatives.
   B. Gather and verify the information.
   C. Consider the consequences of the actions.
   D. Make a decision.

7. Ethical dilemmas most often involve which of the following situations?
   A. A conflict of basic human rights
   B. Violations of the Nurses' Code of Ethics
   C. Nurses who do not understand the ethical code
   D. Patients who wish to die

8. When applying the ethical principle of autonomy to patient care, the nurse should understand that which of the following is applicable to autonomy?
   A. Autonomy is an absolute principle that has no exceptions.
   B. Only patients who are awake and oriented have the right to autonomy.
   C. Under certain conditions, autonomy can be limited.
   D. Autonomy is the same as the principle of nonmaleficence.

9. A patient asks the nurse why he is taking a new medication. The nurse tells the patient that the medication will help him feel better, and not to worry about it. The nurse's response demonstrates which of the following conditions?
   A. Therapeutic communication
   B. Paternalism
   C. Lack of knowledge
   D. Legal obligations

10. The nurse attempts to apply the standard of best interest to a patient who has had a cardiac arrest and is now unconscious. Which of the following conditions is the most important factor for the nurse to consider?
    A. The patient's wishes as expressed before he became unconscious
    B. The family's wishes now that the patient can no longer communicate
    C. The patient's chances for survival after the cardiac arrest
    D. The physician's orders regarding future arrest situations

11. Which of the following punishments distinguishes criminal liability from civil liability?
    A. Personal liability
    B. Financial recovery
    C. Loss of license
    D. Potential loss of freedom

12. Which of the following is an unintentional tort?
    A. Negligence
    B. Outrage
    C. Assault
    D. Privacy invasion

13. The nurse is administering medication to a patient who has tuberculosis. The patient refuses the medication. The nurse understands that which of the following is true regarding the patient's autonomous rights?
    A. Patients can refuse any or all treatments.
    B. Patient's Self-Determination Act guarantees the right to refuse all treatments.
    C. Legal systems can force patients to take medication for contagious diseases.
    D. Health care systems cannot force patients to take medications for contagious diseases.

3
CULTURAL INFLUENCES ON NURSING CARE

▶ VOCABULARY
Match the words on the left with the definitions on the right.

1. _____ Belief
2. _____ Cultural awareness
3. _____ Cultural competence
4. _____ Ethnic
5. _____ Ethnocentrism
6. _____ Generalization
7. _____ Stereotype
8. _____ Value
9. _____ Worldview
10. _____ Custom
11. _____ Religious affiliation
12. _____ Sexual orientation

A. A usual way of acting in a given situation
B. Accepted as true, need not be proven
C. Focuses on history and ancestry
D. Belief that "my way is the only right way"
E. An assumption that needs validation
F. An opinion or belief about someone from an ethnic group
G. Belonging to a subgroup of a larger cultural group
H. Way a person perceives the universe
I. Having knowledge and skills about another culture
J. A principle or belief that has worth to an individual or group
K. Primary characteristics of culture
L. Secondary characteristics of culture

▶ CULTURAL CHARACTERISTICS
Answer the following questions. Discuss with a classmate.

1. What are some examples of primary characteristics of culture? _____

_____

_____

2. What are some examples of secondary characteristics of culture? _____

_____

_____

3. What is meant by traditional health care practitioners? Give an example. _____

_____

_____

4. What are some characteristics of people who are primarily present oriented? Past oriented? Future oriented? _____

_____

_____

► CRITICAL THINKING: IMMIGRANTS

There are no right or wrong answers to the following questions. Share your thoughts with your classmates.

1. Are immigrants taking away from the United States, or are they adding to its richness? Give specific examples and share your reasons for your position. _____

_____

_____

2. Identify difficulties that new immigrants must overcome in the United States. How might you, as a nurse, help immigrants overcome these difficulties? _____

_____

_____

► PERSONAL INSIGHTS

Answer the following questions. Consider how people from other cultures might answer differently.

1. What do you personally do to prevent illness? _____

_____

_____

2. What home remedies do you use when you have a minor illness such as a cold or flu? Do you use over-the-counter medications to treat yourself? How might these over-the-counter medicines cause a problem with prescription medications? ____

_____

_____

3. What significance does food have to you besides satisfying hunger? _____

_____

_____

4. Are you usually on time for social events? For appointments? Why or why not? _____

_____

_____

► CRITICAL THINKING: BATHING

Read the following case study and answer the questions.

An elderly male Arab-American patient refuses to be bathed by a female nurse's aide. He has not been bathed for 3 days, and today he really needs a bath. His family is at his bedside.

1. Why do you think he is refusing his bath? _____

_____

_____

2. What alternatives do you have? _____

_____

_____

3. What is the best solution to the problem? _____

_____

_____

Choose the best answer.

1. A 26-year-old Pueblo Native-American mother arrives at the health clinic to receive treatment for a laceration on her leg. Accompanying her are her two children, who missed their immunization appointments last month because she did not have transportation. As the clinic nurse, what is the best approach to ensure that the children get their immunizations?
    A. Give the immunizations today.
    B. Reschedule the appointment for next month at the regular hours for the immunization clinic.
    C. Reschedule the immunizations when she returns to have her stitches removed.
    D. Ask the community health nurse to go to the home to give the immunizations.

2. Your Guatemalan patient died after a cardiac arrest. His wife is uncontrollably wailing and shouting "Vaya con dios," and is lying on the floor shaking. What action should the nurse take?
    A. Call a cardiac arrest team.
    B. Immediately call for a stretcher and get her off the floor.
    C. Calmly remain beside her and talk to her.
    D. Call the house physician to order a tranquilizer.

3. A Laotian child is brought to the emergency department by the school nurse. She wants the child examined for the possibility of child abuse because he has several circular ecchymotic areas 2 inches in diameter on his back. What action should the intake nurse perform?
    A. Call the child welfare authorities to intervene.
    B. Explain to the school nurse that the bruised areas are consistent with the traditional Chinese practice of cupping. The areas are painless and harmless unless the skin is broken, increasing the chance for infection.
    C. Inform the child's mother that he is in the emergency department.
    D. Report the school nurse for not getting consent from the mother to bring the child to the emergency department.

4. A 42-year-old Arab-American patient has chronic renal failure. He asks the nurse where he can purchase a kidney for transplantation. Which response is best?
    A. Organs cannot be purchased in the United States.
    B. Explain the ethical dilemma in purchasing organs.
    C. Call the hospital administrator.
    D. Give him the area organ procurement telephone number.

5. A 12-year-old child from a traditional Korean-American family is newly diagnosed with diabetes mellitus. His home health nurse is to teach the patient and family diabetic care. Both parents and the child can administer his insulin and recite the signs and symptoms of hypoglycemia and hyperglycemia. They are highly educated and read and speak English well. Which is the best first step in teaching them about a diabetic diet?
    A. Give them a food exchange list for a diabetic diet.
    B. Determine whether they can calculate calories in a sample meal.
    C. Assess dietary food practices.
    D. Have them make an appointment with the consulting dietitian.

6. A 46-year-old Cuban-American high school teacher has been admitted for cancer of the breast. She wants her religious counselor, a Santero, to visit. Which action should the nurse take?
    A. Ask your nursing supervisor to see if it is permitted.
    B. Tell her Santeros are not permitted in the hospital.
    C. Suggest that she see a priest instead.
    D. Tell her it is okay, but the Santero cannot perform animal sacrifice in the hospital for safety reasons.

7. A 62-year-old Peruvian woman is in the operating room having bypass surgery. Eighteen to twenty family members arrive on the unit and wait in her room, which is shared by two other patients. Which is the best solution to this problem?
    A. Allow two family members to wait in the room and send the rest of them to the cafeteria.
    B. Send all of them to the lobby and tell them you will get them when the patient returns to her room.
    C. Allow only her husband and elderly mother to visit.
    D. Assign the patient to a private room and allow the family to wait there.

8. A 42-year-old Appalachian patient is 40 pounds overweight. She admits to baking pies with lard and frying in bacon grease, practices she does not wish to stop. The home health nurse should encourage her to do which of the following?
    A. Do not purchase lard.
    B. Reduce the portion size when she cuts her pies.
    C. Bake two separate pies, one for her and one for her family.
    D. Continue baking with lard, but reduce calories she receives from other foods in her diet.

9. A 41-year-old Appalachian woman has had a mastectomy for cancer of the breast. Her physician recommends radiation therapy. She says, "What is the use? My life is in God's hands anyway." Which of the following responses is appropriate?
   A. Agree with her, but tell her she must go with the radiation or she will die.
   B. Explain that sometimes God wants a person to help himself or herself in addition to His help.
   C. Tell her to think about radiation because the nurse is sure she will give in to it.
   D. Have her ask her physician to give her chemotherapy instead of radiation therapy.

10. A 72-year-old Iranian patient refuses his morning antibiotic, which is scheduled every 8 hours, because he is celebrating Ramadan and has to fast from sun-up to sundown. Which of the following actions should the nurse take?
    A. Explain that the medicine must be taken now to maintain the blood level.
    B. Rearrange his medication schedule so he can take all his medicines between sundown and sun-up.
    C. Omit the medicine and record his refusal on the medication administration record.
    D. Ask his family to encourage him to take the medicine.

4

ALTERNATIVE AND COMPLEMENTARY THERAPIES

▶ VOCABULARY

Match the term with the appropriate definition or statement.

1. _____ Alternative therapy

2. _____ Complementary therapy

3. _____ Homeopathy

4. _____ Naturopathy

5. _____ Ayurvedic

6. _____ Chiropractic

A. Illness is falling out of balance with nature
B. Uses nutrition, herbs, and hydrotherapy
C. Illness is a result of nerve dysfunction
D. Added to a conventional therapy
E. Unconventional therapy
F. "Like cures like"

▶ COMPLEMENTARY THERAPY: PROGRESSIVE MUSCLE RELAXATION

Describe the purpose of progressive muscle relaxation. Write a teaching plan on how to do progressive muscle relaxation. Try teaching it to a family member or friend.

Purpose: _____

_____

_____

Teaching Plan: _____

_____

_____

▶ CRITICAL THINKING

Mrs. Lawless is admitted to your unit with heart failure and fluid overload. As you collect admission data, you find that she is taking feverfew and capsaicin regularly in addition to her prescribed medications for heart failure. When you question her, she says that the salesperson at the health food store told her these herbs were safe to use with her other medications.

1. What is feverfew used for? _____

2. What is capsaicin used for? _____

3. Where can you get information about the safety of taking these herbs with heart failure or with heart failure medications?

_____

4. What should you tell Mrs. Lawless? _____

REVIEW QUESTIONS

Choose the best answer.

1. Which of the following would be considered a complementary therapy?
   A. Using both inhalers and oral medications for asthma
   B. Participating in a cardiac rehabilitation program after having a heart attack
   C. Using echinacea instead of antibiotics for an upper respiratory infection
   D. Using progressive muscle relaxation in addition to muscle relaxants for back pain

2. Which of the following would be considered an alternative therapy?
   A. Using hydrotherapy in place of nonsteroidal anti-inflammatory drugs for arthritis
   B. Visiting a spiritual healer in addition to chemotherapy for cancer treatment
   C. Using antibiotics and bronchodilators for acute bronchitis
   D. Using aspirin for a headache

3. Which of the following statements would indicate to the nurse that the patient needs additional teaching on the use of guided imagery?
   A. "I will focus on my breathing."
   B. "I imagine the ocean, including the smell, the sound, and the feel of the air."
   C. "I will relax all parts of my body."
   D. "I will keep my eyes open until the exercise is complete."

4. Which of the following terms describes traditional western medicine?
   A. Homeopathy
   B. Naturopathy
   C. Allopathy
   D. Ayurveda

5. A 47-year-old woman tells her nurse that her chiropractor is going to do minor surgery to remove a small superficial lump on her neck. Which response by the nurse is best?
   A. "The lump is probably pressing against a nerve; that is why it needs to be removed."
   B. "You need to question your chiropractor's qualifications. Chiropractors do not perform surgery."
   C. "Chiropractors specialize in nerve function; removing the lump will restore normal nerve function."
   D. "Surgery might not be necessary; usually a simple chiropractic adjustment will relieve pressure on a nerve."

6. Which of the following herbal remedies might be effective against viruses and colds?
   A. Echinacea
   B. Feverfew
   C. Chamomile
   D. Ginger

7. A client admitted with chronic pain says he is interested in pursuing an alternative therapy for his pain, but he is unsure how to determine whether it is safe. Which of the following responses by the nurse is best?
   A. "As long as the therapy does not include medication, it should be safe."
   B. "You should talk with your primary care practitioner before trying anything new."
   C. "Be careful, because most alternative therapies have dangerous side effects."
   D. "Traditional analgesics are always the safest bet for chronic pain."

8. A nurse is interested in providing therapeutic touch therapy for her home care patient with severe pain. This will be her first experience with therapeutic touch. Which of the following steps is least appropriate before beginning to provide this new service?
   A. Obtain permission from the patient's physician and home care agency.
   B. Take classes on how to administer therapeutic touch.
   C. Tell the patient he will be able to reduce the number of medications he takes.
   D. Read current research on the use of therapeutic touch.

UNIT TWO

UNDERSTANDING HEALTH AND ILLNESS

CHECKLIST FOR LEARNING SUCCESS

Fluid, Electrolyte, and Acid-base Balance and Imbalance	Nursing Care of Patients Receiving Intravenous Therapy	Nursing Care of Patients with Infections	Nursing Care of Patients in Shock	Nursing Care of Patients in Pain	Nursing Care of Patients with Cancer	Nursing of Patients Having Surgery	Nursing Care of Patients with Emergent Conditions
☐ Fluid balance	☐ Indications for intravenous (IV) therapy	☐ Infectious process	☐ Pathophysiology of shock	☐ Mechanisms of pain transmission	☐ Review of normal anatomy and physiology	☐ Surgery urgency/purpose	☐ Primary survey
☐ Dehydration	☐ IV access	☐ Body's defense mechanisms	☐ Complications from shock	☐ Types of pain	☐ Cancer classification	☐ Preoperative phase	☐ Secondary survey
☐ Fluid overload	☐ Venipuncture steps	☐ Infectious disease	☐ Hypovolemic shock	☐ Nonopioid analgesics	☐ Risk factors for cancer	☐ Preoperative assessment/ admission	☐ Shock
☐ Electrolyte balance	☐ Types of infusions	☐ Community infection control	☐ Cardiogenic shock	☐ Opioid analgesics	☐ Diagnostic tests	☐ Nursing process: Preoperative	☐ Anaphylaxis
☐ Sodium imbalances	☐ Methods of infusion	☐ Bioterrorism	☐ Obstructive shock	☐ Adjuvants	☐ Staging and grading	☐ Intraoperative phase	☐ Major trauma
☐ Potassium imbalances	☐ Types of fluids (tonicity)	☐ Health care agency infection control	☐ Distributive shock	☐ Routes for analgesic administration	☐ Surgery	☐ Postoperative nursing process	☐ Hypothermia
☐ Calcium imbalances	☐ Complications of IV therapy	☐ Antibiotic-resistant infections	☐ Medical-surgical management of shock	☐ Nondrug therapies	☐ Radiation therapy	☐ Postanesthesia Care Unit (PACU)	☐ Frostbite
☐ Magnesium imbalances	☐ Central catheters	☐ Infectious diseases treatment	☐ Nursing process	☐ Pain assessment	☐ Chemotherapy	☐ Respiratory	☐ Hyper-thermia
☐ Acid-base balance	☐ Nutrition support	☐ Nursing process for infection		☐ Patient education	☐ Side effects of therapies	☐ Circulatory	☐ Poisoning and drug overdose
☐ Respiratory acidosis					☐ Nursing care of patients with cancer	☐ Pain	☐ Near-drowning
☐ Metabolic acidosis					☐ Hospice care	☐ Urinary	☐ Psychiatric emergencies
☐ Respiratory alkalosis					☐ Superior vena cava syndrome	☐ Wound care	☐ Disaster response
☐ Metabolic alkalosis					☐ Spinal cord compression	☐ Gastrointestinal (GI)	
					☐ Hypercalcemia	☐ Mobility	
					☐ Pericardial effusion	☐ Patient discharge	
					☐ Disseminated intravascular coagulation (DIC)	☐ Home health care	

5

NURSING CARE OF PATIENTS WITH FLUID, ELECTROLYTE, AND ACID-BASE IMBALANCES

► VOCABULARY
Fill in the blanks with key words from the chapter.

1. The process by which a solute moves across a membrane from an area of higher to an area of lower concentration is

   _____.

2. A fluid that has the same osmolarity as blood is said to be _____.

3. A fluid that has a higher osmolarity than blood is said to be _____.

4. A decrease in blood volume is called _____.

5. Electrolytes in the blood that have a positive charge are called _____.

6. The patient with an excess of sodium in the blood has _____.

7. The patient with not enough potassium in the blood has _____.

8. The patient with not enough calcium in the blood has _____.

9. _____ occurs when the serum pH falls below 7.35.

10. If the pH is too high, the condition is called _____.

► DEHYDRATION
Circle the errors in the following paragraph and write the correct information in the space provided.

   Mrs. White is a 78-year-old woman admitted to the hospital with a diagnosis of severe dehydration. The licensed practical nurse/licensed vocational nurse (LPN/LVN) assigned to Mrs. White is asked to collect data related to fluid status. The LPN expects Mrs. White's blood pressure to be elevated because of the shift of fluid from tissues to her bloodstream. The nurse also finds Mrs. White's skin to be taut and firm, and she notes that the urine is copious and dark amber. She asks Mrs. White if she knows where she is and what day it is because she knows that severe dehydration may cause confusion. In addition, she initiates intake and output measurements because this is the most accurate way to monitor fluid balance.

► ELECTROLYTE IMBALANCES

Match the electrolyte imbalance with its signs and symptoms.

1. _____ Hyponatremia

2. _____ Hyperkalemia

3. _____ Hypokalemia

4. _____ Hypercalcemia

5. _____ Hypocalcemia

A. Osteoporosis, hyperactive reflexes
B. Muscle weakness, weak pulse
C. Muscle weakness, impaired clotting
D. Fluid balance and mental status changes
E. Muscle cramps, irregular heart rate

► CRITICAL THINKING

Read the following case study and answer the questions.

Mr. James is an 89-year-old gentleman admitted to your unit with worsening chronic bronchitis. On admission he is short of breath, but he is able to walk to the bathroom without difficulty. The physician orders bronchodilators, antibiotics, and an intravenous infusion of normal saline at 150 mL per hour. The next day when you return to work, you find Mr. James gasping for breath, coughing, and panicky. You quickly listen to his lungs and hear an increase in moist crackles since yesterday.

1. What additional data do you collect to confirm your suspicion of fluid overload? _____

_____

_____

2. You report your findings to the registered nurse (RN) and collaborate on quickly developing a nursing diagnosis of fluid overload. What factors contributed to this problem? _____

_____

_____

3. The RN pages the physician while you return to check on the patient. What nursing interventions can help until orders are received? _____

_____

_____

4. How will you know when the problem has been resolved? _____

_____

_____

REVIEW QUESTIONS

Choose the best answer.

1. Which of the following intravenous solutions is hypotonic?
   A. Normal saline
   B. 0.45% saline
   C. Ringer's lactate
   D. 5% dextrose in normal saline

2. Which of the following hormones retains sodium in the body?
   A. Antidiuretic hormone
   B. Thyroid hormone
   C. Aldosterone
   D. Insulin

3. Which patient is most at risk for fluid volume overload?
   A. The 40-year-old with meningitis
   B. The 35-year-old with kidney failure
   C. The 60-year-old with psoriasis
   D. The 2-year-old with influenza

4. Which patient should be monitored most closely for dehydration?
   A. The 50-year-old with an ileostomy
   B. The 19-year-old with chronic asthma
   C. The 72-year-old with diabetes mellitus
   D. The 28-year-old with a broken femur

5. Which food should be avoided by the patient on a low-sodium diet?
    A. Apples
    B. Cottage cheese
    C. Chicken
    D. Broccoli

6. Which food is recommended for the patient who must increase intake of potassium?
    A. Bread
    B. Egg
    C. Potato
    D. Cereal

7. Which is the most reliable method for monitoring fluid balance?
    A. Daily intake and output
    B. Daily weight
    C. Vital signs
    D. Skin turgor

8. An elderly nursing home resident who has always been alert and oriented is now showing signs of dehydration and has become confused. Which electrolyte imbalance is most likely involved?
    A. Hyponatremia
    B. Hyperkalemia
    C. Hypercalcemia
    D. Hypomagnesemia

9. Which nursing action is most appropriate for the weak patient with hypocalcemia?
    A. Maintain bed rest.
    B. Encourage fluids.
    C. Ambulate with assistance.
    D. Provide a high-protein diet.

10. Which organ(s) is/are most at risk for dysfunction in a patient with a potassium level is 6.2 mEq/L?
    A. Lungs
    B. Kidneys
    C. Liver
    D. Heart

11. A 19-year-old student develops symptoms of respiratory alkalosis related to an anxiety attack. Which nursing intervention is appropriate?
    A. Make sure his oxygen is being administered as ordered.
    B. Have him breathe into a paper bag.
    C. Place him in a semi-Fowler's position.
    D. Have him do coughing and deep breathing exercises.

12. A patient has chronic respiratory acidosis related to long-standing lung disease. Which of the following problems is the cause?
    A. Hyperventilation
    B. Hypoventilation
    C. Loss of acid by kidneys
    D. Loss of base by kidneys

6

NURSING CARE OF PATIENTS RECEIVING INTRAVENOUS THERAPY

▶ VOCABULARY
Match the following words to their definitions.

1. _____ Intravenous (IV)

2. _____ Cannula

3. _____ Venipuncture

4. _____ Bolus

5. _____ Peripherally inserted central catheter (PICC)

6. _____ Central line

7. _____ Phlebitis

8. _____ Infiltration

A. Inserting a needle into a vein
B. Seepage of IV fluid into tissues
C. Catheter inserted into a centrally located vein with the tip residing in the vena cava
D. Inflammation of a vein
E. Access device inserted into a superficial peripheral vein and advanced into the central system (usually the superior vena cava)
F. An IV needle or catheter
G. Volume of medication injected into a vein
H. Inside the vein

▶ PERIPHERAL VEINS
Label the veins that can be used for IV therapy.

▶ COMPLICATIONS OF IV THERAPY

Fill in the blank with the correct complication.

1. Pain and inflammation at the IV insertion site is called _____.

2. Redness and exudate at the IV insertion site indicate presence of _____.

3. Infiltration of tissue by a vesicant drug is called _____.

4. Dyspnea and crackles can be a sign of _____.

5. A cool, puffy insertion site indicates _____.

6. Fever, chills, and tachycardia indicate a systemic infection called _____.

7. Bloody sputum, chest pain, and a feeling of panic might be present if a _____ _____ has occurred.

8. If the patient develops cyanosis, hypotension, and loss of consciousness, the nurse should suspect _____ _____.

▶ CRITICAL THINKING

Read the following case study and answer the questions.

Mr. Livesay is admitted with cellulitis and is receiving IV fluids by gravity drip. When you check his IV, you find it is not dripping. What assessment can you do to determine the cause of the problem? What is the role of the licensed practical nurse (LPN)? When must the registered nurse (RN) be consulted?

_____

_____

_____

▶ CALCULATION PRACTICE

Calculate the answers to the following problems. (Note: The RN is generally accountable for administering IV fluids and medications. However, it is wise for the LPN/LVN to be aware of how to calculate IV flow rates for patients whose care is delegated to him or her.)

1. June has an IV of 5% dextrose and water to run at 83 mL/hr. How many drops per minute should be set if the tubing delivers 15 drops per milliliter? _____

2. Frank has a piggyback antibiotic of 500 mg in 50 mL of 5% dextrose and water. The medication must infuse over 20 minutes. The tubing drip factor is 10. How many drops per minute? _____

3. Dave has an IV of normal saline ordered at 1 L over 12 hours. How many milliliters per hour should he receive? _____

_____

4. Lucy has an order to administer 800 units of heparin per hour. You have heparin 50,000 units in 500 mL of D5W. You will run it on a controller. How many milliliters should be administered per hour? _____

5. Jack has an order for 1000 mL of normal saline over 24 hours. You use minidrip tubing. How many drops should be administered per minute? _____

Choose the best answer.

1. Which document guides the practice of IV therapy?
   A. Intravenous Standards of Practice
   B. Nurses' Code of Ethics
   C. Intravenous Nursing Society's Mission Statement
   D. American Nurses Association Standards of Medical Surgical Practice

2. The physician orders furosemide (Lasix) 40 mg IV stat for an acutely fluid-overloaded patient. Why was the IV route likely chosen?
   A. Furosemide can be administered only by the IV route.
   B. IV is the route of choice for rapid administration.
   C. IV dosing is more accurate.
   D. IV furosemide has fewer side effects than oral.

3. Which vein should be used first when initiating IV therapy?
   A. Jugular vein
   B. Basilic vein
   C. Brachiocephalic vein
   D. Axillary vein

4. When preparing a site for venipuncture with alcohol, how long must the area be cleaned?
   A. 5 seconds
   B. 10 seconds
   C. 30 seconds
   D. 60 seconds

5. Which of the following complications can occur if a clotted cannula is aggressively flushed?
   A. Pulmonary embolism
   B. Air embolism
   C. Arterial spasm
   D. Extravasation

6. Which of the following symptoms most indicates that an infusion is infiltrated?
   A. Redness at the site
   B. Pain at the site
   C. Puffiness at the site
   D. Exudate at the site

7. A patient has orders to receive 1 L (1000 mL) of 5% dextrose and lactated Ringer's solution to be infused over 8 hours. How many milliliters will be infused per hour?
   A. 80
   B. 100
   C. 125
   D. 150

8. A patient is receiving an IV piggyback antibiotic in 50 mL of 5% dextrose and water, to run over 1 hour. The tubing has a drip factor of 60. How many drops per minute should be set?
   A. 6
   B. 17
   C. 50
   D. 100

9. Which of the following IV solutions is hypertonic?
   A. Normal saline
   B. 5 % dextrose in 0.9 % NaCl
   C. 0.45% NaCl
   D. 0.225% NaCl

10. What is the last step when inserting an IV cannula?
    A. Secure the cannula with tape.
    B. Document the insertion site, date, and type of cannula used.
    C. Assess the site.
    D. Place a sterile dressing over the insertion site.

7

NURSING CARE OF PATIENTS WITH INFECTIONS

▶ VOCABULARY

Define the following terms and use them in a sentence.

Antigen

    Definition: _____

    Sentence: _____

Asepsis

    Definition: _____

    Sentence: _____

Bacteria

    Definition: _____

    Sentence: _____

Nosocomial infection

    Definition: _____

    Sentence: _____

Pathogens

    Definition: _____

    Sentence: _____

Phagocytosis

    Definition: _____

    Sentence: _____

Virulence

    Definition: _____

    Sentence: _____

Viruses

    Definition: _____

    Sentence: _____

▶ PATHOGEN TRANSMISSION

Match the pathogen with its mode of transmission.

1. _____ Chickenpox

2. _____ Malaria

3. _____ Tuberculosis

4. _____ Rocky Mountain spotted fever

5. _____ Meningitis

6. _____ Hepatitis A

7. _____ Measles

8. _____ Influenza

A. Common vehicle
B. Droplet
C. Airborne
D. Vector borne

▶ PATHOGENS AND INFECTIOUS DISEASE

Fill in the word for the definition of pathogens and infectious diseases.

1. _____ Gram-positive bacteria clusters that can cause pneumonia, cellulitis, peritonitis, and toxic shock

2. _____ Gram-positive bacteria chains that can cause pneumonia, meningitis, otitis media, sinusitis, septicemia

3. _____ Infection of the skin or mucous membrane with any species of *Candida*

4. _____ Fungus infection of the skin

5. _____ A systemic fungal respiratory disease caused by *Histoplasma capsulatum*

6. _____ A disease caused by infection with the protozoa *Toxoplasma gondii*

7. _____ Single-celled parasitic organisms that move and live mainly in the soil

8. _____ Small intracellular parasites that can only live inside cells; may produce disease when they enter a cell

9. _____ Parasites that must be inside living cells to reproduce and cause disease

10. _____ Group of plantlike organisms that includes yeast, molds, and mushrooms; rarely pathogenic

▶ CRITICAL THINKING

Read the following case study and answer the questions.

A 72-year-old patient is admitted to a private room with an antibiotic-resistant respiratory tract infection.

1. What equipment is needed for isolation? _____

2. What type of equipment would be used to do assessments and nursing interventions? _____

_____

_____

3. Describe the psychosocial needs of the patient. _____

_____

_____

REVIEW QUESTIONS

Choose the best answer.

1. Which of the following is the most important reason for the nurse to use sterile technique when obtaining a urine specimen for culture and sensitivity?
   A. Protect the nurse from being infected by the patient.
   B. Protect the patient from exposure to other microorganisms.
   C. Prevent the spread of organisms in the urine to others.
   D. Allow for a more accurate diagnosis.

2. When caring for patients, which of the following methods is best for the nurse to use to prevent the spread of infection?
   A. Sterilizing hands with a germicide once a day
   B. Washing hands at the beginning of patient rounds
   C. Washing hands before and after each patient contact
   D. Wearing gloves for all patient care

3. In planning care for a patient, the nurse understands that surgical asepsis is based on which of the following principles?
   A. Destroying organisms before they enter the body
   B. Isolating all patients who have infectious diseases
   C. Destroying bacteria as they leave the body
   D. Maintaining basic cleanliness

4. To plan care for a patient, the nurse understands that which of the following is needed by all pathogenic organisms to multiply?
   A. Moisture
   B. Light
   C. A host
   D. Oxygen

5. To collect a sterile urine specimen, which of the following techniques should the nurse use?
   A. Cleanse the patient's external genitalia before the patient voids.
   B. Have the patient void into a sterile container.
   C. Straight catheterize the patient.
   D. Obtain a midstream voided specimen.

6. Which of the following does the nurse understand is the best time to obtain a sputum specimen?
   A. After eating
   B. Before eating
   C. After waking in the morning
   D. Before going to sleep at night

7. A patient has been diagnosed recently as having an upper respiratory infection. Which of the following symptoms indicates to the nurse that the patient is developing complications?
   A. Scratchy throat
   B. Clear, watery drainage from the nose
   C. Dry cough
   D. High fever

8. The nurse is collecting a culture of wound drainage. The patient asks what a culture is. Which of the following is the best response by the nurse to explain what a culture is?
   A. A culture identifies presence of pathogens.
   B. It measures antibiotic levels.
   C. It identifies an antibiotic's effect on a pathogen.
   D. It determines the appropriate medication dosage.

9. Which of the following is a sign of a local infection?
   A. Warm skin
   B. Clammy skin
   C. Anorexia
   D. Paleness

10. Which of the following is a method of sterile technique?
    A. Use of antiseptics
    B. Steam under pressure cleansing
    C. Frequent hand washing
    D. Use of gloves when coming in contact with body fluids

11. Nosocomial infections are those that are acquired by which of the following?
    A. After another infectious process
    B. From a sexual partner
    C. As a result of hospitalization
    D. From poor habits of hygiene

12. Which of the following antibiotics is commonly used to treat methicillin-resistant *Staphylococcus aureus*?
    A. Gentamycin
    B. Tobramycin
    C. Penicillin
    D. Vancomycin

8

NURSING CARE
OF PATIENTS IN SHOCK

▶ VOCABULARY

Fill in the blank with the word formed by word building.

1. _____ acid—sour + osis—condition

2. _____ an—without + aerobic—presence of oxygen

3. _____ an—without + phylaxis—protection

4. _____ anti—against + a—not + rhythmic—rhythm

5. _____ cardi—heart + genic—originating from

6. _____ cyan—blue coloring + osis—condition

7. _____ dys—difficult or abnormal + rhythmia—rhythm

8. _____ olig—few + uria—urine condition

9. _____ tachy—fast + cardia—heart condition

10. _____ tachy—fast + pnea—breathing

▶ MATCHING

Match the area of the cardiovascular system that contributes to the development of shock with each type of shock.

___ 1. Hypovolemic shock

___ 2. Cardiogenic shock

___ 3. Anaphylactic shock

___ 4. Septic shock

___ 5. Neurogenic shock

___ 6. Obstructive shock

A. Heart
B. Blood vessels
C. Fluid volume

▶ SIGNS AND SYMPTOMS OF SHOCK PHASES

Complete the table.

Signs/Symptoms	Phases		
	Mild/Compensating	**Moderate/Progressive**	**Severe/Irreversible**
Heart rate	Elevated	_____	Slowing
Pulses	_____	Weaker, thready	_____
Blood pressure			
Systolic	Normal	<90 mm Hg *In hypertensive, 25% below baseline	_____
Diastolic	_____	_____	Decreasing to 0
Respirations	_____	Tachypnea	_____
Depth	_____	_____	_____
Temperature	Varies	Decreased *May elevate in septic shock	_____
Level of consciousness	_____	Confused, lethargy	Unconscious, comatose
Skin/mucous membranes	Cool, pale	Cold, moist, clammy, pale	_____
Urine output	_____	_____	15 mL/hr decreasing to anuria
Bowel sounds	_____	Decreasing	_____

▶ CRITICAL THINKING

Identify the phase of shock, category of shock, and initial action to take for the following patients.

1. An 80-year-old woman admitted with a bowel obstruction has minimal urine output. A nasogastric tube has 1500 mL of bloody aspirate returned on insertion. She becomes comatose. Vital signs are as follows: Blood pressure 80 with the Doppler, pulse 140 and thready, respirations 8, and temperature 94° F (34° C).

   Stage: _____

   Category of Shock: _____

   Initial Action: _____

2. A 56-year-old patient with chronic renal failure is agitated. Her blood pressure is 100/92, pulse 110, respirations 18, and temperature 102° F (39° C).

   Stage: _____

   Category of Shock: _____

   Initial Action: _____

3. A 50-year-old patient with chronic renal failure is hypotensive after receiving dialysis and is presently receiving a fluid challenge of 1000 mL 0.9 percent normal saline over 4 hours. Her lung sounds are now full of crackles. Her heart rhythm is irregular. Jugular vein distention and ankle edema are present. Blood pressure has dropped from 96/50 to 80/40 in 1 hour, pulse 108, respirations 24, and temperature 95° F (35° C). She is confused.

   Stage: _____

   Category of Shock: _____

   Initial Action: _____

Choose the best answer.

1. The nurse assesses a patient with chronic renal failure who has just returned from completing a hemodialysis session and reviews the patient's previous data. Assessment data before dialysis is as follows: Blood pressure 150/88, pulse 90, respirations 18, temperature 98.9° F (37° C), and weight 168. Assessment data after dialysis is as follows: Blood pressure 100/54, pulse 110, respirations 18, temperature 99° F (37° C), and weight 161. Which of the following actions should the nurse take after comparing the data?
   A. Monitor intravenous infusion of 5 percent dextrose/0.9 percent normal saline.
   B. Provide a quiet environment.
   C. Have the physician notified.
   D. Verify the patient's weight.

2. A 47-year-old patient is admitted with hypovolemic shock from trauma injuries in an automobile accident. The patient remains oliguric 2 days later. Which of the following assessments of the patient indicates to the nurse that the patient is experiencing a complication of shock that requires follow-up treatment?
   A. Hematocrit 42 percent (N = 38 to 47 percent)
   B. Creatinine 2.2 mg/dL (N = 0.6 to 1.3 mg/dL)
   C. Blood urea nitrogen 24 mg/dL (N = 6 to 25 mg/dL)
   D. Hemoglobin 13.4 g/dL (N = 13.5 to 18 g/dL)

3. The nurse is caring for a patient with a bowel obstruction. The nurse would be correct in interpreting which of the following as an indication of mild shock?
   A. Blood pressure 88/50 mm Hg
   B. Pulse 110
   C. Lethargy
   D. Urine 18 mL/hr

4. The nurse is caring for a postoperative patient following a splenectomy. The nurse would be correct in interpreting which of the following as an indication of moderate shock?
   A. Blood pressure 86/52 mm Hg
   B. Pulse 100
   C. Cool, pale skin
   D. Urine 40 mL/hr

5. The nurse is caring for a patient with gastrointestinal bleeding who has an intravenous infusion of 0.9 percent normal saline at 50 mL/hr. The patient has a large, red, bloody stool and complains of dizziness. The nurse assists the patient back to bed and obtains blood pressure 90/52, pulse 118, and respirations 22. Which of the following actions should the nurse take next?
   A. Continue monitoring vital signs.
   B. Inform the registered nurse.
   C. Decrease the intravenous flow rate.
   D. Elevate the head of the bed.

6. Which of the following medications would the nurse anticipate the physician would order to increase blood pressure for a patient with septic shock?
   A. Atropine
   B. Dopamine
   C. Digoxin
   D. Nitroglycerin

7. Which of the following is a nursing intervention to assess for inadequate peripheral tissue perfusion in a patient in shock?
   A. Monitor apical pulse.
   B. Assess capillary refill.
   C. Assess sacral edema.
   D. Monitor level of consciousness.

8. Which of the following does the nurse understand is the primary reason that respirations increase in mild shock?
   A. Anxiety causes hyperventilation.
   B. Retention of carbon dioxide is decreased.
   C. Normal oxygen levels are maintained
   D. Cardiac output is increased.

9. Which of the following types of shock does the nurse understand causes the skin to be cold and moist?
   A. Mild
   B. Compensating
   C. Progressive
   D. Irreversible

10. The nurse is caring for a hypertensive patient whose blood pressure is usually 156/86. Which of the following blood pressures is considered a progressive shock blood pressure finding for this patient?
   A. 90/44
   B. 140/80
   C. 114/64
   D. 130/72

11. Which of the following outcomes for the nursing diagnosis Deficient knowledge is appropriate for the patient recovering from shock?
   A. Accepts responsibility for shock
   B. States understanding of shock
   C. Interacts with others
   D. Verbalizes fears

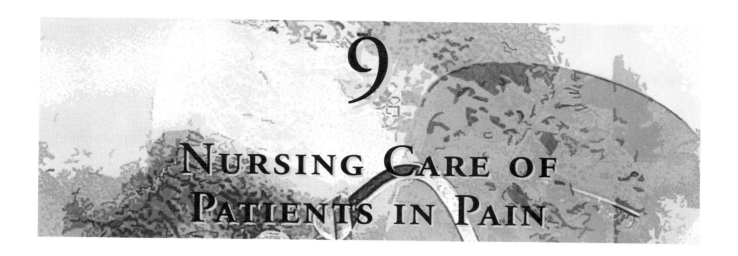

9
NURSING CARE OF
PATIENTS IN PAIN

▶ VOCABULARY
Match the word to its definition.

1. _____ Addiction

2. _____ Tolerance

3. _____ Ceiling effect

4. _____ Pain

5. _____ Prostaglandin

6. _____ Adjuvants

7. _____ Opioid

8. _____ Patient-controlled anesthesia (PCA)

9. _____ Endorphins

10. _____ Analgesics

A. Whatever the experiencing person says it is
B. Endogenous chemicals that act like opioids
C. Larger dose of analgesic required to relieve same pain
D. Psychological dependence
E. Self-administered analgesics
F. Dose of analgesic limited by side effects
G. Medications that relieve pain
H. Drugs that are used to potentiate analgesics
I. Neurotransmitter released during pain
J. A morphine-like drug

▶ CULTURAL COMPETENCE
You are working on a medical unit in a large metropolitan area. Your patients come from varied cultural backgrounds. What differences in pain expressions might you expect to see in patients from the following cultures?

Native-American _____

European-American _____

African-American _____

Hispanic-American _____

Asian-American _____

▶ CRITICAL THINKING

Read the following case study and answer the questions.

Miss Murphy is a 32-year-old admitted to your unit following an emergency appendectomy at 8:00 AM. When you enter her room at 2 PM, she is sitting up in bed smiling and visiting with her family. She tells you she is hurting and asks for a pain shot. You check her medication record and find orders for morphine 5 to 10 mg IM q4h as needed (PRN) for pain.

1. List at least seven areas you will assess related to her pain. _____

_____

_____

_____

2. Based on your assessment, you decide to administer 10 mg of morphine. What class of drugs does morphine belong to? What

is its mechanism of action? _____

_____

_____

_____

3. What is the most effective medication schedule you can implement today? _____

_____

_____

4. What side effects will you watch for? _____

_____

_____

5. How will you know if the medication has been effective? _____

_____

_____

6. The next morning you decide to administer Tylenol No. 3 for Miss Murphy's pain, but it is not effective. Why do you think

it did not help? _____

_____

_____

7. What nondrug therapies might be appropriate for Miss Murphy? What technique has already been effective for her? _____

_____

_____

REVIEW QUESTIONS

Choose the best answer.

1. Which of the following definitions of pain is most appropriate?
   A. Knifelike sensation along a nerve pathway
   B. Burning sensation that accompanies severe injury or trauma
   C. Injured tissues responding with release of neurotransmitters that cause a sensation of pressure or discomfort
   D. Whatever the experiencing person says it is, occurring whenever the experiencing person says it does

2. Which of the following terms describes a feeling of threat to one's self-image or life that may accompany pain?
   A. Fear
   B. Anxiety
   C. Suffering
   D. Panic

3. Which of the following is a common side effect of opioid administration?
    A. Constipation
    B. Respiratory depression
    C. Tachycardia
    D. Addiction

4. Which is the most accurate way to assess the severity of a patient's pain?
    A. Observe for moaning or other physical signs.
    B. Watch for elevated blood pressure and pulse.
    C. Have the patient rate pain on a standard pain scale.
    D. Monitor the frequency with which the patient requests pain medication.

5. Which of the following statements best explains why a patient can be laughing and talking yet still be in pain?
    A. Most patients try to deny their pain because pain is socially unacceptable.
    B. Distraction can help relieve pain when used in conjunction with analgesics.
    C. Most patients who are laughing and talking are not in pain.
    D. Laughing prolongs the effects of opioids in the body.

6. Which type of pain may be accompanied by changes in vital signs?
    A. Acute pain
    B. Chronic nonmalignant pain
    C. Cancer pain

7. An 82-year-old male patient has been receiving meperidine (Demerol) IM for chronic back pain. After several weeks he becomes very irritable, which is unlike him. Which response by the nurse is best?
    A. Understand that chronic pain can cause a patient to become irritable.
    B. Obtain an order for a sedative to administer with the meperidine.
    C. Ask him if there is something bothering him that he would like to talk about.
    D. Consult with the registered nurse or physician about possible toxic effects of normeperidine.

8. Which of the following should be assessed and documented before administering an opioid analgesic?
    A. Liver and kidney function studies
    B. Blood glucose level
    C. Pain level and respiratory rate
    D. Physical cause of pain

9. Which drug can be given to reverse the effects of an opioid overdose?
    A. Naloxone (Narcan)
    B. Methadone (Dolophine)
    C. Hydrocodone with acetaminophen (Vicodin)
    D. Phenytoin (Dilantin)

10. A 42-year-old woman has chronic pain for which no cause can be found. Her physician orders a placebo. Which response by the nurse is best?
    A. "We will give the placebo and document her response."
    B. "I know if the placebo helps her pain, then her pain is not real."
    C. "Doctor, I am not comfortable administering this placebo without the patient's consent."
    D. "Doctor, may we alternate the placebo with her opioid order?"

11. A patient has a PCA pump following surgery on his spine. He appears to be in pain, but is too drowsy to push the button on the pump. Which response by the nurse is correct?
    A. Push the button for the patient.
    B. Instruct the patient's wife to push the button, but only every 10 minutes.
    C. Assess the patient's vital signs.
    D. Increase the dose of medication delivered in each injection.

12. A known cocaine abuser is admitted following a motorcycle accident. He calls you into his room and says, "I need something for this pain. Now." Which assumption by the nurse is best?
    A. The patient is withdrawing from cocaine and needs an opioid to prevent withdrawal symptoms.
    B. The patient is in pain and needs an analgesic.
    C. The patient is trying to establish control over his situation.
    D. The patient is faking pain to gain access to opioids.

10
NURSING CARE OF PATIENTS WITH CANCER

▶ VOCABULARY
Fill in the blank.

1. Loss of hair is called _____.

2. Loss of appetite is called _____.

3. Leuko_____ places the patient at risk of infection.

4. Dry mouth is called _____.

5. Treatment aimed at maintaining comfort is called _____ therapy.

6. _____ is the use of drugs to combat cancer.

7. Substances that poison cells are called _____.

8. _____ is the term used to describe new growth.

9. When cancer _____, it travels to a new site.

10. A tumor that is not cancerous is called _____.

▶ CELLS
Label each statement as true or false.

1. _____ Chromosomes are made of DNA and protein.

2. _____ A gene is the code for one DNA molecule.

3. _____ Messenger RNA carries the genetic code to the cell membrane.

4. _____ A genetic change in a cell is called a mutation.

5. _____ Transfer RNA brings amino acids to the proper sites on the DNA.

6. _____ Mutations are how cells become malignant.

7. _____ In any human cell, most of the genes are always active.

8. _____ The chromosome number for a human cell is 48.

9. _____ The process of mitosis produces two identical cells with 23 chromosomes each.

10. _____ Mitosis is necessary only for growth of the body.

▶ BENIGN VERSUS MALIGNANT TUMORS

Compare the characteristics of benign and malignant tumors. List as many characteristics as you can remember.

_____

_____

_____

_____

_____

▶ CRITICAL THINKING

Delmae is a 48-year-old restaurant worker undergoing chemotherapy following a right modified mastectomy. List two or three nursing interventions for each of the side effects she can expect to experience.

1. Leukopenia: _____

   _____

2. Thrombocytopenia: _____

   _____

3. Anemia: _____

   _____

4. Stomatitis: _____

   _____

5. Nausea and vomiting: _____

   _____

6. Alopecia: _____

   _____

REVIEW QUESTIONS

Choose the best answer.

1. Genes are made of which of the following?
   A. Chromosomes
   B. DNA
   C. RNA
   D. Protein

2. Which of the following best describes osmosis?
   A. The diffusion of any substance
   B. The diffusion of water
   C. The filtration of water
   D. The active transport of water

3. Which of the following is the term used for a group of similar cells found on an external or internal body surface?
   A. Skin
   B. Mucous membrane
   C. Epithelial tissue
   D. Connective tissue

4. Which statement best describes cancer cells?
   A. They are well organized.
   B. They have a specific function.
   C. They cease to grow and divide.
   D. They are confused.

5. Which of the following foods can increase cancer risk?
   A. Broccoli, cauliflower
   B. Butter, ice cream
   C. Chicken, fish
   D. Cakes, breads

6. A patient is admitted with suspected lung cancer and asks, "How will my physician know for sure if I have cancer?" Which of the following responses is best?
   A. "Your physician will do cultures of your sputum."
   B. "An x-ray examination will be done to confirm the diagnosis."
   C. "A biopsy is the only way to know for sure."
   D. "Your physician will do a bronchoscopy to look at the cancer."

7. A 47-year-old woman has mucositis related to radiation therapy. Which of the following nursing interventions will help relieve her symptoms?
    A. Provide frequent mouth care.
    B. Offer cold liquids often.
    C. Provide high-carbohydrate foods.
    D. Offer juices frequently.

8. The nurse is caring for a patient with a radioactive implant. Which of the following actions is appropriate?
    A. Avoid entering the patient's room for 24 hours.
    B. Limit the amount of time spent with the patient.
    C. Avoid touching the patient.
    D. Place a "contaminated" sign on the patient's bed.

9. A 67-year-old patient is receiving chemotherapy following surgery for prostate cancer. Which of the following problems indicates that he is experiencing thrombocytopenia?
    A. Fever
    B. Petechiae
    C. Pain
    D. Vomiting

10. How can the nurse best prevent complications in the patient with leukopenia?
    A. Wash hands frequently.
    B. Avoid injections.
    C. Allow no visitors.
    D. Offer fresh fruits and vegetables.

11. A patient has severe pain related to bone cancer. You note that she does not ask for pain medication when she is watching television. Which of the following statements best explains this?
    A. Distraction is a good pain relief method and can prevent the need for analgesics.
    B. She probably asks for pain medication when she is not watching television because she is bored or depressed.
    C. Her pain must be psychosomatic because it is relieved by television.
    D. Distraction can be a helpful intervention when used in addition to analgesics.

12. A 43-year-old patient with terminal cancer is referred to hospice for support. How can hospice help the patient and his family?
    A. Hospice nurses can help administer curative chemotherapy.
    B. Hospice supports research efforts in finding cancer cures.
    C. Hospice can help the patient's family keep the patient comfortable until his death.
    D. Hospice can help the patient find financial resources for cancer treatment.

11

NURSING CARE OF PATIENTS HAVING SURGERY

▶ VOCABULARY
Fill in the blank.

1. _____ are physicians who perform surgical procedures.

2. The three surgical phases are referred to collectively by the word _____.

3. The _____ phase begins with the admission of the patient to the postanesthesia care unit (PACU) and continues until the patient's recovery is completed.

4. _____ is the period when an anesthetic is first given until full anesthesia is reached.

5. The _____ phase begins with the decision to have surgery and ends with transfer of the patient to the operating room.

6. The _____ phase begins when the patient is transferred to the operating room and ends when the patient is admitted to the PACU.

7. An _____ agent is medication (such as narcotics, muscle relaxants, or antiemetics) used with the primary anesthetic agents.

8. The sudden bursting open of a wound's edges that may be preceded by an increase in serosanguineous drainage is referred to as _____.

9. _____ are physicians who administer anesthesia.

10. _____ causes a loss of sensation and allows the surgical procedure to be done safely.

11. _____ occurs from hypoventilation or mucus obstruction that prevents some alveoli from opening and being fully ventilated.

12. _____ is the removal of necrotic and infected tissue.

13. _____ is a body temperature that is below normal range.

14. _____ is the viscera spilling out of the abdomen.

▶ SURGERY URGENCY LEVELS
Match the surgery urgency level to the appropriate definition or example. The level may be used more than once.

1. _____ Surgery needed when any delay jeopardizes the patient's life or limb

2. _____ Fracture repair

3. _____ Surgery needed within 24 to 30 hours

4. _____ Extremity emboli

A. Optional surgery
B. Elective surgery
C. Urgent surgery
D. Emergency surgery

5. _____ Surgery planned and scheduled without immediate time constraints

6. _____ Surgery done at request of patient

7. _____ Hernia repair

8. _____ Rhinoplasty

9. _____ Infected gallbladder

10. _____ Cosmetic surgery

► NOURISHING THE SURGICAL PATIENT

Find the seven errors and insert the correct information.

Healing requires increased vitamin A for collagen formation, vitamin B_{12} for blood clotting, and magnesium for tissue growth, skin integrity, and cell-mediated immunity. Carbohydrates are essential for controlling fluid balance and manufacturing antibodies and white blood cells. Hypoalbuminemia, low urine albumin, impedes the return of interstitial fluid to the venous return system, decreasing the risk of shock. A serum zinc level is a useful measure of protein status.

► MEDICATIONS

Indicate whether the statement is true or false and correct the false statement.

1. _____ All medications that patients are taking must be reviewed preoperatively.

2. _____ Most anticoagulants, such as warfarin (Coumadin), do not need to be stopped before surgery.

3. _____ Diabetic patients on insulin are told to take their normal insulin dose the day of surgery.

4. _____ Blood glucose monitoring for diabetic patients is ordered on admission.

5. _____ If a patient is on chronic oral steroid therapy it cannot be abruptly stopped when nil per os (NPO).

6. _____ Surgery is not a great stressor for the body.

7. _____ Chronic oral steroid therapy should be continued via the parenteral route if the patient is NPO.

8. _____ Circulatory collapse can develop if steroids are not stopped abruptly.

► INTRAOPERATIVE NURSING DIAGNOSES AND OUTCOMES

Write a patient objective (goal) for each nursing diagnosis.

1. Risk for injury related to pressure points from positioning, chemicals, electrical equipment, and effect of being anesthetized

   _____

   _____

2. Risk for impaired skin integrity related to chemicals, pressure points from positioning, and immobility _____

   _____

   _____

3. Risk for Deficient fluid volume related to being NPO and blood loss _____

   _____

   _____

4. Risk for infection related to incision and invasive procedures _____

   _____

   _____

5. Pain related to pressure points from positioning, incision, and surgical procedure _____

_____

_____

▶ WOUND HEALING PHASES
Complete the table.

Phase	Time Frame	Wound Healing	Patient Effect
Phase I	_____	_____	Fever, malaise
Phase II	_____	Granulation tissue forms	_____
Phase III	_____	Collagen deposited	_____
Phase IV	Months to 1 year	_____	

▶ CRITICAL THINKING
Read the case study and answer the questions.

Mrs. Vell, 74, is scheduled for a total hip replacement because of osteoarthritis. She is seen in the preadmission testing department 1 week before surgery.

1. Why is Mrs. Vell in preadmission testing? _____

_____

2. What testing may be done in preadmission testing? _____

_____

3. What teaching should the nurse do in preadmission testing? _____

_____

4. What are the responsibilities of the admitting nurse to prepare Mrs. Vell for surgery? _____

_____

5. What is the role of the holding area nurse? _____

_____

6. What is the role of the licensed practical nurse/licensed vocational nurse (LPN/LVN) in the operating room? _____

_____

7. What are the two prioritized primary responsibilities of the postanesthesia care nurse? _____

_____

8. Explain why postoperative care for this patient must include pain control, deep breathing and coughing, leg exercises, activity, leg abduction, and drain care. _____

REVIEW QUESTIONS

Choose the best answer.

1. Which of the following is a priority LPN/LVN patient care role in the preoperative phase?
   A. Obtaining preoperative orders
   B. Explaining the surgical procedure
   C. Offering emotional support
   D. Providing informed consent

2. The LPN/LVN is caring for a patient in the preoperative period who, even after verbalizing concerns and having questions answered, states, "I know I am not going to wake up after surgery." Which of the following is the best action for the LPN/LVN to take?
   A. Reassure patient everything will be all right
   B. Inform the registered nurse
   C. Explain the national surgery death rate
   D. Ask the family to comfort the patient

3. The nurse is reviewing the medication history of a new preoperative patient who is NPO. The nurse notes that the patient has been on long-term oral steroid therapy. The nurse understands that which of the following is the reason that steroids cannot be abruptly stopped?
   A. Higher steroid levels are needed during stress
   B. Malignant hyperthermia will result
   C. Malignant hypertension will occur
   D. Respiratory failure will result

4. When teaching the preoperative patient who is elderly, which of the following is a teaching strategy that improves learning?
   A. Sit in front of window in bright sunlight
   B. Use small, white-on-black printed materials
   C. Speak in high tone
   D. Eliminate background noise

5. When the patient's signature is witnessed by the nurse on the surgical consent, which of the following does the nurse's signature indicate?
   A. The nurse obtained informed consent.
   B. The nurse provided informed consent.
   C. The nurse answered all surgical procedure questions.
   D. The nurse verified that the patient signed the consent.

6. Which of the following is an intraoperative outcome for a patient undergoing an inguinal hernia repair?
   A. Verbalizes fears
   B. Maintains skin integrity
   C. Demonstrates leg exercises
   D. Explains coughing and deep breathing exercises

7. Which of the following is a discharge criterion from the PACU for a patient following surgery?
   A. Oxygen saturation above 90%
   B. Oxygen saturation below 90%
   C. Intravenous (IV) narcotics given less than 15 minutes ago
   D. IV narcotics given less than 30 minutes ago

8. Which of the following is one of the discharge criteria from ambulatory surgery for patients following surgery?
   A. Able to drive self home
   B. Has home telephone
   C. Understands discharge instructions
   D. IV narcotics given less than 30 minutes before discharge

9. Several hours after returning from surgery, the nurse tells the patient that she is ordered to be ambulated. The patient asks, "Why?" Which of the following complications would the nurse correctly explain can be prevented by early postoperative ambulation?
   A. Increased peristalsis
   B. Coughing
   C. Pneumonia
   D. Wound healing

10. Which of the following actions should the nurse take to maintain patient safety when ambulating a patient for the first time post operatively?
   A. Use one person to assist patient.
   B. Use two people to assist patient.
   C. Encourage patient to "dangle" self 1 hour before ambulation.
   D. Give narcotic 15 minutes before ambulation.

11. The nurse is caring for a patient with a bowel resection. Which of the following would indicate that the patient's gastrointestinal tract is resuming normal function?
   A. Firm abdomen
   B. Excessive thirst
   C. Presence of flatus
   D. Absent bowel sounds

12. The patient is dangling at the bedside and states, "Oh, my stomach is tearing open." Which of the following actions should the nurse immediately take when dehiscence occurs?
   A. Have patient sit upright in a chair.
   B. Slow intravenous fluids.
   C. Have patient lie down.
   D. Obtain a sterile suture set.

13. When the LPN/LVN is assisting the patient to use an incentive spirometer, which of the following actions by the patient indicates that the patient needs further teaching on how to use the spirometer?
   A. Taking two normal breaths before use
   B. Inhaling deeply to reach target
   C. Sitting upright before use
   D. Exhaling deeply to reach target

14. After surgery the nurse notes that the patient's urine is dark amber and concentrated. Which of the following does the nurse understand may be the reason for this?
   A. The sympathetic nervous system saves fluid in response to stress of surgery.
   B. The sympathetic nervous system diureses fluid in response to stress of surgery.
   C. The parasympathetic nervous system saves fluid in response to stress of surgery.
   D. Parasympathetic nervous system saves fluid in response to stress of surgery.

15. The patient develops a low-grade fever 18 hours postoperatively and has diminished breath sounds. Which of the following actions is most appropriate for the nurse to take to help reduce the fever and prevent complications?
   A. Administer antibiotics.
   B. Encourage coughing and deep breathing.
   C. Administer acetaminophen (Tylenol).
   D. Decrease fluid intake.

12

NURSING CARE OF PATIENTS WITH EMERGENT CONDITIONS

▶ VOCABULARY

Match the word with its definition.

1. _____ Skin scraped away because of injury

2. _____ Disease caused by organism entering body through an open wound resulting in convulsions, muscle spasms, stiffness of the jaw, coma, and death

3. _____ Insufficient intake of oxygen

4. _____ Inadequate and progressively failing tissue perfusion that can result in cellular death

5. _____ Irregular tear of the skin

6. _____ Loss of water and electrolytes through heavy sweating, causing hypovolemia

7. _____ Tearing away or crushing of body limbs

8. _____ Frozen body parts that are white or yellow-white

A. Asphyxia
B. Tetanus
C. Abrasion
D. Laceration
E. Shock
F. Amputation
G. Heat exhaustion
H. Frostbite

▶ PRINCIPLES FOR TREATING SHOCK

Indicate whether the statement is true or false, and correct the false statement.

1. Maintain an open airway and give oxygen as ordered. _____

2. Control external bleeding by indirect pressure. _____

3. Elevate the upper extremities 10 to 12 inches. _____

4. If possible, keep the patient supine. _____

5. Accurately record vital signs. _____

6. Give the patient oral fluids. _____

7. Administer intravenous fluids as ordered. _____

▶ SIGNS AND SYMPTOMS OF INCREASED INTRACRANIAL PRESSURE

Indicate whether the sign is an early sign or a late sign for increased intracranial pressure.

1. _____ Abnormal posturing

2. _____ Altered level of consciousness

3. _____ Amnesia

A. Early sign
B. Late sign

4. _____ Changes in respiratory pattern

5. _____ Changes in speech

6. _____ Decreased pulse rate

7. _____ Dilated nonreactive pupils

8. _____ Drowsiness

9. _____ Headache

10. _____ Nausea and vomiting

11. _____ Unresponsiveness

12. _____ Widening pulse pressure

▶ ASSESSMENT OF MOTOR FUNCTION
Complete the table.

If the patient is unable to	The lesion is above the level of
_____	C-5 to C-7
Extend and flex legs	_____
Flex foot, extend toes	_____
_____	S-3 to S-5

▶ HYPERTHERMIA
Indicate whether the sign is an early sign or a late sign of hyperthermia caused by exposure to a hot environment.

1. _____ Core body temperature 100.4° F to 102.2° F (38° C to 39° C)

2. _____ Diaphoresis

3. _____ Hot, dry, flushed skin

4. _____ Hypotension

5. _____ Pulse rate more than 100

6. _____ Increasing body core temperature of 106° F (41° C) or more

7. _____ Cool, clammy skin

8. _____ Altered mental status

9. _____ Coma or seizures

10. _____ Dizziness

A. Early sign
B. Late sign

▶ CRITICAL THINKING
Read the case study and answer the questions.

Mr. Ricks, age 66, retired 1 year ago and made plans to travel with his wife. His wife unexpectedly died from a myocardial infarction 2 months ago. Mr. Ricks now lives alone. He has been withdrawn and rarely leaves the house since his wife's funeral. His son, Ted, who lives in another state, arrives for a weekend visit and is concerned about his father's behavior. Mr. Ricks has not bathed and is wearing soiled clothing. The refrigerator is bare and he keeps the curtains drawn. He continually paces and says, "I want to die." Ted takes his father to the local emergency room.

1. Why may Mr. Ricks be exhibiting this behavior change? _____

_____

_____

2. What symptoms of an acute psychiatric episode is Mr. Ricks exhibiting? _____

_____

3. Why should Mr. Ricks be referred for treatment? _____

_____

4. What nursing diagnoses apply to Mr. Ricks? _____

_____

5. What nursing interventions are appropriate for Mr. Ricks initially? _____

_____

REVIEW QUESTIONS

Choose the best answer.

1. A patient who experiences anaphylactic shock after receiving a medication is most likely to experience which of the following symptoms?
   A. Chest pain
   B. Hot, dry skin
   C. Difficulty breathing
   D. Fever

2. The nurse is assessing a patient's extremity, which may be fractured. Which of the following is the nurse's purpose in checking capillary refill during the assessment?
   A. To evaluate arterial blood flow in an extremity
   B. To assess venous blood flow in an extremity
   C. To measure oxygen saturation of the blood
   D. To assess peripheral edema

3. The nurse anticipates that treatment for a semiconscious patient who has ingested 50 tablets of alprazolam (Xanax), a noncaustic substance, would include which of the following?
   A. Administering an antiemetic
   B. Activated charcoal
   C. Forced vomiting
   D. Forcing fluids

4. The nurse is planning care for Mr. Stevens, who has hyperthermia. Which of the following is an outcome criterion for hyperthermia?
   A. Core body temperature less than 94° F (34.4° C)
   B. Patient alert and oriented
   C. Skin cool and moist to touch
   D. Core body temperature greater than 101° F (38.3° C)

5. The physician orders haloperidol (Haldol) 3 mg intramuscularly for a patient who is experiencing a psychiatric crisis. Haloperidol 5 mg/mL is available. How many milliliters should the nurse give?
   A. 0.3 mL
   B. 0.5 mL
   C. 0.6 mL
   D. 1.3 mL

6. The nurse is assessing a patient who has lost a large volume of blood from a laceration. Which of the following pulse findings would indicate to the nurse that the patient is in shock?
   A. Normal, bounding pulse
   B. Slow, strong pulse
   C. Rapid, thready pulse
   D. Slow, bounding pulse

7. The nurse is admitting a trauma patient to the emergency department. As the nurse uses the primary survey, which of the following is given first priority?
   A. Circulation
   B. Breathing
   C. Airway
   D. Disability

8. The nurse is caring for a patient who is bleeding from the radial artery and has lost a large volume of blood from a laceration. The nurse is applying direct pressure to the radial artery and has elevated the arm, but the wound continues to bleed. Which of the following actions should the nurse take next?
   A. Apply pressure to the carotid artery.
   B. Apply pressure to the brachial artery.
   C. Apply pressure to the femoral artery.
   D. Apply pressure to the temporal artery.

UNIT THREE

UNDERSTANDING LIFE SPAN INFLUENCES ON HEALTH AND ILLNESS

13
INFLUENCES ON HEALTH AND ILLNESS

▶ VOCABULARY
Unscramble the word that fits the definition.

1. Short-term intermittent rest provided to care givers—*serptei crea* _____

2. Perception that one's own actions will not affect an outcome—*wporelsesesns* _____

3. Condition of long duration—*rhcnoic* _____

4. Life principles that pervade one's being—*sitrpiauilty* _____

5. State in which person sees no alternatives or choices—*pohelesnsses* _____

6. Disease that can be expected to cause patient to die—*retmnial lilenss* _____

7. A certain life time frame containing tasks an individual needs to accomplish for high-level wellness—*evdlepoemnatl taseg*

_____ _____

▶ CHRONIC ILLNESS AND THE ELDERLY
Find and correct the seven errors.

The elderly constitute one of the smallest age-groups living with chronic illness. Elderly spouses or older family members rarely have to care for a chronically ill family member. Children of elders who themselves are reaching their forties are being expected to care for their parents. These elderly caregivers do not experience chronic illness themselves. For elderly spouses, it is usually the less ill spouse who provides care to the other spouse. The elderly family unit is at great risk for ineffective coping or further development of health problems. Nurses should assess ill members of the elderly family to ensure that their health needs are being met.

Elderly adults are not concerned about becoming dependent and a burden to others. They may become depressed and give up hope if they feel that they are a burden to others. Establishing long-term goals or self-care activities that allow them to participate or have small successes are important nursing actions that can decrease their self-esteem.

▶ DYING AND GRIEVING

Indicate whether the statement is true or false, and correct false statement.

1. _____ Denial prevents hope after being informed that death may occur.

2. _____ Anger reflects the question, "Why me?"

3. _____ In bargaining, a deal is made with the doctor if the patient is allowed to live just a little longer.

4. _____ Depression indicates that the patient is sad and feels that nothing more can be done.

5. _____ With acceptance, the patient withdraws.

▶ CRITICAL THINKING

Read the case study and answer the questions.

Mrs. Martin is hospitalized for an exacerbation of her multiple sclerosis. She tells the nurse she is tired of being ill and is not getting any better. She says, "When I am in the hospital, I cannot attend church, which is my only enjoyment." Later in the day, Mrs. Martin is tearful and withdrawn when the nurse makes rounds.

1. What further data collection should the nurse obtain to meet Mrs. Martin's needs? _____

_____

2. What possible nursing diagnoses would be appropriate for Mrs. Martin? _____

_____

3. What interventions could the nurse use to meet Mrs. Martin's goal? _____

_____

4. How would the nurse know that Mrs. Martin's goal had been met? _____

_____

REVIEW QUESTIONS

Choose the best answer.

1. As the nurse assesses a patient's developmental stage, which of the following does the nurse understand is Erikson's developmental stage for the older adult?
    A. Generativity versus self-absorption
    B. Identity versus role confusion
    C. Intimacy versus isolation
    D. Integrity versus despair

2. The nurse is developing a plan of care for a patient, age 68, focusing on preventive health care. While planning his care, the nurse understands that aging processes are most affected by which of the following factors?
    A. Stress management
    B. Financial issues
    C. Age at retirement
    D. Hobbies

3. A patient, age 64, is active and wants to learn how to promote her health. Which of the following actions by the nurse supports the patient's desire to actively promote her health?
    A. Assign responsibilities for the patient's care to her family.
    B. Select a family physician for the patient.
    C. List health care activities for the patient to carry out.
    D. Ask the patient to select desired health care activities.

4. The home care nurse is caring for a patient with emphysema who seems depressed. Which of the following nursing interventions increases the patient's participation in self-care and assists with improving the patient's depression?
    A. Being a caretaker instead of a partner
    B. Assisting the patient instead of doing everything for the patient
    C. Performing activities of daily living (ADLs) for the patient instead of empowering the patient
    D. Doing everything for the patient instead of assisting the patient

5. The nurse is caring for a patient who is recovering from a stroke. Which of the following nursing interventions during rehabilitation will most increase the patient's self-esteem?
   A. Offering praise for small patient efforts
   B. Offering praise for major patient efforts
   C. Performing ADLs for the patient
   D. Assisting patient at first sign of difficulty with ADLs

6. Which of the following nursing actions might be most helpful for psychosocial intervention for the patient who is withdrawn, depressed, or tense because of isolation resulting from a chronic illness?
   A. Avoiding the use of humor
   B. Reading comics or jokes from magazines
   C. Maintaining a serious demeanor
   D. Limiting conversation to a minimum

7. Which of the following results for caregivers of chronically ill patients when respite care is not available?
   A. Personal time increases
   B. Rest time increases
   C. Financial costs decrease
   D. Stress increases

8. Which of the following is a health promotion method useful for the chronically ill patient?
   A. Making the choices for the patient
   B. Setting the goals for the family
   C. Setting the goals for the patient
   D. Allowing the patient to make informed decisions

9. In contributing to the chronically ill patient's plan of care, which of the following is an appropriate nursing intervention for the nurse to include to empower the patient?
   A. Provide educational information
   B. Limit visiting hours for family members
   C. Ask family members to provide care
   D. Set the goals for the patient and family

10. As the nurse assesses a patient who is terminally ill, which of the following is a sign of impending death in the patient?
    A. Disorientation
    B. Increased body temperature
    C. Insomnia during the night
    D. Polyuria

11. Which of the following does the nurse understand is a benefit of decreased food and fluid intake with impending death?
    A. Body uses excess energy
    B. Metabolism increases
    C. Natural analgesia may result
    D. Peristalsis increases

12. While providing care for a patient who is terminally ill, the nurse understands which of the following senses is the last to leave?
    A. Taste
    B. Smell
    C. Touch
    D. Hearing

13. Which of the following does the nurse understand is an example of a chronic illness?
    A. Peripheral vascular disease
    B. Cellulitis
    C. Peritonitis
    D. Bowel obstruction

14. Which of the following is a primary task that patient's who are chronically ill need to perform and so should be included in the patient's plan of care?
    A. Being willing and able to carry out the medical regimen
    B. Reducing social activities to compensate for limitations
    C. Learning how to play the sick role
    D. Refusing to accept negative changes

15. Which of the following does the nurse understand is a congenital chronic illness?
    A. Head injury
    B. Malabsorption syndrome
    C. Chronic obstructive pulmonary disease
    D. Arthritis

16. The nurse is caring for a patient with Huntington's disease. The family asks what the cause of the illness is. Which of the following responses is most appropriate by the nurse?
    A. Genetic
    B. Congenital
    C. Acquired

14

NURSING CARE OF ELDERLY PATIENTS

► VOCABULARY

Fill in the blank with the word for the definition.

1. _____ _____ _____ _____ Behaviors that are performed in the care and maintenance of self and surroundings

2. _____ Irregular heart rhythm

3. _____ Opacity of the lens of the eye, its capsule, or both

4. _____ State of feeling or mind

5. _____ Accidental drawing of foreign substances into the airway

6. _____ Collection of excess fluid in body tissues

7. _____ A group of eye diseases characterized by increased intraocular pressure

8. _____ The act or process of coughing up materials from the air passageways leading to the lungs

9. _____ A condition of sluggish or difficult bowel action/evacuation

10. _____ The body's attempts to maintain a balance whenever a change occurs

11. _____ Abnormal accumulation of fibrosis connective tissue in skin, muscle, or joint capsule that prevents normal mobility

12. _____ _____ An open sore or lesion of the skin that develops because of prolonged pressure against an area

13. _____ Excessive urination at night

14. _____ _____ External variables that determine the occurrence and rate of structural and functional declines in the human body over time

15. _____ _____ Age-related breakdown of the macular area of the retina of eye, disrupting central vision

16. _____ A condition in which there is a reduction in the mass of bone per unit volume

17. _____ _____ None or minimal stimulation of senses that creates potential for maladaptive coping

18. _____ _____ Highest level of patient activity considering the patient's condition

19. _____ _____ A process to orient a person to names, dates, time, and other pertinent information through use of repeating messages

20. _____ _____ Excessive stimulation of the senses that creates the potential for maladaptive coping

▶ AGING CHANGES

Match the aging change with the effect of the change.

1. _____ Increased conduction time

2. _____ Decreased blood vessel elasticity

3. _____ Leg veins dilate, valves less efficient

4. _____ Basal metabolic rate slows

5. _____ Decreased cardiac output

6. _____ Decreased insulin release

7. _____ Irregular heartbeats

8. _____ Altered adrenal hormone production

9. _____ Decreased gag reflex

10. _____ Decreased peristalsis

11. _____ Reduced liver enzymes

12. _____ Decreased saliva

13. _____ Delayed gastric emptying

14. _____ Decreased bladder size and tone, changes from pear to funnel shaped

15. _____ Decreased kidney concentrating ability

16. _____ Less sodium saved

17. _____ Reduced renal blood flow

18. _____ Decreased immune function

19. _____ Body content water loss

20. _____ Decreased sebaceous/sweat gland

21. _____ Reduced cell replacement

22. _____ Muscle responses slowed

23. _____ Decreased brain blood flow

24. _____ Less vaginal lubrication

25. _____ Decreased sensation

26. _____ Decreased lung capacity

A. Heart rate slows, unable to increase quickly
B. Less oxygen delivered to tissues
C. Increased blood pressure and cardiac workload
D. Poor heart oxygenation
E. Varicose veins, fluid accumulation in tissues
F. Possible weight gain
G. Decreased ability to respond to stress
H. Hyperglycemia
I. Appetite may be reduced
J. Dry mouth, altered taste
K. Increased aspiration risk
L. Frequency of urination
M. Reduced drug metabolism/detoxification
N. Reduced appetite, constipation
O. Nocturia
P. Risk of dehydration
Q. Decreased renal clearance of all medications
R. Greater infection and cancer risk
S. Slower healing process
T. Dryness of the skin
U. Decreased temperature regulation
V. Response time increased
W. Short-term memory loss
X. Risk of injury, burns
Y. Dyspnea with activity
Z. Painful intercourse

▶ COMMUNICATING WITH THE HEARING IMPAIRED

Indicate whether the statement is true or false, and correct false statements.

1. _____ Ensure that hearing aids are turned on and have working batteries.

2. _____ The speaker should turn to the side so the speaker's profile is visible to patient.

3. _____ Speak toward the patient's impaired side of hearing.

4. _____ Speak in a clear, moderate-volume, low-pitched tone.

5. _____ Do not shout because doing so distorts sounds.

6. _____ Recognize that high-frequency tones and consonant sounds are lost last—s, z, sh, ch, d, g.

7. _____ Eliminate background noise because it distorts sounds.

▶ MEDICATIONS
Find the six errors and correct them.

Older patients are less susceptible to drug-induced illness and adverse medication side effects for various reasons. They take few medicines for the one chronic illness that they have. Different medications interact and produce side effects that can be dangerous. Over-the-counter medicines that older patients take, as well as the self-prescribed extracts, elixirs, herbal teas, cultural healing substances, and other home remedies commonly used by individuals of their age cohort, do not influence other medications.

If an older patient crushes a large enteric-coated pill so it can be taken in food and is easily swallowed, it enhances the enteric protection and can inadvertently cause damage to the stomach and intestinal system. Some patients unintentionally skip prescribed doses in an effort to save money. When prescribed doses are not being taken as expected, problems do not clear up as quickly and new problems may result. The nurse should educate the older patient and the patient's family. Patients need to know what each prescribed pill is for, when it is prescribed to be taken, and how it should be taken.

▶ CRITICAL THINKING
Read the following case study and answer the questions. This is a values clarification exercise.

While making 10 PM rounds in the extended care facility, the nurse looks into Mr. B's room to find Mr. B and a female resident from down the hall together, sleeping soundly in Mr. B's bed with the side rails up. Mr. B and the female resident are both 63 years of age. Mr. S, who is Mr. B's roommate, is sound asleep alone in his own bed.

1. What are your initial feelings about this situation? _____

_____

2. What influences your feelings? _____

_____

3. What is the first thing that you would do after this discovery? _____

_____

4. What issues did you consider before making this decision? _____

_____

5. How will you interact with these patients in the future? _____

_____

REVIEW QUESTIONS

Choose the best answer.

1. A 72-year-old patient has been seeing a doctor for treatment of glaucoma for the last 5 years. Which of the following symptoms does the nurse expect the patient to relate when discussing the symptoms of late disease?
   A. Headaches more severe in the evening
   B. Blurred vision when attempting to focus
   C. Morning headaches that disappear after rising
   D. Increased sensitivity to light in the early morning

2. As the nurse performs an oral assessment on an 84-year-old patient, which of the following is an expected finding within the patient's mouth caused by advancing age?
   A. Loss of teeth
   B. Hardness of the gums
   C. Increased production of saliva
   D. Decreased taste sensitivity for salt

3. As the nurse assesses an elderly patient, which of the following is recognized as an aging change in the cardiovascular system?
   A. Increased cardiac output
   B. Increased peripheral vascular resistance
   C. Increased resting heart rate
   D. Increased cardiac reserve

4. Which of the following does the nurse understand is the rationale for dangling a 70-year-old patient at the bedside before helping the patient to stand upright?
   A. To provide a heightened awareness of body position
   B. To accommodate a less efficient circulatory system
   C. To strengthen legs
   D. To reduce anxiety about getting up

5. As the nurse provides care to an elderly patient with an intravenous (IV) infusion, the nurse understands that it is essential for older patients who are receiving IV fluids to be monitored closely to prevent which of the following?
   A. Circulatory distress, which can occur quickly if fluid input exceeds fluid output
   B. Dislodging of the IV, which often occurs in older patients
   C. Venous distention, which occurs if the flow rate is not calibrated accurately
   D. Increased urinary output, which may occur with IV fluids

6. The nurse is talking with a patient who is hard of hearing and is having the most difficulty with high-pitched tones. To increase the patient's hearing, which of the following should the nurse do when speaking with the patient?
   A. Speak slowly with emphasis on important words.
   B. Double the voice volume.
   C. Whisper responses in close proximity to the patient's ear.
   D. Use a modulated voice and talk normally in either ear.

7. The nurse understands that wax buildup in an older patient's ears can cause which type of hearing loss?
   A. Sensorineural
   B. Bone conduction
   C. Perceptive
   D. Neural

8. The nurse understands that which of the following factors is most often the cause of sexual dysfunction for older people?
   A. Physical factors
   B. Psychological factors
   C. Social factors
   D. Environmental factors

9. A nurse is working in an extended care facility. Which of the following nursing behaviors demonstrates the nurse's respect for the older patient's sexuality?
   A. Providing privacy time for a patient by enclosing the bed with the curtain and ensuring that the patient is undisturbed for an hour
   B. Entering a patient's room without knocking when a visitor is present
   C. Walking in on a patient and visitor during an embrace to prepare medications
   D. Changing the subject when a patient expresses feelings toward a friend

10. Which of the following actions should be taken to help an older person prevent osteoporosis?
    A. Decrease dietary intake of calcium.
    B. Encourage regular exercise.
    C. Increase dietary intake of salt.
    D. Increase dietary protein intake.

UNIT FOUR

UNDERSTANDING THE CARDIOVASCULAR SYSTEM

Review of Anatomy and Physiology	Major Disorders	Nursing Assessment	Diagnostic Tests	Common Interventions
☐ Cardiovascular:	☐ Cardiovascular:	☐ Medical history	☐ Noninvasive	☐ Exercise
☐ Structures	☐ Hypertension	☐ Medications	☐ Electrocardiogram ambulatory	☐ Smoking cessation
☐ Function	☐ Inflammatory	☐ Family history	☐ Exercise tolerance testing	☐ Diet
☐ Aging effects	☐ Infectious	☐ Health promotion	☐ Echocardiogram	☐ Lifestyle and cardiac care
	☐ Occlusive	☐ Vital signs	☐ Tilt table test	☐ Antiembolism devices
	☐ Valvular	☐ Physical assessment	☐ Radioisotope imaging	☐ Cardioversion/defibrillation
	☐ Dysrhythmias		☐ Blood studies	☐ Pacemakers
	☐ Heart failure		☐ Cardiac enzymes	☐ Angioplasty
			☐ Cardiac troponin	☐ Valvuloplasty
			☐ Lipids	☐ Surgery
			☐ Invasive	☐ Cardiac rehabilitation
			☐ Angiography	
			☐ Cardiac catheterization	

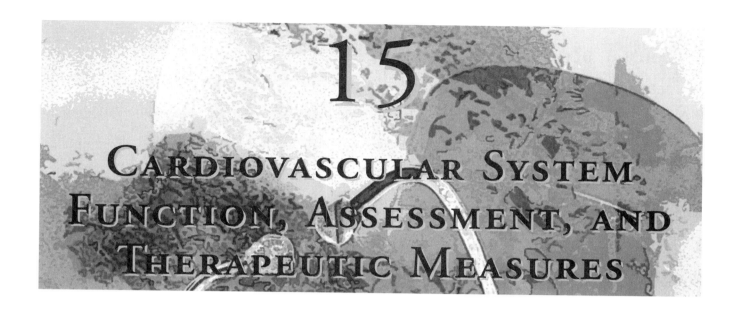

15

CARDIOVASCULAR SYSTEM FUNCTION, ASSESSMENT, AND THERAPEUTIC MEASURES

▶ **STRUCTURES OF THE CARDIOVASCULAR SYSTEM**
Label the following structures.

► CARDIAC BLOOD FLOW

Number the following in proper sequence with respect to the flow of blood through the heart and to and from the lungs and body. Begin at the caval veins.

A. _____ Superior and inferior caval veins

B. _____ Left ventricle

C. _____ Right atrium

D. _____ Right ventricle

E. _____ Body

F. _____ Lungs

G. _____ Pulmonary artery

H. _____ Pulmonary veins

I. _____ Aorta

J. _____ Left atrium

K. _____ Mitral valve

L. _____ Aortic valve

M. _____ Tricuspid valve

N. _____ Pulmonic valve

► VOCABULARY

Complete the crossword puzzle.

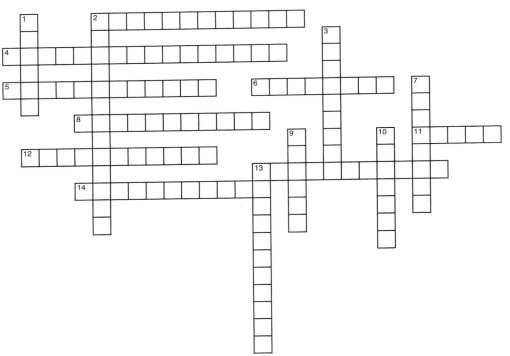

ACROSS

2. Calf pain
4. Thickening and hardening of the blood vessels
5. Resulting from inadequate venous drainage
6. Obstruction of circulation resulting in decreased blood supply
8. Pain on passive dorsiflexion of the foot; a sign of thrombosis
11. Adventitious venous or arterial sound heard on auscultation
12. Disturbance in heart rhythm
13. Abnormal sensation (e.g., burning or prickling)
14. Heart rate lower than 60 beats per minute

DOWN

1. Vibration felt by examiner related to incompetent heart valve
2. Body temperature that varies with the environmental temperature
3. Loss or impairment of a motor or sensory function
7. Rounding of ends and swelling of fingers
9. Indicative of mitral stenosis
10. Venous return to heart stretching ventricle
13. Subjective sensation of rapid or irregular heartbeat

► AGING AND THE CARDIOVASCULAR SYSTEM

Find the 11 errors and insert the correct information.

It is believed that the 'aging' of blood vessels, especially arteries, begins in adulthood. Average resting blood pressure tends to decrease with age and may contribute to stroke or right-sided heart failure. The thicker-walled veins, especially those of the legs, may also weaken and stretch, making their valves incompetent.

With age, the heart lining becomes less efficient, and there is an increase in both maximum cardiac output and heart rate. The health of the myocardium depends on the lungs' blood supply. Hypertension causes the right ventricle to work harder, so it may atrophy. The heart valves may become thinner from fibrosis, leading to heart murmurs. Dysrhythmias become more common in the elderly as the cells of the conduction pathway become more efficient.

► CARDIOVASCULAR SYSTEM

Fill in the blanks.

1. The function of the _____ _____ is to carry oxygen and nutrients to the tissues and remove waste products.

2. The _____ function is to pump blood.

3. The peripheral _____ is composed of arteries, veins, _____ and lymph vessels.

4. With aging, the walls of blood vessels _____ .

5. The heart sound _____ occurs at the beginning of systole when the atrioventricular valves close, and the sound *dupp* occurs at the start of _____ when the semilunar valves close.

6. Palpation of pulse quality is recorded as _____ 0; weak, thready 1+; _____ 2+; bounding 3+.

7. Tests to assess _____ function may include x-ray examination, electrocardiogram (ECG), stress test, echocardiogram, thallium scan, dipyridamole thallium scan, multiple gated acquisition (MUGA), serum troponin I, creatine kinase-myoglobin (CK-MB), lactate dehydrogenase (LDH), myoglobin, cardiac _____, and angiography.

8. Six Ps characterize _____ vascular disease: _____, pulselessness, pallor, _____, paresthesia, and paralysis.

9. Tests to assess peripheral _____ disease are plethysmography, Doppler ultrasound, pressure measurement, stress testing, _____, and arteriography.

► ACUTE CARDIOVASCULAR NURSING ASSESSMENT

Identify a word that is obtained during a history that matches the given assessment statement.

1. _____ Assessed before medication administration, test dyes

2. _____ Modifiable risk factor for cardiovascular disorders

3. _____ Location: chest, calf; radiation: arms, jaw neck

4. _____ Sign resulting from right-sided heart failure

5. _____ Lungs sounds with left-sided heart failure

6. _____ Symptom of dysrhythmias

7. _____ Effect of decreased cardiac output

8. _____ Classic symptom of acute heart failure

► CRITICAL THINKING

Make a cognitive map for a patient who is to undergo a cardiac catheterization. A cognitive map helps you visualize the patient's needs. Think of possible categories of needs of this patient and then complete activities and needs under each category. Some categories have been given to get you started, but you may think of others to include. You can get even more detailed and create subcategories for each activity or need. A cognitive map has no defined ending point.

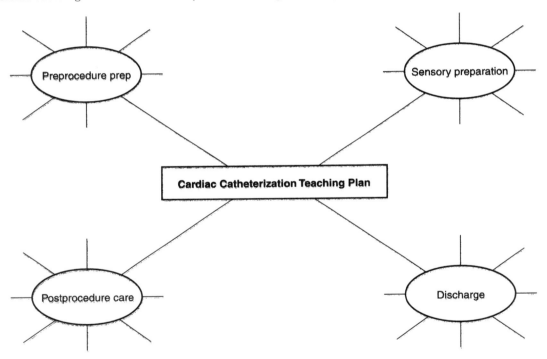

REVIEW QUESTIONS

Choose the best answer.

1. Each normal heartbeat is initiated by which of the following?
    A. Sinoatrial node in the wall of the right atrium
    B. Bundle of His in the interventricular septum
    C. Cardiac center in the medulla
    D. Sympathetic nerves from the spinal cord

2. During one cardiac cycle which of the following occurs?
    A. Ventricles contract first, followed by the atria
    B. Atria contract first, followed by the ventricles
    C. Atria and ventricles contract simultaneously
    D. Ventricles contract twice for every contraction of the atria

3. Which of the following detects changes in blood pressure?
    A. Pressoreceptors in the medulla
    B. Blood vessels in the medulla
    C. Pressoreceptors in the carotid and aortic sinuses
    D. Coronary vessels in the myocardium

4. Epinephrine increases blood pressure because it does which of the following?
    A. Increases water resorption by the kidneys
    B. Causes vasodilation in the skin and viscera
    C. Decreases heart rate and force of contraction
    D. Increases heart rate and force of cardiac contraction

5. When blood pressure decreases, the kidneys help raise it by secreting which of the following?
    A. Renin
    B. Epinephrine
    C. Aldosterone
    D. Erythropoietin

6. Which of the following prevents the backflow of blood in veins?
    A. Precapillary sphincters
    B. Middle layer
    C. Smooth muscle layer
    D. Valves

7. A patient has had a bilateral mastectomy, so the nurse obtains blood pressures readings from the patient's legs. Which of the following does the nurse understand is the usual difference between blood pressure readings in the leg and the arm?
    A. 10 mm Hg higher
    B. 10 mm Hg lower
    C. 15 mm Hg higher
    D. 15 mm Hg lower

8. The nurse obtains a lower blood pressure on a patient's left arm than the right arm. As a result, which of the following extremities should the nurse use for ongoing blood pressure measurement?
    A. Left arm
    B. Right arm
    C. Right leg
    D. Either arm

9. The nurse is checking a patient's blood pressure for orthostatic hypotension. The nurse understands that normally when the patient stands, the blood pressure drops by which of the following amounts?
    A. Up to 15 mm Hg
    B. Up to 20 mm Hg
    C. Up to 25 mm Hg
    D. Up to 30 mm Hg

10. While the nurse checks the patient's blood pressure for orthostatic hypotension, the patient's heart rate increases. The nurse understands that normally when the patient stands, the heart rate does which of the following?
    A. Drops up to 10 beats per minute
    B. Drops up to 20 beats per minute
    C. Increases up to 20 beats per minute
    D. Increases up to 30 beats per minute

11. The nurse is examining a patient's legs for data collection and notes that there is bilateral decreased hair distribution, thick, brittle nails, and shiny, taut, dry skin. The nurse understands that this can indicate which of the following?
    A. Increased arterial blood flow
    B. Decreased arterial blood flow
    C. Increased venous blood flow
    D. Decreased venous blood flow

12. The nurse is explaining to a patient that for his thallium stress test dipyridamole (Persantine), a coronary vasodilator, will be given. Which of the following purposes will the nurse explain as the reason that this medication is being given?
    A. To decrease blood flow to cardiac cells
    B. To increase blood flow that occurs with exercise
    C. To prevent a clot from forming during the test
    D. To reduce systemic vascular resistance

13. For which of the following dysrhythmias will the nurse anticipate a patient's need for a permanent pacemaker?
    A. Ventricular fibrillation
    B. Asymptomatic bradycardia
    C. Atrial fibrillation
    D. Third degree heart block

16

NURSING CARE OF PATIENTS WITH HYPERTENSION

▶ VOCABULARY

Match the word with its definition.

1. _____ Atherosclerosis

2. _____ Peripheral vascular resistance

3. _____ Normotensive

4. _____ Isolated systolic hypertension

5. _____ Hypertension

6. _____ Diastolic blood pressure

7. _____ Cardiac output

8. _____ Systolic blood pressure

9. _____ Secondary hypertension

10. _____ Primary hypertension

11. _____ Plaque

A. Most common form of arteriosclerosis, in which fats are deposited on arterial walls
B. Amount of blood the heart pumps out each minute
C. Amount of pressure exerted on the wall of the arteries when the ventricles are at rest; the bottom number in a blood pressure reading
D. Abnormally elevated blood pressure
E. Systolic pressure is 160 mm Hg or more, but the diastolic pressure is less than 95 mm Hg
F. Normal blood pressure
G. Opposition to blood flow through the vessels
H. Deposit of fatty material in the artery
I. Abnormally elevated blood pressure, the cause of which is unknown; also called essential hypertension
J. High blood pressure that is a symptom of a specific cause, such as a kidney abnormality
K. Maximal pressure exerted on the arteries during contraction of the left ventricle of the heart; top number of a blood pressure reading

▶ DIURETICS

Select the letter that identifies the type of each diuretic.

1. _____ Spironolactone (Aldactone)

2. _____ Bumetanide (Bumex)

3. _____ Chlorothiazide (Diuril)

4. _____ Triamterene (Dyrenium)

5. _____ Furosemide (Lasix)

6. _____ Amiloride (Midamor)

7. _____ Metolazone (Zaroxolyn)

8. _____ Hydrochlorothiazide (HydroDIURIL, HCTZ)

A. Thiazide or thiazide-like
B. Loop
C. Potassium sparing

► HYPERTENSION RISK FACTORS

Indicate whether the statement is true or false.

1. _____ Constant stress can cause hypertension.

2. _____ There is a link between a high-fat diet, obesity, and hypertension.

3. _____ High calcium, potassium, and magnesium levels are important risk factors for the development of hypertension.

4. _____ People who are not active on a regular basis are at an increased risk of developing hypertension.

5. _____ A diet high in salt is also high in vitamins and minerals.

► STAGES OF HYPERTENSION AND RECOMMENDATIONS FOR FOLLOW-UP

Indicate whether the statement is true or false, and correct the false statements.

1. _____ The recommended follow-up for a systolic blood pressure of 130 to 139 is 2 years.

2. _____ The recommended follow-up for a systolic blood pressure of less than 130 is 2 years.

3. _____ The recommended follow-up for a systolic blood pressure more than 180 is now.

4. _____ The recommended follow-up for a systolic blood pressure of 160 to 179 is 2 months.

5. _____ The recommended follow-up for a systolic blood pressure of 140 to 159 is 2 months.

6. _____ The recommended follow-up for a diastolic blood pressure of 90 to 99 is 1 month.

7. _____ The recommended follow-up for a diastolic blood pressure of more than 110 is now.

8. _____ The recommended follow-up for a diastolic blood pressure of 100 to 109 is 2 months.

9. _____ The recommended follow-up for a diastolic blood pressure less than 85 is 2 years.

10. _____ The recommended follow-up for a diastolic blood pressure of 85 to 89 is 1 year.

► CRITICAL THINKING

Read the case study and answer the questions.

Mrs. Laura Martin, age 42, is seen in the hypertension clinic for a follow-up visit for hypertension. Her blood pressure is 160/92 mm Hg and she is diagnosed with hypertension. The physician encourages lifestyle modification and prescribes an angiotensin-converting enzyme inhibitor.

1. What additional information should the nurse collect to develop a teaching plan for lifestyle modifications and the medication? _____

_____

2. Develop a teaching plan for Mrs. Martin's needs based on the data collected (see Answers for feedback). _____

_____

3. What interventions will help Mrs. Martin reach her goal for controlling her hypertension? _____

_____

4. How will you know when Mrs. Martin has reached her goals? _____

_____

REVIEW QUESTIONS

Choose the best answer.

1. The nurse is developing a teaching plan for a patient. Which of the following is a nonmodifiable risk factor for the development of hypertension?
   A. Race
   B. High cholesterol
   C. Cigarette smoking
   D. Sedentary lifestyle

2. If the systolic blood pressure is elevated and the diastolic blood pressure is normal, the nurse recognizes that a patient is most likely to have which type of hypertension?
   A. Primary
   B. Secondary
   C. Isolated systolic
   D. Malignant

3. The patient asks the nurse, "What is hypertension?" Which of the following is the best response to explain hypertension?
   A. It is measured as the heart pumps blood into the arteries.
   B. It is higher than normal on two separate occasions.
   C. It is regulated by stress, activity, and emotions.
   D. It is determined by peripheral vascular resistance.

4. Which of the following is information the nurse would be correct in giving the patient about smoking and its effect on blood pressure?
   A. It is associated with stage III hypertension.
   B. It does not affect blood pressure regulation.
   C. It vasodilates the peripheral blood vessels.
   D. It causes sustained blood pressure elevations.

5. Which of the following medications should the nurse explain may cause headache as a side effect?
   A. Furosemide (Lasix)
   B. Atenolol (Tenormin)
   C. Clonidine (Catapres)
   D. Adalat (Procardia)

6. The nurse understands that a patient with blood pressure readings of 164/102 and 176/100 on two separate occasions would be classified in which hypertension category?
   A. Stage I
   B. Stage II
   C. Stage III

7. A patient has been prescribed bumetanide (Bumex) every morning for control of hypertension. Which of the following statements indicates correct knowledge of the treatment regimen?
   A. "I can travel to Florida and sunbathe all day."
   B. "Now I can eat whatever I want, whenever I want."
   C. "I'll take my medication in the morning, every morning."
   D. "I won't need medication once my pressure goes down."

8. Which common side effect of metolazone (Zaroxolyn) should the nurse instruct a patient to report to the health care provider?
   A. Numb hands
   B. Muscle weakness
   C. Gastrointestinal distress
   D. Nightmares

9. The nurse understands that which of the following best describes the action of enalapril maleate (Vasotec)?
   A. It decreases levels of angiotensin II.
   B. It adjusts the extracellular volume.
   C. It dilates the arterioles and veins.
   D. It decreases cardiac output.

10. The nurse understands that which of the following is a side effect most likely to be reported by patients receiving enalapril maleate (Vasotec)?
    A. Acne
    B. Diarrhea
    C. Cough
    D. Heartburn

11. The nurse understands that which of the following best describes the action of propranolol (Inderal)?
    A. It increases heart rate.
    B. It decreases cardiac output.
    C. It decreases fluid volume.
    D. It increases cardiac contractility.

12. What instruction should the nurse give to the patient taking propranolol (Inderal) for hypertension?
    A. Have potassium level checked.
    B. Report any changes in appetite.
    C. Do not stop medication abruptly.
    D. Resume usual daily activities.

13. Which of the following nursing diagnoses is the focus of care for a patient with hypertension?
    A. Activity intolerance
    B. Ineffective airway clearance
    C. Impaired physical mobility
    D. Deficient knowledge

14. Which of the following statements, if made by a patient with hypertension, indicates to the nurse a need for more teaching?
    A. "High blood pressure may affect the kidneys and eyes."
    B. "Most people with hypertension watch their diet."
    C. "Medication will no longer be needed when I feel better."
    D. "Many people do not know when their blood pressure is high."

15. A patient teaching plan should include which of the following lifestyle modifications to help control hypertension?
    A. Regular aerobic exercise
    B. Low-tar cigarettes
    C. Three alcoholic beverages per day
    D. Daily multivitamin supplements

17

NURSING CARE OF PATIENTS WITH INFLAMMATORY AND INFECTIOUS CARDIOVASCULAR DISORDERS

► VOCABULARY
Identify the word that is formed by the word building.

1. _____ choreia—dance

2. _____ peri—around + kardia—heart + itis—inflammation

3. _____ myo—muscle + kardia—heart + itis—inflammation

4. _____ petecchia—skin spot

5. _____ peri—around + kardia—heart + kentesis—puncture

6. _____ kardia—heart + tamponade—plug

7. _____ kardia—heart + myo—muscle + pathy—disease

8. _____ kardia—heart + mega—large

9. _____ my—muscle + ectomy—cutting out

10. _____ thromb—lump (clot) + phleb—vein + itis—inflammation

► INFLAMMATORY AND INFECTIOUS CARDIOVASCULAR DISORDERS
Match the word with its definition.

1. _____ Solid, liquid, gaseous masses of undissolved matter traveling with the current in a blood or lymphatic vessel

2. _____ Gram-positive bacteria whose group A causes disease

3. _____ Inflammation of the heart lining caused by microorganisms

4. _____ Standardized test for reporting prothrombin to prevent variability in testing results and provide uniformity in monitoring therapeutic levels for coagulation

5. _____ Severe damage to the heart from rheumatic fever

A. Infective endocarditis
B. Emboli
C. International normalized ratio
D. Rheumatic heart disease
E. Beta-hemolytic streptococci

▶ RHEUMATIC FEVER AND RHEUMATIC HEART DISEASE

Find the 12 errors and insert the correct information.

Rheumatic fever causes a streptococcal infection such as a sore throat. Rheumatic fever signs and symptoms include polyarthritis, subcutaneous nodules, cholera with rapid, controlled movements, carditis, fever, arthralgia, and pneumonia. The joints become inflamed all at once, resulting in polyarthritis. The minor joints are most commonly affected, but this inflammation causes permanent damage. Subcutaneous nodules that are small, firm, and painful, develop over bony prominences. A throat culture diagnoses rheumatic fever. Chronic rheumatic carditis can be a complication of rheumatic fever. The heart valves and their structures can be scarred and damaged. These changes may occur immediately after an episode of rheumatic fever and can lead to heart failure. Rheumatic fever can be prevented by detecting and treating streptococcal infections promptly with aspirin. The signs and symptoms of a pharynx streptococcal infection include sudden sore throat, low-grade fever, chills, throat redness with exudate, sinus or ear infection, and lymph node enlargement. Nursing care focuses on relieving the patient's pain and anxiety, maintaining normal cardiac function, and educating the patient about rheumatic heart disease.

▶ THROMBOPHLEBITIS

Complete the rationale and evaluation of the nursing care plan for a patient with thrombophlebitis.

Nursing Diagnosis

ACUTE PAIN RELATED TO INFLAMMATION OF VEIN

Interventions	Rationale	Evaluation
Assess pain using rating scale such as 0 to 10.		
Provide analgesics and nonsteroidal antiinflammatory drugs (NSAIDs) as ordered.		
Apply warm, moist soaks.		
Maintain bed rest with leg elevation above heart level.		

Nursing Diagnosis

DEFICIENT KNOWLEDGE RELATED TO LACK OF KNOWLEDGE ABOUT DISORDER AND TREATMENT

Interventions	Rationale	Evaluation
Explain condition, symptoms, and complications.		
Explain medications, therapies ordered, monthly lab test monitoring, and need for Medic Alert identification.		
Teach patient not to massage extremity.		

▶ DIAGNOSTIC TESTS FOR INFECTIVE ENDOCARDITIS

Match the test with its finding that is indicative of infective endocarditis.

Test

1. _____ White blood cell count with differential
2. _____ Blood cultures
3. _____ Erythrocyte sedimentation rate
4. _____ Rheumatoid factor
5. _____ Electrocardiogram
6. _____ Chest x-ray examination
7. _____ Echocardiogram
8. _____ Cardiac catheterization

Finding

A. Abnormal heart and valve function
B. Dysrhythmias
C. Elevated
D. Heart failure
E. Identifies causative organism
F. Positive
G. Slight elevation
H. Vegetations on heart valves

▶ CRITICAL THINKING

Read the case study and answer the questions.

Mr. Evans, 68, is admitted to the hospital for heart failure resulting from hypertrophic cardiomyopathy. He has dyspnea, fatigue, and angina. His lung sounds reveal crackles.

A. What is the pathophysiology of hypertrophic cardiomyopathy? _____

B. What occurs with ventricular size and ventricular filling with blood in hypertrophic cardiomyopathy? _____

C. What diagnostic test will show hypertrophic cardiomyopathy and left-sided heart failure? _____

D. Why is digoxin contraindicated for Mr. Evans? _____

E. Why would a myectomy be helpful? _____

F. Why should Mr. Evans be taught to avoid (a) dehydration and (b) exertion? _____

G. Why is it important for the family to learn cardiopulmonary resuscitation (CPR)? _____

REVIEW QUESTIONS

Choose the best answer.

1. A patient visits the doctor for a severe sore throat and fever. As the nurse plans the patient's care, the nurse understands that it is important to perform which of the following diagnostic tests to help prevent cardiac complications?
   A. Chest x-ray examination
   B. Throat culture
   C. White blood cell count
   D. Erythrocyte sedimentation rate

2. Which of the following does the nurse understand usually precedes rheumatic fever?
   A. A viral infection
   B. A fungal infection
   C. A staphylococcal infection
   D. A beta-hemolytic streptococci infection

3. A patient with a history of endocarditis is undergoing a bowel resection. The nurse explains that the prophylactic antibiotics prevent which of the following?
   A. Endocarditis
   B. Peritonitis
   C. Vegetative emboli
   D. Inflammation

4. A patient has a positive Homans' sign. Which of the following does the nurse understand explains why ambulation and performing the Homans' sign is now contraindicated?
   A. They can cause calf swelling.
   B. They can cause patient pain.
   C. They can cause an emboli.
   D. They may cause a clot to form.

5. A patient develops a postoperative deep vein thrombosis and is started on intravenous heparin. Which of the following laboratory tests is monitored during the heparin therapy?
   A. Plasma fibrinogen
   B. Prothrombin time (PT)
   C. Partial thromboplastin time (PTT)
   D. International normalized ratio (INR)

6. The nurse is caring for a patient on warfarin (Coumadin) with an elevated INR level. Which of the following would be ordered as the antidote for warfarin?
   A. Vitamin K
   B. Vitamin B_{12}
   C. Calcium chloride
   D. Protamine sulfate

7. Which of the following is a desired outcome for the nursing diagnosis of acute pain for a patient with acute thrombophlebitis?
   A. States anxiety is decreased.
   B. States pain is satisfactorily relieved.
   C. Is able to participate in desired activities.
   D. Reports ability to ambulate without pain.

8. The nurse is reviewing the patient's daily PT and INR levels. The PT level is 24 (normal = 9.5 to 11.3 seconds). Which of the following actions should the nurse take?
   A. Give the next dose of warfarin when it is ordered to be given.
   B. Inform physician before the next dose of warfarin is given.
   C. Stop the heparin infusion.
   D. Continue monitoring heparin infusion.

9. A patient, who had a hysterectomy 2 days ago, reports tenderness in her left calf. The nursing assessment reveals the following: left calf 17.5″, right calf 14″, left thigh 32″, right thigh 28″, and a shiny, warm, and reddened left leg. Which of the following interventions should be given priority in the patient's plan of care?
   A. Maintain bed rest.
   B. Encourage ambulation tid.
   C. Apply bilateral antiembolism stockings.
   D. Encourage bilateral leg exercises.

10. The nurse is caring for a patient receiving warfarin therapy. Which of the following findings is essential to report to the physician?
    A. TCT 9 (thrombin clotting time) (normal = 10 to 15 seconds)
    B. PT 26 (normal = 9.5 to 11.3 seconds)
    C. PTT 29 (normal = 30 to 45 seconds)
    D. INR 2.2 (normal = 2 to 3 seconds)

11. A patient has end-stage dilated cardiomyopathy. He comes to the emergency department with dyspnea. He says he went to bed and awoke with a feeling of suffocation. He says it was frightening. Which of the following responses by the nurse is most appropriate?
    A. "You must have been dreaming."
    B. "Reclining decreases the heart's ability to pump blood."
    C. "Sleeping increases heart rate, which increases the body's need for oxygen."
    D. "Reclining increases fluid returning to the heart, which builds up fluid in the lungs."

12. The nurse is caring for a patient, age 68, who is receiving digoxin (Lanoxin) 0.125 mg qd for cardiac myopathy. Which of the following assessments of the patient would indicates that he is experiencing a side effect of digoxin that requires follow-up?
    A. Skin flushing
    B. Anorexia
    C. Hypertension
    D. Constipation

13. The physician writes a "now" order for codeine 45 mg intramuscular (IM) for a patient with thrombophlebitis. The nurse has on hand codeine 60 mg/2 mL. Which of the following doses should be given?
    A. 1.45 mL
    B. 1.50 mL
    C. 1.75 mL
    D. 2.15 mL

14. A patient, age 46, is admitted for observation following an auto accident. He hit the steering wheel and has a chest contusion. As the nurse assesses him for a pericardial friction rub, she understands that which of the following causes a pericardial friction rub?
    A. Inflamed cardiac tricuspid and mitral valves
    B. Decreased cardiac output
    C. Increased pulmonary pressures
    D. Friction of inflamed pericardial and epicardial layers

15. As the nurse assesses the patient, the nurse understands that which of the following is the most common symptom of pericarditis?
    A. Dyspnea
    B. Intermittent claudication
    C. Chest pain
    D. Calf pain

18

NURSING CARE OF PATIENTS WITH OCCLUSIVE CARDIOVASCULAR DISORDERS

▶ VOCABULARY

Match the word with its definition.

1. _____ Arteriosclerosis

2. _____ Atherosclerosis

3. _____ Stenosis

4. _____ Ischemia

5. _____ Skin breakdown as a result of chronic venous insufficiency

6. _____ High-density lipoprotein

7. _____ Collateral circulation

8. _____ Percutaneous transluminal coronary angioplasty

9. _____ Chest pain caused by decreased blood supply to the heart

10. _____ Chest pain that usually subsides with rest

11. _____ Chest pain that increases in frequency and is not affected by rest

12. _____ Tortuous and bulging veins, usually in lower extremity

13. _____ Disease causing venospasms when exposed to cold

14. _____ A bulging or dilation of an artery

15. _____ Death of a portion of the myocardium

16. _____ Laboratory value that determines degree of damage to the heart

17. _____ A moving clot

18. _____ A stationary clot

19. _____ Intermittent claudication

20. _____ Obstructed blood flow in the coronary arteries

A. Varicose veins
B. Procedure that compresses plaque against wall of artery
C. Unstable angina
D. Hardening of arteries
E. Angina pectoris
F. Coronary artery disease
G. Stable angina
H. Raynaud's disease
I. Plaque buildup within arterial wall
J. Lack of blood supply
K. Aneurysm
L. Vessels grow to compensate for blocked blood flow
M. Narrowing of a vessel
N. Myocardial infarction
O. Embolism
P. "Good" cholesterol
Q. Thrombus
R. Venous stasis ulcer
S. Troponin I
T. Exertional calf pain that ceases with rest

▶ ATHEROSCLEROSIS

Answer the following questions.

1. What is the pathophysiology of atherosclerosis? _____

_____

_____

2. What are modifiable risk factors that contribute to atherosclerosis? _____

_____

_____

3. Develop a teaching plan for one of the modifiable risk factors for atherosclerosis. _____

_____

_____

▶ MYOCARDIAL INFARCTION

Find the 23 errors and insert the correct information.

Myocardial infarction (MI) is the death of a portion of the pericardial sac caused by blockage or spasm of a coronary artery. When the patient has an MI, the affected part of the muscle becomes damaged and no longer functions properly. Ischemic injury takes a few minutes before complete necrosis and infarction take place. The ischemic process affects the subendocardial layer, which is the least sensitive to hypoxia. Myocardial contractility is depressed, so the body attempts to compensate by triggering the parasympathetic nervous system. This causes a decrease in myocardial oxygen demand. After necrosis, the contractility function of the muscle is temporarily lost. If treatment is initiated after several signs of an MI, the area of damage can be minimized. If prolonged ischemia occurs, the size of the infarction can be small.

The area that is affected by an MI depends on which coronary artery is involved. The left anterior descending (LAD) branch of the left main coronary artery is the area that feeds the lateral wall. The right coronary artery (RCA) feeds the anterior wall and parts of the atrioventricular node and the sinoatrial node. An occlusion of the RCA leads to an inferior MI and abnormalities of impulse conduction and formation. The left circumflex coronary artery feeds the inferior wall and part of the posterior wall of the heart.

Pain is the least common complaint. The pain does not radiate. Other symptoms may include restlessness; a feeling of impending doom; nausea; diaphoresis; and cold, clammy, ashen skin. The only symptom that might be present in the elderly patient is vomiting.

The three strong indicators of an MI are patient history, abnormal electrocardiographic (ECG) reading, and high triglyceride levels.

Initially, patients are kept on bed rest to increase myocardial oxygen demand. Patients are medicated promptly when complaining of chest pain. Meperidine (Demerol) is the most widely used narcotic for several reasons. It helps decrease anxiety, increases respirations, and has a vasoconstrictive effect on coronary arteries. Oxygen is given usually at 1 L/hr via nasal cannula. Nitroglycerin sublingual, topical, or by intravenous drip can also be administered. Thrombolytic therapy is a frequent option for preventing a clot that can occlude a coronary artery.

A nursing care plan should include factors that may contribute to decreased cardiac workload. Changes in diet, stress reduction, regular exercise program, cessation of smoking, and following a medication schedule require extensive patient and family teaching.

▶ PHARMACOLOGICAL TREATMENT

Match the medication to the appropriate description.

1. _____ A calcium channel blocker
2. _____ Beta blocker
3. _____ Drug of choice for anginal attacks
4. _____ Does not dissolve existing clots
5. _____ Drug used to lower cholesterol
6. _____ Decreases platelet aggregation
7. _____ Long-acting nitrate
8. _____ Thrombolytic therapy agent
9. _____ Decreases blood viscosity

A. Nitroglycerin
B. Cholestyramine (Questran)
C. Propranolol (Inderal)
D. Nifedipine (Procardia)
E. Streptokinase
F. Dipyridamole (Persantine)
G. Heparin
H. Pentoxifylline (Trental)
I. Isosorbide dinitrate (Isordil)

▶ CRITICAL THINKING

Read the following case study and answer the questions.

Mr. Edwards is a 43-year-old man with a history of peripheral vascular disease and hypertension. He smokes two packs of cigarettes per day. He complains of calf pain during minimal exercise that decreases with rest.

1. Which of the following nursing diagnoses would be the most appropriate relating to his symptoms?
   A. Ineffective tissue perfusion related to compromised circulation
   B. Fatigue related to pain on exertion
   C. Impaired mobility relating to stress associated with pain
   D. Self-care deficit related to pain and muscle spasms

2. Explain what happens when intermittent claudication occurs. _____
   _____
   _____

3. Why does rest decrease the pain? _____
   _____
   _____

4. Describe how smoking contributes to decreased circulation. _____
   _____
   _____

REVIEW QUESTIONS

Choose the best answer.

1. A patient who has been scheduled for a stress ECG asks why this ECG is needed. Which of the following is the nurse's best response?
   A. It can predict whether the patient may soon have a heart attack.
   B. It verifies how much more physically fit the patient needs to become.
   C. It determines the patient's potential target heart rate.
   D. It shows how the heart performs during exercise.

2. During a stress ECG, a patient reports chest pain and the test is stopped. When the patient is asked to undergo a heart catheterization, the patient appears very apprehensive and worried. Which of the following is the most appropriate action for the nurse to take to reduce the patient's anxiety?
   A. Explain how coronary artery disease is treated.
   B. Avoid discussing the heart catheterization until the patient has relaxed.
   C. Explain how well others have done after having this procedure.
   D. Listen to the patient express feelings about the condition.

3. Before a cardiac catheterization and coronary arteriogram, it is essential that the nurse ask a patient if he or she is allergic to iodine or which of the following?
   A. Eggs
   B. Codeine
   C. Shellfish
   D. Penicillin

4. Which of the following statements by a patient demonstrates to the nurse that the patient understands when to replace nitroglycerin tablets?
   A. Pills no longer tingle when used.
   B. Pills disintegrate when touched.
   C. Pills smell like vinegar.
   D. Pills become discolored.

5. After hospitalization for a myocardial infarction, a patient is placed on a low-sodium diet. In discussing foods allowed on this diet, the nurse should tell the patient that this list includes which of the following?
   A. Hot dogs
   B. Fresh vegetables
   C. Milk and cheese
   D. Canned soups

6. A patient, hospitalized with an MI, suddenly begins to have severe respiratory distress with frothy sputum. These signs indicate that the patient probably has developed which of the following?
   A. Pneumonia
   B. Cardiac tamponade
   C. Pulmonary edema
   D. Pneumothorax

7. As the nurse assesses a patient for decreased circulation in the lower extremities, which of the following findings would indicate adequate circulation?
   A. Loss of hair on the extremity
   B. Capillary refill less than 3 seconds
   C. Diminished pulses in the extremity
   D. Thickened nails of the extremity

8. The percentage of calories from fat in the diet should be limited to no more than which of the following to help prevent atherosclerosis?
   A. 10 percent
   B. 25 percent
   C. 30 percent
   D. 45 percent

9. The nurse understands that pain associated with coronary artery disease occurs from which of the following?
   A. Lack of nutrients to the heart
   B. Interrupted electrical activity to the areas of the heart
   C. Lack of sufficient oxygen to the myocardium
   D. Overexertion of heart muscle due to the workload

10. Which of the following does the nurse correctly include in a teaching plan as a modifiable risk factor for coronary artery disease?
    A. Hypertension
    B. Race
    C. Age
    D. Gender

11. Which of the following should the nurse correctly include in a teaching plan as a saturated fat?
    A. Cottonseed oil
    B. Coconut oil
    C. Safflower oil
    D. Sunflower oil

12. Which of the following clinical manifestations is *not* a symptom of acute venous insufficiency?
    A. Full superficial veins
    B. An aching, cramping type of pain
    C. Initial absence of edema
    D. Cool and cyanotic skin

13. The nurse understands that which of the following is the most characteristic symptom of Buerger's disease?
    A. Numbness
    B. Pain
    C. Cramping
    D. Swelling

14. A patient has been diagnosed with Raynaud's disease and asks the nurse what occurs with this disease. The most appropriate response by the nurse is which of the following?
    A. Arterial vessel occlusion is caused by many clots that develop in the heart and are carried to the bloodstream.
    B. Arteriolar vasoconstriction occurs, most often on the fingertips with symptoms of coldness, pain, and pale skin.
    C. Peripheral vasospasm occurs in the lower limbs as a result of valve damage from long-standing venous stasis.
    D. Thrombosis related to prolonged vasoconstriction caused by overexposure to the cold occurs.

19

NURSING CARE OF PATIENTS WITH CARDIAC VALVULAR DISORDERS

▶ VOCABULARY
Fill in the blank with the word that is formed by the word building.

1. _____ annulus—ring + plasty—formed

2. _____ commissura—joining together + tome—incision

3. _____ in—not + sufficiens—sufficient

4. _____ re—again + gurgitare—to flood

5. _____ stenos—narrow

6. _____ valvula—leaf of a folding door + plasty—formed

▶ MITRAL VALVE PROLAPSE
Find the eight errors and insert the correct information in the space provided.

During ventricular diastole, when pressures in the left ventricle rise, the leaflets of the mitral valve normally remain open. In mitral valve prolapse (MVP), however, the leaflets bulge backward into the left ventricle during systole. Often there are functional problems seen with MVP. However, if the leaflets do not fit together, mitral stenosis can occur with varying degrees of severity.

MVP tends to be hereditary, and the cause is known. Infections that damage the mitral valve may be a contributing factor. It is the most common form of valvular heart disease and typically occurs in men age 20 to 55. Most patients with MVP have symptoms. Symptoms that may occur include chest pain, dysrhythmias, palpitations, dizziness, and syncope. No treatment is needed unless symptoms are present. Stimulants and caffeine should be avoided to prevent symptoms. Information on endocarditis prevention is essential.

▶ VALVULAR DISORDERS

Indicate whether the statement is true or false, and correct false statements.

1. _____ Stenosis is widening of the opening of a heart valve.

2. _____ Stenosis inhibits the forward flow of blood.

3. _____ Regurgitation, or insufficiency, is failure of the valve to close completely.

4. _____ Regurgitation inhibits backflow of blood.

5. _____ Rheumatic heart disease and congenital defects are primary causes of valvular disease.

6. _____ The primary valves affected by disease are the tricuspid and pulmonic valves.

7. _____ Compensatory mechanisms in valvular disease are dilation to handle the increased blood volume and hypertrophy to increase the strength of contractions.

8. _____ Symptoms of valvular disease often occur early and reflect decreased cardiac output and pulmonary congestion: fatigue, dyspnea, orthopnea, cough.

9. _____ In severe valvular disease, heart failure occurs, and symptoms reflect the backup of blood from the failing chamber.

10. _____ In acute valve disorders, symptoms of shock are seen.

11. _____ Valve disease diagnosis is made with electrocardiogram (ECG), chest x-ray examination, echocardiogram, and cardiac catheterization.

12. _____ Valvuloplasty uses a balloon to separate the valve leaflets.

13. _____ Commissurotomy narrows the valve opening.

14. _____ Annuloplasty surgically repairs the valve.

15. _____ Patient teaching for valvular disorder includes understanding the importance of prophylactic antibiotics before all invasive procedures.

▶ CRITICAL THINKING

Read the case study and answer the questions.

Mrs. Murphy, 72, has aortic stenosis and is scheduled for an aortic valve replacement. She reports fatigue and dyspnea with exertion.

1. What may be the cause of Mrs. Murphy's aortic stenosis? _____

_____

2. When obtaining Mrs. Murphy's medical history, what should the nurse ask that is relevant to the cause of aortic stenosis?

_____

3. How does the heart compensate for aortic stenosis? _____

4. What should the nurse anticipate may occur in severe aortic stenosis? _____

5. Why is angina a common symptom of aortic stenosis? _____

6. What medication might the nurse expect to be ordered preoperatively? _____

7. Why does Mrs. Murphy's chest x-ray examination show an enlarged heart? _____

_____

8. Why is aortic stenosis treated with valvular replacement? _____

REVIEW QUESTIONS

Choose the best answer.

1. Which of the following does the nurse understand occurs in aortic stenosis?
   A. Aortic valve does not close tightly.
   B. Emptying of blood from left ventricle is impaired.
   C. Blood backflows into the left atrium.
   D. Emptying of the left atrium is impaired.

2. The nurse understands that which of the following occurs in mitral regurgitation?
   A. Backflow of blood into the left atrium
   B. Backflow of blood into the right atrium
   C. Impaired emptying of the right ventricle
   D. Impaired emptying of the left ventricle

3. Which of the following compensatory mechanisms does the nurse understand occurs with ventricular valve disorders?
   A. Decreased atrial kick
   B. Atrial hypertrophy
   C. Ventricular hypertrophy
   D. Systolic hypertension

4. Which of the following does the nurse understand causes fatigue in patients with chronic aortic stenosis?
   A. Atrial fibrillation
   B. Left ventricular failure
   C. Decreased pulmonary blood flow
   D. Increased coronary artery blood flow

5. Which of the following medications does the nurse anticipate that the patient will be given to prevent complications associated with decreased cardiac output?
   A. Furosemide (Lasix)
   B. Cephalexin (Keflex)
   C. Penicillin (Bicillin)
   D. Warfarin (Coumadin)

6. Which of the following diagnostic tests does the nurse understand measures the pressures in the cardiac chambers?
   A. ECG
   B. Exercise stress test
   C. Echocardiogram
   D. Cardiac catheterization

7. Which of the following should the nurse include in the plan of care as a patient outcome for deficient knowledge related to mitral stenosis?
   A. Clear breath sounds, no edema or weight gain
   B. Normal changes in vital signs with less fatigue during self-care
   C. Verbalizes knowledge of disorder
   D. States fear is reduced

8. The nurse is caring for a patient, age 70, who has a nursing diagnosis of deficient knowledge related to furosemide administration. Which of the following interventions is essential to include when planning a teaching session to promote successful learning?
   A. Assess patient's learning priorities.
   B. Tell patient what he needs to learn first about furosemide.
   C. Assess patient's dietary intake of potassium.
   D. Give patient a written test at the end of the teaching session.

9. A patient, age 65, is being discharged after a mechanical valve replacement for aortic stenosis. Which of the following should he be taught regarding his warfarin therapy?
   A. Wear Medic Alert identification.
   B. Increase intake of green leafy vegetables.
   C. Keep yearly blood test appointments.
   D. Use a straight razor when shaving.

10. The nurse is teaching a patient with heart failure how to avoid activity that results in Valsalva's maneuver. Which of the following statements by the patient indicates to the nurse that the teaching has been effective?
    A. "I will breathe normally when moving."
    B. "I will use a straw to drink oral fluids."
    C. "I will take fewer but deeper breaths."
    D. "I will clench my teeth when moving."

11. The nurse is planning care for a patient with chronic mitral regurgitation. Which of the following is the nurse correct in assessing to determine the cause of dyspnea and cough in patients with chronic mitral regurgitation?
    A. Cardiac rhythm
    B. Heart tones
    C. Peripheral edema
    D. Lung sounds

20
NURSING CARE OF PATIENTS WITH CARDIAC DYSRHYTHMIAS

▶ VOCABULARY

Match the words and definitions.

1. _____ Amplitude
2. _____ Atrial depolarization
3. _____ Atrial systole
4. _____ Bigeminy
5. _____ Cardioversion
6. _____ Complete heart block
7. _____ Contractility
8. _____ Decompensation
9. _____ Defibrillate
10. _____ Inherent
11. _____ Ischemia
12. _____ Isoelectric line
13. _____ Multifocal
14. _____ Quadrigeminy
15. _____ Right bundle branch block
16. _____ Trigeminy
17. _____ Unifocal
18. _____ Ventricular diastole
19. _____ Ventricular escape rhythm
20. _____ Ventricular repolarization
21. _____ Ventricular systole

A. Beat occurring every fourth complex, as in premature ventricular contractions (PVCs)
B. Belonging to anything naturally
C. Coming or originating from one site
D. Condition in which there is a complete dissociation between atrial and ventricular systoles
E. Contraction of the atria
F. Contraction of the two ventricles
G. Defect in heart conduction system in which right bundle does not conduct impulses normally
H. Elective procedure in which synchronized shock of 25 to 50 joules is delivered to restore normal sinus rhythm
I. Electrical activation of the atria
J. Electrical tracing is at zero and is neither positive nor negative
K. Failure of the heart to maintain adequate circulation
L. Force with which left ventricular ejection occurs
M. Local and temporary deficiency of blood supply resulting from obstruction of the circulation to another part
N. Occurring every third beat, as in PVCs
O. Occurs every second beat, as in PVCs
P. Originating from many foci or sites
Q. Period of relaxation of the ventricle
R. Reestablishment of the polarized state of the muscle after contraction
S. Size or fullness of voltage
T. Naturally occurring rhythm of the ventricles when the rest of the conduction system fails
U. Use of electrical device to apply counter-shocks to the heart through electrodes placed on the chest wall to stop fibrillation

▶ COMPONENTS OF A CARDIAC CYCLE
Label the components of a cardiac cycle.

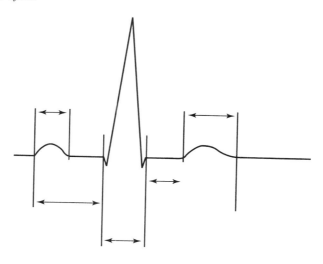

▶ HEART RATE
Count the heart rate using the 6-second method.

1.

Heart rate = _____

2.

Heart rate = _____

3.

Heart rate = _____

▶ CARDIAC CONDUCTION

Match the words and definitions.

1. _____ Sinoatrial node
2. _____ Atrioventricular node
3. _____ Normal sinus rhythm
4. _____ Right atrium
5. _____ Right ventricle
6. _____ Left atrium
7. _____ Left ventricle
8. _____ Bradycardia
9. _____ Tachycardia
10. _____ Q wave
11. _____ P wave
12. _____ R wave
13. _____ S wave
14. _____ T wave
15. _____ U wave
16. _____ Premature
17. _____ Sinus tachycardia
18. _____ Sinus bradycardia
19. _____ Premature atrial contraction
20. _____ Atrial fibrillation
21. _____ Premature ventricular contraction
22. _____ Ventricular tachycardia
23. _____ Ventricular fibrillation
24. _____ Asystole

A. Rate less than 60
B. No QRS complexes seen—straight line
C. An early beat
D. An early beat that has a P wave and a normal QRS complex
E. Where an impulse originates
F. A chaotic pattern—no visible cardiac cycles
G. No identifiable P waves with a normal QRS complex; irregularly, irregular
H. Wave that precedes a QRS complex
I. Where an impulse is delayed before going to the Purkinje fibers
J. An early beat with no P wave and a wide, bizarre QRS complex
K. Successive beats of three or more wide, bizarre QRS complexes
L. Rhythm with normal P waves, QRS, T waves with a heart rate of 60 to 100 beats per minute
M. The first negative deflection of a QRS complex
N. A small wave seen after the T wave
O. The first positive deflection on a QRS complex
P. Rhythm with normal P waves, QRS, T waves with a heart rate of less than 60 beats per minute
Q. The chamber of the heart that pumps the blood to the rest of the body
R. Chamber that receives blood returning to the heart
S. Rhythm with normal P waves, QRS, T waves with a heart rate of more than 100 beats per minute
T. The wave that follows the QRS complex
U. The chamber that receives blood from the pulmonary veins
V. The downward deflection after the R wave
W. Heart rate of more than 100 beats per minute
X. Chamber that propels blood into the pulmonary artery

▶ ELECTROCARDIOGRAM INTERPRETATION

Analyze the electrocardiogram (ECG) rhythms using the five-step interpretation process.

A.

1. Rhythm: _____

2. Heart rate: _____

3. P waves: _____

4. PR interval: _____

5. QRS interval: _____

6. ECG interpretation: _____

B.

1. Rhythm: _____

2. Heart rate: _____

3. P waves: _____

4. PR interval: _____

5. QRS interval: _____

6. ECG interpretation: _____

► CRITICAL THINKING

Read the case study and answer the questions.

Mrs. Samuels is admitted to the hospital for chest pain. Tests are run, and her ECG shows bigeminal PVCs of more than 6 per minute that are close to her T wave. Her potassium level is 3.0 mEq/L. She is short of breath on exertion. Her blood pressure is 104/56, her pulse is 72, and her respirations are 16.

1. What should the nurse do first? _____

2. What actions should the nurse take regarding the dysrhythmia? _____

3. What might some of the causes be for this dysrhythmia? _____

4. What additional symptoms might the nurse anticipate? _____

5. What type of orders should the nurse expect from the doctor? _____

REVIEW QUESTIONS

Choose the best answer.

1. The nurse understands that which of the following defines a cardiac cycle?
   A. Circulation of the blood through the body
   B. Circulation of the blood through the heart
   C. Depolarization and repolarization of heart chambers
   D. Pumping action of the heart

2. When a life-threatening dysrhythmia is seen on a cardiac monitor, which of the following is the nurse's first appropriate action?
   A. Notify the physician immediately.
   B. Assess the patient.
   C. Administer the appropriate medication for the noted dysrhythmia.
   D. Obtain vital signs.

3. The heart receives blood returning from the body through which of the following?
   A. Pulmonary vein
   B. Aorta
   C. Vena cavae
   D. Right coronary artery

4. Which of the following separates the right side of the heart from the left?
   A. Valve
   B. Pericardium
   C. Chamber
   D. Septum

5. Which of the following chambers of the heart is largest and has the thickest myocardium?
   A. Left ventricle
   B. Right ventricle
   C. Right atrium
   D. Left atrium

6. Which of the following represents the resting state of the ventricle on the ECG?
   A. U wave
   B. QRS complex
   C. P wave
   D. T wave

7. Which of the following is the inherent rate for the atrioventricular node?
   A. 20 to 40 beats per minute
   B. 40 to 60 beats per minute
   C. 60 to 100 beats per minute
   D. More than 100 beats per minute

8. The nurse understands that rhythms arising from the primary pacing node of the heart are referred to as which of the following?
   A. Escape beats
   B. Bundle branch blocks
   C. Sinus rhythms
   D. Ectopic rhythms

9. The nurse is teaching a patient about digoxin. Which of the following would the nurse be correct in including in the teaching plan as the action of digoxin?
   A. Decreases ectopic beats.
   B. Increases force of contractions.
   C. Increases heart rate.
   D. Raises blood pressure.

10. The nurse is providing care to a patient with atrial fibrillation. Which of the following is a possible serious complication of atrial fibrillation for which the nurse should be alert?
    A. Formation of a thrombus
    B. Swelling of hands and feet
    C. Cardiac tamponade
    D. Coronary occlusion

11. Which of the following treatments is appropriate for a patient with atrial fibrillation?
    A. Xylocaine (Lidocaine) and oxygen
    B. Nitroglycerin and bed rest
    C. Disopyramide (Norpace) and isoproterenol (Isuprel)
    D. Digoxin (Lanoxin) and cardioversion

12. The nurse is caring for a patient who has had a run of three or more PVCs together. The nurse should document this as which of the following?
    A. Ventricular tachycardia
    B. Bigeminy
    C. Trigeminy
    D. Multifocal PVCs

13. The nurse is caring for a patient in ventricular tachycardia who is hemodynamically stable, which of the following is the first choice of treatment?
    A. Cardioversion
    B. Pacemaker
    C. Defibrillation
    D. Antiarrhythmic intravenous medication

14. The nurse is caring for a patient whose ECG monitor shows a total absence of electrical impulse. The nurse does not detect a pulse. The nurse documents this as which of the following rhythms?
    A. Agonal
    B. Ventricular standstill
    C. Asystole
    D. Sinus arrest

15. A patient with a cardiac disorder is having increased PVCs and feels "anxious." After assessment and vital signs, what is the next action for the nurse to take?
    A. Order an ECG and cardiac enzymes.
    B. Call the physician.
    C. Elevate the head of the bed and start oxygen at 2 L/min.
    D. Put the bed in Trendelenburg's position.

21

NURSING CARE OF PATIENTS WITH HEART FAILURE

▶ VOCABULARY

Fill in the blank with the appropriate word found in the word list.

Afterload
Cor pulmonale
Hepatomegaly
Orthopnea
Paroxysmal nocturnal dyspnea

Peripheral vascular resistance
Preload
Pulmonary edema (Acute Heart Failure)
Splenomegaly

1. _____ _____ is the acute inability of the heart to pump enough blood to meet the body's oxygen and nutrient needs.

2. _____ _____ occurs when the right side of the heart fails because of an increased work-load caused by pulmonary disease.

3. Organ enlargement that may occur with right-sided heart failure is known as _____ and _____.

4. The goal of treatment for heart failure is to improve the heart's pumping ability and decrease the heart's workload by re-ducing _____ _____ _____.

5. _____ _____ _____ causes supine patients to awaken suddenly with a feeling of suffocation.

6. The end-diastole stretch in the ventricles produced by ventricular volume is _____.

7. The tension in the ventricular wall during systole necessary to overcome vascular resistance is _____.

8. _____ is dyspnea that occurs when the patient lies down.

► FLUID ACCUMULATION PATTERNS

Label the backward accumulation of fluid and shade areas of fluid congestion.

The heart pumps blood in a closed circuit. If one side of the heart fails to adequately pump blood forward, it pools and backs up from the failing chamber. On the drawing, use arrows to mark the path of the backward accumulation of fluid from the side of the heart that is failing. Shade in areas where fluid congestion occurs.

To increase your understanding of where the backward accumulation of fluid occurs from a certain side of the heart, use blue shading to illustrate the side with deoxygenated blood accumulation. Use red shading for the side with oxygenated blood accumulation.

► SIGNS AND SYMPTOMS OF HEART FAILURE

In heart failure, certain signs and symptoms occur based on the side of the heart that is failing as a pump. Match the following sign or symptom to the failing side of the heart that is causing it.

1. _____ Dry cough

2. _____ Peripheral edema

3. _____ Crackles

4. _____ Hepatomegaly

5. _____ Jugular vein distention

6. _____ Dyspnea

7. _____ Splenomegaly

8. _____ Orthopnea

L. Left-sided heart failure
R. Right-sided heart failure

► CRITICAL THINKING

Read the following case study and answer the questions.

Mr. Donner, age 72, is admitted to the cardiac unit for increasing dyspnea on exertion and fatigue.

Subjective Data

History of heart failure for 2 years
Unable to walk one block without increasing dyspnea
Sleeps at 60-degree angle in reclining chair
Increasing fatigue during the last 2 weeks

Objective Data

BP 140/78, P 108, R 24, T 98.8° F (37.1° C)
Jugular vein distention at 45 degrees
Has frequent dry cough
Bilateral crackles in lung bases
Nonpitting edema
Diagnostic studies
Chest x-ray examination: left and right ventricular hypertrophy, bilateral fluid in lower lung lobes

1. Explain the cause of Mr. Donner's fatigue, cough, and shortness of breath. _____
_____

2. Which of Mr. Donner's signs and symptoms are from left-sided heart failure and which are from right-sided heart failure?

3. Left: _____

   Right: _____

4. Explain the purpose of each of the following therapies. How would they be beneficial in treating Mr. Donner's heart failure?

   A. Furosemide (Lasix) 40 mg PO bid: _____

   B. Digitalis 0.125 mg PO qd: _____

   C. 2 g sodium diet: _____

   D. Oxygen 4 L/min: _____

4. Mr. Donner suddenly becomes dyspneic and anxious, has moist crackles throughout his lungs, and pink frothy sputum. Explain what is happening. _____
_____

5. Explain the purpose of each of the following therapies. How are they beneficial in treating Mr. Donner's acute heart failure?

   A. High Fowler's position: _____

   B. Oxygen 6 L/min: _____

   C. Furosemide (Lasix) 40 mg IVP: _____

   D. Digitalis 0.125 mg IVP: _____

   E. Morphine 2 mg IVP: _____

6. List two priority nursing diagnoses and goals for Mr. Donner's chronic heart failure. _____
_____

7. What are Mr. Donner's health learning needs to manage his chronic condition? _____
_____

REVIEW QUESTIONS

Choose the best answer.

1. A patient is admitted to a medical unit with a diagnosis of heart failure. The patient reports that she has had increasing fatigue during the past 2 weeks. Which of the following is the most likely cause of this fatigue?
   A. Dyspnea
   B. Decreased cardiac output
   C. Dry cough
   D. Orthopnea

2. A patient asks the nurse what her diagnosis of heart failure means. Which of the following is the nurse's best response?
   A. "Your heart briefly stops."
   B. "Your heart has an area of muscle that is dead."
   C. "Your heart is pumping too much blood."
   D. "Your heart is not an efficient pump."

3. A patient's chest x-ray examination indicates fluid in both lung bases. Which of the following signs or symptoms present during the nurse's assessment most reflects these x-ray examination findings?
   A. Fatigue
   B. Peripheral edema
   C. Bilateral crackles
   D. Jugular vein distention

4. To monitor the severity of a patient's heart failure, which of the following assessments is the most appropriate for the nurse to include as a daily assessment in the plan of care?
   A. Weight
   B. Calorie count
   C. Appetite
   D. Abdominal girth

5. A patient is being given digoxin (Lanoxin) to treat her heart failure. Which of the following doses is a usual adult daily dosage of digoxin (Lanoxin)?
   A. 0.005 mg
   B. 0.025 mg
   C. 0.25 mg
   D. 2.5 mg

6. Which of the following signs indicates to the nurse that digoxin (Lanoxin) has been effective for a patient?
   A. Urine output decreases
   B. Urine output increases
   C. Heart rate higher than 95
   D. Heart rate lower than 50

7. When the nurse is reviewing a patient's daily laboratory test results, which of the following electrolyte imbalances should the nurse recognize as predisposing the patient to digoxin toxicity?
   A. Hypokalemia
   B. Hyperkalemia
   C. Hyponatremia
   D. Hypernatremia

8. For a patient who is being discharged on digoxin, the nurse should include which of the following in an explanation to the patient on the signs and symptoms of digoxin toxicity?
   A. Poor appetite
   B. Constipation
   C. Halos around lights
   D. Fast heart rate

9. The patient is being discharged on furosemide (Lasix). The nurse evaluates the patient as understanding her medication teaching if she states that she will have which of the following laboratory tests monitored as ordered?
   A. "I will have my urine sodium checked."
   B. "I will have my calcium level checked."
   C. "I will have my prothrombin time checked."
   D. "I will have my potassium level checked."

10. Which of the following does the nurse understand is the primary reason a patient with pulmonary edema is given morphine sulfate?
    A. To reduce anxiety
    B. To relieve chest pain
    C. To strengthen heart contractions
    D. To increase blood pressure

11. If a patient has elevated pulmonary vascular pressures, the nurse understands that the patient is most likely to develop which of the following physiological cardiac changes?
    A. Left atrial atrophy
    B. Right atrial atrophy
    C. Left ventricular hypertrophy
    D. Right ventricular hypertrophy

12. The nurse evaluates that furosemide IV is effective in treating pulmonary edema if which of the following patient signs or symptoms is resolved?
    A. Pedal edema
    B. Jugular vein distention
    C. Pink, frothy sputum
    D. Bradycardia

13. A patient is being taught the action of digoxin, which is an inotropic agent. The nurse defines an inotropic agent as a medication that has which of the following actions?
    A. Decreases heart rate.
    B. Increases heart rate.
    C. Increases conduction time.
    D. Strengthens heart contraction.

14. For a patient receiving furosemide, the nurse evaluates the medication as being effective if which of the following effects occurs?
    A. Urine output increased
    B. Serum potassium decreased
    C. Heart rate increased
    D. Pulse pressure increased

15. When caring for an anxious patient with dyspnea, which of the following nursing actions is most helpful to include in the plan of care to relieve anxiety?
    A. Increasing activity levels
    B. Staying at patient's bedside
    C. Pulling the privacy curtain
    D. Closing the patient's door

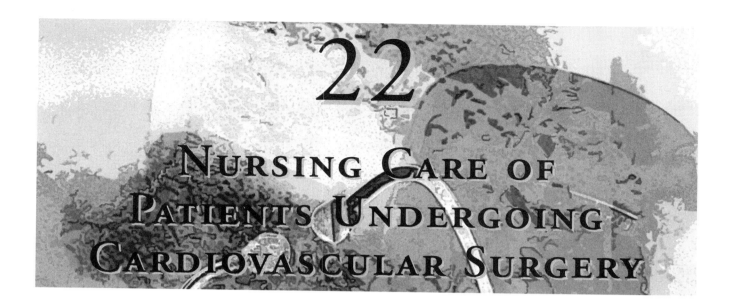

22

NURSING CARE OF PATIENTS UNDERGOING CARDIOVASCULAR SURGERY

► VOCABULARY

Match each word with its definition.

1. _____ Branch of the gastroduodenal artery used as graft material in reoperations

2. _____ Formed when an artery and a vein are directly anastomosed

3. _____ To connect or join two normally distinct structures

4. _____ When valve cusps are incised with a knife or broken apart with a dilator

5. _____ Increase in number of leukocytes in the blood

6. _____ Suture or ring placed around the valve opening to improve closure of the leaflets

7. _____ Incision into the membrane surrounding the heart

8. _____ Destruction of blood cells

9. _____ Condition in which there is altered level of consciousness and confusion caused by medication, hypoxia, or edema of brain tissue

10. _____ Abnormal sensations resulting from nerve irritation or injury

A. Pericardiotomy
B. Anastomose
C. Commissurotomy
D. Annuloplasty
E. Hemolysis
F. Leukocytosis
G. Paresthesia
H. Encephalopathy
I. Gastroepiploic
J. Arteriovenous (AV) fistula

► CARDIAC SURGERY

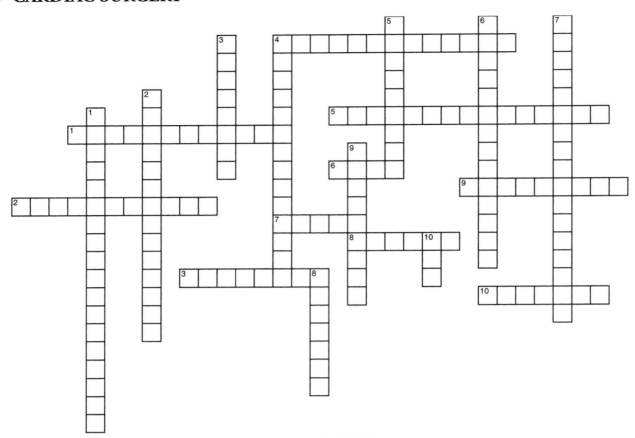

ACROSS

1. A complication of mechanical valves in which prevention is the best measure
2. The most common pulmonary complication after cardiac surgery
3. A sac formation caused by a weakened muscle wall in a blood vessel or the heart
4. Frustrating and stressful to the ventilated patient after surgery
5. Life-threatening gastrointestinal complication
6. A highly subjective postoperative nursing diagnosis
7. How many types of cardiac valves are there?
8. Plan for _____-minute intervals of uninterrupted sleep for the patient
9. Another name for a nonpenetrating cardiac injury
10. _____ levels increase in response to stress

DOWN

1. Common preoperative nursing diagnosis
2. A diffuse neurological complication of cardiac surgery
3. The most common cardiovascular complication after surgery
4. When valve cusps are broken or incised
5. Long-term anticoagulant therapy is not used with this type of valve replacement
6. _____ syndrome is when a patient arouses normally and is oriented yet has periods of confusion
7. A gastrointestinal complication that can affect pulmonary status
8. A benign primary cardiac tumor
9. The vein most frequently used for cardiac revascularization
10. Alternative form of nutritional support used postoperatively

► PREOPERATIVE CARDIAC SURGERY ADMISSION TESTING

Indicate the routine tests that are done preoperatively for cardiac surgery.

1. _____ 12-Lead electrocardiogram

2. _____ Abdominal x-ray examination

3. _____ Complete blood cell count

4. _____ Coagulation studies

5. _____ Chemistry profile

6. _____ Thallium stress test

7. _____ Venogram

8. _____ Crossmatch for blood

9. _____ Liver function studies

10. _____ Urinalysis

▶ CARDIOPULMONARY BYPASS
Find the eight errors and insert the correct information.

Using the cardiopulmonary bypass (CPB) pump can present its own unique set of complications. Before going on the pump, the patient is coagulated with heparin until the prothrombin time (PTT) is one to two times greater than normal. The effects of the heparin are reversed with vitamin K, the antidote for heparin, immediately after coming off the pump. However, heparin is absorbed and stored in organs and tissue and can be sporadically released hours after surgery, thus predisposing the patient to excessive clotting. Air embolism is a risk that is increased by the pump being primed with lactated Ringer's solution. The priming solution increases circulating volume, which then results in a shifting of fluid from the interstitial tissue and edema formation. These fluid shifts can continue up to 6 hours after surgery and can cause hypertension.

▶ CRITICAL THINKING
Read the case study and answer the questions.

Mr. Barnes, a 75-year-old widower, is admitted preoperatively for a mitral valve replacement. He has a history of insulin-dependent diabetes and chronic obstructive pulmonary disease. His son and daughter live out of state but will be arriving this evening. During your assessment, he is calm, answering and asking questions appropriately.

1. What additional preoperative test might you expect Mr. Barnes to have in addition to the routine tests? _____

2. When would you begin preoperative teaching? _____

3. If Mr. Barnes asks specific questions regarding postoperative care, would you provide the specific information? _____

4. What might you expect to occur postoperatively regarding Mr. Barnes' insulin requirements and why? _____

5. What might you expect to occur regarding Mr. Barnes' pulmonary status and why? _____

REVIEW QUESTIONS

Choose the best answer.

1. A patient asks what the CPB pump does. Which of the following is a function of the CPB pump that the nurse should include in the explanation to the patient?
   A. Removes the end products of metabolism
   B. Removes carbon dioxide and put oxygen in the blood
   C. Cleanses the blood of all medications
   D. Depletes the blood supply to the body

2. Once the patient is placed on the CPB pump, the circulatory flow is altered. Which of the following is the direction of blood flow from the CPB pump when the patient is on the CPB pump?
   A. Vena cava to the right atrium to the right ventricle to the pulmonary artery to the CPB
   B. Aorta to the periphery to the vena cava to the CPB pump
   C. Aorta to the left atrium to the left ventricle to the periphery to the vena cava to the CPB pump
   D. Pulmonary vein to the left atrium to the left ventricle to the aorta to the CPB pump

3. The nurse understands that lactated Ringer's priming solution for the CPB pump causes which of the following patient effects?
   A. Hypertension and headaches
   B. Electrolyte imbalance and alkalosis
   C. Hemodilution and weight gain
   D. Shock and confusion

4. A patient is scheduled for a mitral commissurotomy. Which of the following is the nurse's understanding of the procedure?
   A. A portion of the valve is replaced with a mechanical device.
   B. A metal ring is sewn around the mitral valve for support.
   C. The joining edges of the valve cusps are sewn together for support.
   D. The valve cusps are incised with a knife or broken apart with a dilator.

5. A patient asks about the most common complication that occurs after cardiac surgery. The nurse's reply is which of the following?
   A. Hypertension
   B. Tamponade
   C. Dysrhythmias
   D. Bleeding

6. The nurse is caring for a patient who has undergone a cardiac transplant. The nurse is aware that signs of rejection are most likely to occur during what time frame postoperatively?
   A. Immediately after surgery
   B. 10 months after surgery
   C. 1 year after surgery
   D. 2 years after surgery

7. Mr. Rims is admitted with a large sutured laceration on his forehead after being an unrestrained driver in a motor vehicle accident. Mr. Rims has been reporting midsternal chest discomfort since arriving at the hospital without nausea, dyspnea, or diaphoresis. Which of the following conditions might Mr. Rims' symptoms indicate?
   A. Subdural hematoma
   B. Ruptured bladder
   C. Fractured ribs
   D. Cardiac contusion

8. The nurse understands that when a patient has a cardiac contusion, the risk is high for developing which of the following conditions?
   A. Sternal fracture
   B. Myocardial infarction
   C. Tamponade
   D. Pneumothorax

9. If a patient develops cardiac tamponade, what should the nurse anticipate the plan of treatment will be?
   A. Pericardiocentesis
   B. Chest tube insertion
   C. Surgery to wire the sternum
   D. Intravenous nitroglycerin

10. Patients sustaining a severe cardiac contusion should be monitored for which of the following life-threatening complications?
    A. Thrombocytopenia
    B. Angina
    C. Aortic stenosis
    D. Cardiac rupture

11. Incisional bleeding or oozing following a carotid endarterectomy may lead to which of the following conditions for which the nurse should monitor?
    A. Hypovolemia leading to shock
    B. Anemia with light-headedness
    C. Hematoma formation with tracheal compression
    D. Hypovolemia and wound separation

12. The nurse is documenting the assessment of a patient's hemodialysis blood access in which an artery and a vein have been directly anastomosed. Which of the following terms would the nurse be correct in documenting for this blood access?
    A. AV shunt
    B. AV fistula
    C. AV malformation
    D. AV graft

13. When the nurse is assessing peripheral pulses, which of the following is not included in the assessment?
    A. Presence or absence
    B. Location and quality
    C. Reperfusion pressure
    D. Occlusion pressure

14. Which of the following does the nurse understand is the most common pulmonary complication after cardiac surgery?
    A. Atelectasis
    B. Pneumothorax
    C. Pneumonia
    D. Phrenic nerve paralysis

15. Which of the following nursing interventions is appropriate for the nurse to include in the plan of care for a patient with atelectasis?
    A. Anticipation of chest tube placement
    B. Coughing and deep breathing every 1 to 2 hours
    C. Prolonged mechanical ventilation
    D. Administering prescribed antibiotics

UNIT FIVE

UNDERSTANDING THE HEMATOPOIETIC AND LYMPHATIC SYSTEMS

CHECKLIST FOR LEARNING SUCCESS

Review of Anatomy and Physiology	Major Disorders	Nursing Assessment	Diagnostic Tests	Interventions	Common Medications
☐ Blood components ☐ Functions of different blood cells ☐ Lymphatic system	☐ Anemias ☐ Disseminated intravascular coagulation ☐ Idiopathic thrombocytopenic purpura ☐ Hemophilia ☐ Leukemia ☐ Multiple myeloma ☐ Hodgkin's disease ☐ Lymphoma	☐ Signs and symptoms of bleeding ☐ Lymph nodes ☐ Skin	☐ Complete blood cell count ☐ White blood cell differential ☐ Coagulation studies ☐ Bone marrow biopsy	☐ Blood product administration ☐ Chemotherapy ☐ Thrombocytopenia precautions ☐ Infection precautions ☐ Bone marrow transplant	☐ Iron ☐ Colony stimulating factors ☐ Chemotherapy ☐ Clotting factors

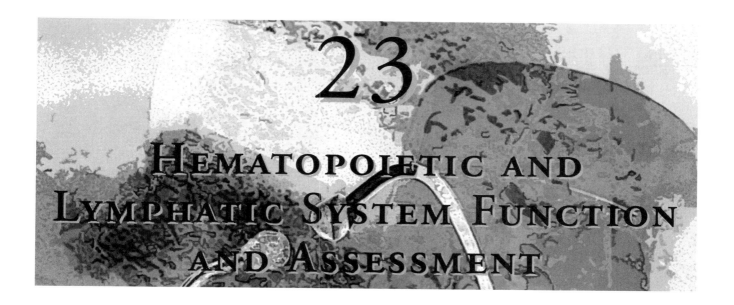

23
HEMATOPOIETIC AND LYMPHATIC SYSTEM FUNCTION AND ASSESSMENT

► VOCABULARY
Fill in the blank with the appropriate word.

1. _____ is a blue-black discoloration from hemorrhage under the skin.

2. _____ is the term used to describe swelling from blockage of lymph circulation.

3. Tiny hemorrhages into the skin creating a polka-dot appearance are called _____.

4. _____ is caused by hemorrhages into the skin, mucous membranes, or internal organs.

5. The patient with _____ has an increased risk for bleeding because of a lack of platelets.

► LYMPHATIC SYSTEM
Match each part of the lymphatic system with its proper description.

1. _____ Lymph capillaries
2. _____ Lymph nodules
3. _____ Thoracic duct
4. _____ Lymph nodes
5. _____ Valves

A. Destroy pathogens in the lymph from the extremities before the lymph is returned to the blood
B. Collect tissue fluid from intercellular spaces
C. Prevent backflow of lymph in larger lymph vessels
D. Destroy pathogens that penetrate mucous membranes
E. Empties lymph from the lower body and upper left quadrant into the left subclavian vein

► STRUCTURES OF THE LYMPHATIC SYSTEM

Label the following structures.

► HEMATOPOIETIC SYSTEM

Match each term with its definition.

1. _____ Albumin

2. _____ Macrophages

3. _____ Calcium ions

4. _____ Intrinsic factor

5. _____ Hemoglobin

6. _____ Basophils

7. _____ Red bone marrow

8. _____ Stem cell

9. _____ Megakaryocyte

10. _____ Lymphocytes

A. May become any kind of blood cell
B. Essential for chemical clotting
C. Contain heparin and histamine
D. A hematopoietic tissue
E. May become cells that produce antibodies
F. Large phagocytic cells
G. Prevents digestion of vitamin B_{12}
H. Its fragments become platelets
I. Carries oxygen in red blood cells
J. Pulls tissue fluid into capillaries to maintain blood volume

► CRITICAL THINKING

Read the case study and answer the questions.

Mr. Foster is receiving a unit of packed red blood cells. You assist with identification of the patient before it starts. The registered nurse then delegates monitoring of his vital signs every half hour to you.

1. Why should Mr. Foster be monitored for each of the following symptoms?

A. Fever _____

B. Back pain _____

C. Respiratory distress _____

D. Crackles _____

E. Hives _____

2. Mr. Foster's respiratory rate increases from 16 to 20 breaths per minute. What do you do? _____

_____

_____

3. The physician asks that the transfusion be slowed down. How many hours can the blood hang before it must be stopped?

_____

REVIEW QUESTIONS

Choose the best answer.

1. Blood plasma transports all *except* which of the following?
   A. Oxygen
   B. Nutrients
   C. Carbon dioxide
   D. Hormones

2. What is the mineral necessary for chemical clotting?
   A. Iron
   B. Sodium
   C. Potassium
   D. Calcium

3. Through which of the following does lymph return to the blood?
   A. Carotid arteries
   B. Aorta
   C. Inferior vena cava
   D. Subclavian veins

4. Which of the following is a normal hemoglobin value?
   A. 38% to 48%
   B. 12 to 18 g/100 mL
   C. 48 to 54 mg %
   D. 27 to 36 g/dL

5. Which laboratory study is monitored for the patient receiving heparin therapy?
   A. International normalized ratio (INR)
   B. Prothrombin time
   C. Partial thromboplastin time
   D. Bleeding time

6. Which blood product replaces missing clotting factors in the patient who has a bleeding disorder?
   A. Platelets
   B. Packed red blood cells
   C. Albumin
   D. Cryoprecipitate

7. A patient is on warfarin (Coumadin) therapy and has an INR of 1.6. Which action by the nurse is appropriate?
   A. Observe the patient for abnormal bleeding.
   B. Notify the physician and expect an order to increase the warfarin dose.
   C. Advise the patient to double today's dose of warfarin.
   D. Administer vitamin K per protocol.

8. You are asked to initiate an intravenous needle for a blood transfusion. What gauge needle do you choose?
   A. 18
   B. 22
   C. 24
   D. 28

9. A patient receiving a transfusion of packed red blood cells complains of chest and back pain. How do you respond?
   A. Do a complete physical assessment.
   B. Ask the patient to describe his pain.
   C. Call the registered nurse STAT to stop the transfusion.
   D. Administer his analgesic, as needed (PRN).

10. You are assisting the physician with a bone marrow biopsy. Which of the following interventions is most important for the nurse to do before the procedure?
    A. Explain the procedure to the patient's family.
    B. Administer an analgesic to the patient.
    C. Observe the patient for bleeding.
    D. Drape the biopsy site.

24

NURSING CARE OF PATIENTS WITH HEMATOPOIETIC DISORDERS

▶ VOCABULARY

Label each statement true or false.

1. _____ Anemia is a reduction in white blood cells.

2. _____ Hemolysis is the destruction of red blood cells.

3. _____ Pancytopenia is reduced numbers of all blood cells.

4. _____ Ecchymosis and petechiae are symptoms of abnormal bleeding.

5. _____ Polycythemia is the production of new and different blood cells.

6. _____ Phlebotomy is the excision of a vessel.

7. _____ Disseminated intravascular coagulation results from accelerated clotting throughout the circulation.

8. _____ Thrombocytopenia is a reduction in platelets.

9. _____ Hemarthrosis is bleeding into the muscles.

10. _____ Leukemia literally means "white blood."

▶ CRITICAL THINKING

Read the case study and answer the questions.

Mr. Frantzis is a 60-year-old gentleman in the acute stage of chronic lymphocytic leukemia. He is admitted to a nursing home because he has no family to help care for him. He has had chemotherapy in the past but has decided against further treatment. You are assigned to his care today. You find him pale and weak, with no energy to get out of bed. He also complains of pain in his chest.

1. Mr. Frantzis says he is too weak to get up for breakfast. What do you do? _____

_____

_____

2. How do you follow up on the pain in his chest? _____

_____

3. The nursing assistant assigned to Mr. Frantzis has a runny nose. How do you respond? _____

_____

4. Mr. Frantzis calls you "Jennifer" when you enter his room, but that is not your name. How do you respond? _____

_____

5. You note bleeding from Mr. Frantzis' gums. What care can you provide? _____

_____

_____

▶ SICKLE CELL ANEMIA

Fill in the signs and symptoms of sickle cell anemia.

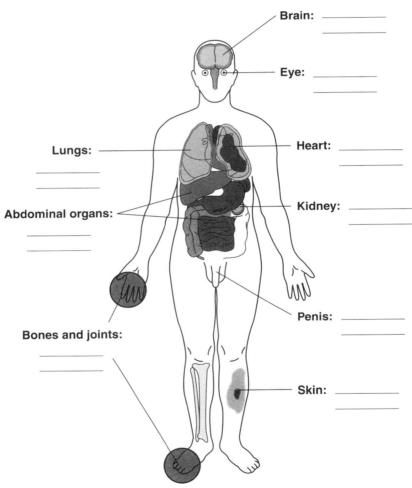

REVIEW QUESTIONS

Choose the best answer.

1. A 16-year-old girl has iron deficiency anemia. Which of the following foods will best help her get the iron she needs?
   A. Fresh fruits
   B. Lean red meats
   C. Dairy products
   D. Breads and cereals

2. A patient admitted with gastrointestinal tract bleeding has a hemoglobin level of 6 g/dL. She asks the nurse why she feels short of breath. Which response is best?
   A. "Anemia prevents your lungs from absorbing oxygen effectively."
   B. "You do not have enough hemoglobin to carry oxygen to your tissues."
   C. "You don't have enough blood to feed your cells."
   D. "You have lost a lot of blood, and that has damaged your lungs."

3. A 50-year-old African-American gentleman is diagnosed with anemia. Where can the nurse assess for pallor?
   A. Scalp
   B. Axillae
   C. Chest
   D. Conjunctivae

4. Which of the following is an early sign of anemia?
   A. Palpitations
   B. Glossitis
   C. Pallor
   D. Weight loss

5. A 17-year-old African-American boy is admitted in sickle cell crisis. Which of the following events most likely contributed to the onset of the crisis?
   A. He started a new job last week.
   B. He walked home in a cold rain yesterday.
   C. He had seafood for dinner last night.
   D. He has not exercised for a week.

6. A patient has hand-foot syndrome related to his sickle cell anemia. What findings does the nurse expect to see as the patient is assessed?
   A. Unequal growth of fingers and toes
   B. Webbing between fingers and toes
   C. Purplish discoloration of hands and feet
   D. Deformities of the wrists and ankles

7. The nurse has taught a patient with thrombocytopenia how to prevent bleeding. Which of the following is the best evidence that the teaching has been effective?
   A. The patient states that he will be careful to avoid injury.
   B. The patient can list signs and symptoms of bleeding.
   C. The patient uses an electric razor instead of his safety razor.
   D. The patient states when he should call the doctor.

8. A patient with a history of hemophilia A arrives in the emergency department complaining of a "funny feeling" in his elbow. The patient states that he thinks he is bleeding into the joint. Which response by the nurse is correct?
   A. Perform deep palpation on the patient's elbow to assess for swelling.
   B. Notify the physician immediately and expect an order for factor VIII.
   C. Prepare the patient for an x-ray examination to determine whether bleeding is occurring.
   D. Apply heat to the patient's elbow and wait for the physician.

9. For which of the following problems is the patient with multiple myeloma most at risk?
   A. Uncontrolled bleeding
   B. Respiratory distress
   C. Liver engorgement
   D. Pathological fractures

10. Which of the following interventions can help minimize complications related to hypercalcemia?
   A. Encourage 3 to 4 L of fluid daily.
   B. Have the patient cough and deep breathe every 2 hours.
   C. Place the patient on bed rest.
   D. Apply heat to painful areas.

25

NURSING CARE OF PATIENTS WITH LYMPHATIC DISORDERS

► VOCABULARY
Fill in the blanks with the appropriate terms.

1. Cancer of the lymph system is called _____.

2. _____ _____ are the filtering structures of the body's immune system.

3. Abnormalities in _____ cells and _____ cells can result in lymphoma.

4. Enlargement of the spleen is called _____.

5. Removal of the spleen is called _____.

► HODGKIN'S DISEASE
Circle the errors in the following paragraph and write in the correct information.

Joe is a 28-year-old construction worker diagnosed with stage I Hodgkin's disease. He initially went to his physician because of a painful lump in his neck. He is also experiencing high fevers and weight loss. The diagnosis was confirmed in laboratory test by the presence of Reed-Steinway cells. He expresses his fears to his nurse, who tells him that Hodgkin's disease is not really cancer, and that it is often curable. Joe takes a leave from work and begins palliative radiation therapy.

REVIEW QUESTIONS

Choose the best answer.

1. A 36-year-old mother of three has a new diagnosis of lymphoma. She is experiencing fatigue. Which of the following is the best way to monitor her fatigue?
   A. Observe her activity level.
   B. Monitor for changes in vital signs.
   C. Monitor hemoglobin and hematocrit values.
   D. Have her rate her fatigue on a scale of 0 to 10.

2. Patients with lymphoma are at risk for infection. Which of the following activities increases this risk?
   A. Going to church
   B. Taking a walk outside
   C. Cleaning the house
   D. Watching television

3. The patient is having difficulty coping with her new diagnosis of lymphoma. Which response is most helpful?
   A. "Don't worry. You'll be okay."
   B. "The treatments you are receiving will make you feel better very soon."
   C. "Who do you usually go to when you have a problem?"
   D. "Have you made end-of-life decisions?"

4. A 42-year-old man is admitted for a splenectomy. Why is an injection of vitamin K ordered before surgery?
   A. To correct clotting problems
   B. To promote healing
   C. To prevent postoperative infection
   D. To dry secretions

5. Which of the following conditions places a patient at risk for respiratory complications following his splenectomy?
   A. A low platelet count
   B. An incision near his diaphragm
   C. Early ambulation
   D. Early discharge

6. Patients are at risk for overwhelming postsplenectomy infection (OPSI) following splenectomy. Which of the following symptoms alerts the nurse to this possibility?
   A. Bruising around the operative site
   B. Irritability
   C. Pain
   D. Fever

7. What discharge teaching is most important to help the patient who has had a splenectomy prevent infection?
   A. Avoid showering for 1 week.
   B. Sleep in a semi-Fowler's position.
   C. Receive vaccines against infection.
   D. Stay on antibiotics for life.

Unit Six

Understanding the Respiratory System

Checklist for Learning Success

Review of Anatomy and Physiology and Aging Changes	Major Disorders	Nursing Assessment	Diagnostic Tests	Interventions
☐ Lungs and bronchial tree	☐ Upper respiratory infections	☐ Adventitious lung sounds	☐ Red blood cell count	☐ Breathing exercises
☐ Mechanisms of breathing	☐ Influenza	☐ Dyspnea	☐ White blood cell count	☐ Cough and deep breathe (C & DB)
☐ Acid-base balance	☐ Cancer of larynx	☐ Activity tolerance	☐ Sputum culture and sensitivity (C & S)	☐ Oxygen therapy
☐ Aging changes	☐ Pneumonia		☐ Oxymetry	☐ Nebulized mist treatments
	☐ Tuberculosis		☐ Arterial blood gases	☐ Metered dose inhalers
	☐ Pleural effusion		☐ Chest x-ray	☐ Chest physiotherapy
	☐ Chronic bronchitis		☐ Pulmonary function test	☐ Incentive spirometry (IS)
	☐ Asthma		☐ Bronchoscopy	☐ Chest tubes
	☐ Emphysema			☐ Tracheostomy
	☐ Cystic fibrosis			☐ Mechanical ventilation
	☐ Pulmonary embolism			☐ Noninvasive positive pressure ventilation (NIPPV)
	☐ Pneumothorax			☐ Thoracic surgery
	☐ Respiratory failure			
	☐ Lung cancer			

26

RESPIRATORY SYSTEM FUNCTION AND ASSESSMENT

▶ VOCABULARY

Complete the sentences with words provided below.

Adventitious	Apnea	Barrel chest
Crepitus	Dyspnea	Respiratory excursion
Thoracentesis	Tidaling	Tracheostomy
Tracheotomy		

1. A patient with a low oxygen saturation may develop _____.

2. _____ may develop if air leaks into tissues from a chest tube site.

3. A _____ may be necessary for severe pleural effusion.

4. The patient with air trapping may develop a _____ _____.

5. The nurse can measure _____ to check chest expansion.

6. Crackles are an example of a/an _____ sound.

7. A patient who is choking may need an emergency _____.

8. The _____ in the water-seal chamber shows that the chest tube is intact.

9. _____ is the absence of respirations.

10. Jennifer has the inner cannula of her _____ tube removed and cleaned every 8 hours.

▶ ANATOMY

Number the following structures in the order in which air flows through them.

_____ Nose	_____ Nasal cavities	_____ Trachea
_____ Larynx	_____ Oropharynx	_____ Secondary bronchi
_____ Primary bronchi	_____ Bronchioles	_____ Alveoli
_____ Laryngopharynx	_____ Nasopharynx	

▶ VENTILATION

Number the events of breathing in proper sequence beginning with the medulla.

_____ The medulla generates motor impulses.

_____ The chest cavity is enlarged in all directions.

_____ The diaphragm and external intercostal muscles contract.

_____ Intrapulmonic pressure decreases.

_____ Motor impulses travel along the phrenic and intercostal nerves.

_____ The chest wall expands the parietal pleura, which expands the visceral pleura, which in turn expands the lungs.

_____ Air enters the lungs until intrapulmonic pressure equals atmospheric pressure.

▶ ADVENTITIOUS LUNG SOUNDS

Match the adventitious lung sound to its description.

1. _____ Coarse crackles

2. _____ Fine crackles

3. _____ Wheezes

4. _____ Stridor

5. _____ Pleural friction rub

6. _____ Diminished

A. Velcro being torn apart
B. Faint lung sounds
C. Leather rubbing together
D. Loud crowing noise
E. Moist bubbling
F. High-pitched violins

▶ CHEST DRAINAGE

Label the parts of the chest drainage system and explain the function of each.

▶ THE RESPIRATORY SYSTEM

Label the parts.

► CRITICAL THINKING

Read the case study and answer the questions.

Bill, a licensed practical nurse (LPN), is collecting admission data on Mr. Howe, who has been admitted for dyspnea and weight loss. While questioning Mr. Howe, Bill learns that he has had progressive weight loss over the past several months and that he has a productive cough. He also complains of waking up at night "wringing wet," and his wife has to change the bed sheets.

1. What additional questions should Bill ask about Mr. Howe's cough? _____

_____

_____

2. What disorder is suggested by Mr. Howe's symptoms? _____

_____

_____

3. What diagnostic tests do you expect to see ordered? _____

_____

_____

4. Mr. Howe is scheduled for a bronchoscopy. What preprocedure care does Bill provide? Postprocedure? _____

_____

_____

REVIEW QUESTIONS

Choose the best answer.

1. Which of the following structures covers the larynx during swallowing?
    A. Hydroid cartilage
    B. Vocal cords
    C. Soft palate
    D. Epiglottis

2. Where are the respiratory centers located in the brain?
    A. Cerebral cortex and cerebellum
    B. Medulla and pons
    C. Hypothalamus and cerebral cortex
    D. Hypothalamus and temporal lobes

3. What is the purpose of the serous fluid between the pleural membranes?
    A. Enhance exchange of gases
    B. Facilitate coughing
    C. Destroy pathogens
    D. Prevent friction

4. Within the alveoli, surface tension is decreased and inflation is possible because of the presence of which substance?
    A. Tissue fluid
    B. Surfactant
    C. Pulmonary blood
    D. Mucus

5. What is the function of the nasal mucosa?
    A. Assist with gas exchange
    B. Sweep mucus and pathogens to the trachea
    C. Warm and moisten the incoming air
    D. Increase the oxygen content of the air

6. Deteriorating cilia in the respiratory tract predispose the elderly to which of the following problems?
    A. Chronic hypoxia
    B. Pulmonary hypertension
    C. Respiratory infection
    D. Decreased ventilation

7. Which of the following lung sounds is a violin-like sound?
    A. Crackles
    B. Wheezes
    C. Friction rub
    D. Crepitus

8. An LPN checks the oxygen saturation on a patient with chronic lung disease. The result is 72 percent. She notes that the patient has removed her oxygen cannula, and it is lying on the bed. Which of the following actions is appropriate next?
    A. Call the registered nurse stat.
    B. Put the oxygen cannula back on the patient.
    C. Do a nebulized mist treatment.
    D. No action necessary; this is a normal saturation.

9. The purpose of pursed-lip breathing is to promote which of the following?
   A. Carbon dioxide excretion
   B. Carbon dioxide retention
   C. Oxygen excretion
   D. Oxygen retention

10. Which of the following positions will help increase oxygen saturation in the patient with lung disease?
    A. Prone
    B. Supine with head on pillow
    C. Trendelenburg
    D. Side lying with good lung dependent

11. What care should the nurse provide for the patient with a transtracheal catheter?
    A. Assist with cleaning the catheter two to three times a day.
    B. Provide supplemental oxygen via mask at all times.
    C. Help remove the catheter at night for sleeping.
    D. Assist to connect the catheter to a humidification source.

12. What is the purpose of chest physiotherapy?
    A. Help the patient strengthen chest muscles.
    B. Humidify thick respiratory secretions.
    C. Promote lung expansion.
    D. Help the patient expectorate secretions.

13. The nurse notes that the suction-control chamber on a chest-drainage system is bubbling vigorously. Which intervention is appropriate?
    A. Check the system for leaks.
    B. Replace the drainage system with a new one.
    C. Reduce the level of wall suction.
    D. Increase the water level in the suction control chamber.

27

NURSING CARE OF PATIENTS WITH UPPER RESPIRATORY TRACT DISORDERS

► VOCABULARY

Unscramble the letters of the following words to fill in the blanks in the statements below.

hiitsrin
pixessait
laiohnpstry
aadihpysg
daxueet
cayetorlemeng

1. The patient who has had his or her larynx removed is called a _____ .

2. A nosebleed is called _____ .

3. _____ is the term used to describe drainage or pus.

4. A "nose job" is called _____ .

5. Difficulty swallowing is called _____ .

6. _____ is the correct term for a runny nose.

► NASAL SURGERY

Read the case study and answer the accompanying questions.

Mr. Jones has a submucous resection done for a deviated nasal septum.

1. Following surgery, you note that Mr. Jones is swallowing repeatedly while he sleeps. What do you do? _____

_____

_____

2. Before discharge you explain to Mr. Jones that he should not do anything that can increase bleeding, such as sneezing, coughing, or straining to have a bowel movement. He says, "How can I avoid doing those things? It sounds impossible." How do you respond? _____

_____

3. Mr. Jones asks if he can use aspirin for pain. What do you say? _____

_____

▶ CRITICAL THINKING

Read the case study and answer the questions that follow.

Your son comes down with influenza. He is feverish, tired, and has a sore throat and headache. The physician did a throat culture and told you it is viral. She told you to put your son to bed and give him fluids and acetaminophen.

1. Why didn't the physician order antibiotics? _____

_____

2. How will fluids help? _____

_____

3. When should you give the acetaminophen? _____

_____

4. Your daughter develops the same symptoms. Is it necessary to take her to the physician? _____

_____

5. Your elderly grandmother was visiting when your son first developed symptoms. She is now calling to say she has gotten the

   flu, and her chest hurts. She asks what she should do. What should you tell her? _____

_____

REVIEW QUESTIONS

Choose the best answer.

1. A patient visits her nurse practitioner (NP) after she has had a cold for a week and is now experiencing a severe headache and fever. Her NP diagnoses a sinus infection. Which of the following additional symptoms is the patient likely to exhibit?
   A. Facial tenderness
   B. Chest pain
   C. Photophobia
   D. Ear drainage

2. In addition to antibiotics, which of the following recommendations can the nurse make to increase comfort in a patient experiencing sinusitis?
   A. Coughing and deep breathing
   B. Sinus irrigation
   C. Rest and a room humidifier
   D. Percussion and postural drainage

3. When evaluating the effectiveness of nursing interventions for sinusitis, which of the following does the nurse assess?
   A. White blood cell count
   B. Dyspnea level
   C. Capillary refill
   D. Comfort level

4. A 58-year-old man is diagnosed with cancer of the larynx. Which of the following are early symptoms of this cancer?
   A. Anemia and fatigue
   B. Crackles and stridor
   C. A noticeable lump in the neck
   D. Dysphagia or hoarseness

5. Which of the following nursing actions takes priority following laryngectomy surgery?
   A. Keeping tissues at the bedside for a productive cough
   B. Assessing the patient's acceptance of his laryngectomy
   C. Maintaining a patent airway
   D. Controlling postoperative pain

6. Which of the following communication methods is not an option for a patient following laryngectomy surgery?
   A. Placing a finger over the stoma
   B. Using a special valve that diverts air into the esophagus
   C. Using a picture board
   D. Learning esophageal speech

7. A narcotic analgesic is ordered for postoperative pain. Why are narcotics given in low doses to the laryngectomy patient?
   A. They depress the respiratory rate and cough reflex.
   B. They increase respiratory tract secretions.
   C. They have a tendency to cause stomal edema.
   D. They can cause addiction.

8. The nurse teaches a patient how to live with a new tracheostomy. Which of the following instructions is appropriate?
    A. "Never suction your tracheostomy; you might damage your trachea."
    B. "You should not feel bad about the tracheostomy—you should feel lucky to be alive."
    C. "Be sure to protect your tracheostomy from pollutants such as powders, hair, and chemicals."
    D. "You shouldn't need to clean your tracheostomy; it can be cleaned each time you visit your doctor."

9. A 17-year-old student enters the emergency department with a nosebleed that won't quit. Which of the following positions is recommended for the patient with a nosebleed?
    A. Lying down with feet elevated
    B. Sitting up with neck extended
    C. Lying down with a small pillow under the head
    D. Sitting up leaning slightly forward

10. The physician orders local application of epinephrine 1:1000 solution to treat a nosebleed. The patient asks how this will help. Which of the following responses by the nurse is best?
    A. "It will raise your blood pressure, which is necessary because of blood loss."
    B. "It will dilate your bronchioles and make your breathing easier."
    C. "It will help your blood to clot."
    D. "It will constrict your vessels and slow down the bleeding."

28

NURSING CARE OF PATIENTS WITH LOWER RESPIRATORY TRACT DISORDERS

▶ VOCABULARY
Complete the crossword puzzle.

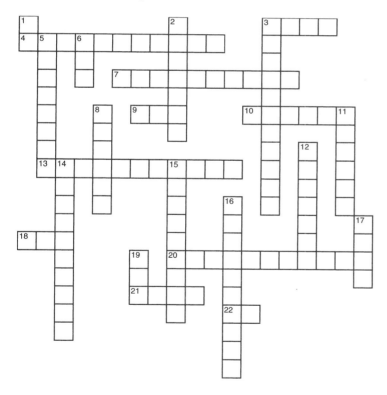

ACROSS

3. Also called "white lung"
4. Chest collapses during inspiration during this type of respiration
7. Bloody sputum
9. Abbreviation for inhaler
10. Respiratory membrane secretion
13. Incision into the chest
18. Abbreviation for inhaled nebulized medication
20. Treatment for repeat pneumothorax
21. Blister on lung
22. Abbreviation for tuberculosis

DOWN

1. Abbreviation for "front to back" when referring to the chest
2. Term used to describe hormones produced by tumors
3. Medication that relieves coughing
5. Treatment in addition to standard therapy
6. Abbreviation for laboratory tests done to measure oxygenation
8. Unable to react, as in skin testing
11. Continuous asthma is called _____ asthmaticus
12. Drainage on infected tonsils
14. Blood in the chest
15. Rapid respirations
16. Firm raised area in positive tuberculosis skin test
17. Smoking is a _____ factor for cancer
19. An abbreviation for dyspnea

▶ RESPIRATORY MEDICATIONS

Match the medication with its action.

1. _____ Prednisone

2. _____ Albuterol (Ventolin)

3. _____ Theophylline (Theo-Dur)

4. _____ Cromolyn sodium (Intal)

5. _____ Guaifenesin (Humibid)

6. _____ Zafirlukast (Accolate)

7. _____ Codeine

A. Expectorant
B. Potent antiinflammatory
C. Leukotriene inhibitor (reduces inflammation in asthma)
D. Beta-adrenergic bronchodilator
E. Methylxanthine bronchodilator
F. Stabilizes mast cells to prevent asthma
G. Antitussive

▶ CRITICAL THINKING

Read the case study and answer the questions.

Edith is a 56-year-old homemaker admitted to the hospital with emphysema and acute dyspnea. She is a smoker with a 48 pack-year history.

1. What data do you collect for Edith's admission database? _____

_____

_____

2. What does a 48 pack-year history mean? _____

_____

3. Explain the pathophysiology involved in emphysema. How does the disease cause dyspnea? _____

_____

_____

4. What do you expect Edith's lungs to sound like when you auscultate? _____

_____

_____

5. Why is it important for Edith to receive no more than 2 L of oxygen per minute? _____

_____

_____

6. Why might Edith be at risk for pneumothorax? _____

_____

_____

7. What position will help Edith's shortness of breath? Why? _____

_____

_____

8. How can you encourage Edith to stop smoking? _____

_____

_____

Choose the best answer.

1. A 72-year-old chemist has left lower lobe pneumonia. His nurse checks his oxygen saturation and the result is 86 percent. Which of the following actions by the nurse is best?
   A. Call the physician for an order for oxygen.
   B. No action necessary; this is a normal SaO_2.
   C. Call the respiratory therapist stat for assistance.
   D. Walk the patient in the hall and recheck his O_2 saturation.

2. Which of the following explanations by the nurse will help a patient understand what to expect during a bronchoscopy?
   A. "The physician will place a small tube through your nose or mouth and into the bronchi to look at your airways."
   B. "You will breathe a radioactive substance that will show diseased areas in your lungs."
   C. "You will need to drink a thick white liquid, which will be opaque on the x-rays."
   D. "A dye will be injected to help visualize the structures of the bronchioles. Do you have any allergies?"

3. Which of the following nursing actions is appropriate when a patient returns to his or her room after a bronchoscopy?
   A. Order a meal because the patient has been nil per os (NPO) for 8 hours.
   B. Encourage fluids to flush dye from the patient's system.
   C. Monitor the patient for return to consciousness.
   D. Check for a gag reflex before allowing the patient to drink.

4. A patient is diagnosed with a primary bronchogenic carcinoma. Which of the following factors increase the risk of lung cancer?
   A. Living in a cold climate; having pets
   B. Smoking; chemical exposure at work
   C. Living in crowded conditions; lack of sunlight
   D. Eating foods high in beta carotene and fiber

5. A patient with a new diagnosis of lung cancer decides to have radiation therapy. Which of the following expectations of this treatment is most appropriate?
   A. Complete cure of the cancer
   B. Increased comfort
   C. Prevention of the need for oxygen
   D. Prevention of cancer spread

6. A newly diagnosed patient asks what asthma is. Which of the following explanations by the nurse is correct?
   A. Your airways are inflamed and spastic.
   B. You have fluid in your lungs that is causing shortness of breath.
   C. Your airways are stretched and nonfunctional.
   D. You have a low-grade infection that keeps your bronchial tree irritated.

7. Which of the following is the best explanation of emphysema for a newly diagnosed patient?
   A. "You have inflamed bronchioles, which causes a lot of secretions."
   B. "Your lungs have lost some of their elasticity, and air gets trapped."
   C. "The blood supply to your lungs is destroyed, so you can't absorb oxygen."
   D. "You have large dilated sacs of sputum in your lungs."

8. A patient is treated with intravenous (IV) methylprednisolone (Solu-Medrol) for emphysema. What is the purpose of corticosteroid treatment in lung disease?
   A. Dry secretions.
   B. Treat the infection that causes an exacerbation.
   C. Improve the oxygen-carrying capacity of hemoglobin.
   D. Reduce airway inflammation.

9. How many liters per minute of oxygen should be administered to the patient with emphysema?
   A. 2 L/min
   B. 6 L/min
   C. 10 L/min
   D. 95 L/min

10. Which of the following medications can be used to quickly reduce shortness of breath in a crisis situation for a patient with end-stage respiratory disease?
    A. Oral cortisone
    B. Intramuscular meperidine (Demerol)
    C. IV morphine
    D. IV propanolol (Inderal)

11. Which of the following positions is best for a chest-drainage system when the patient is being transported by wheelchair?
    A. Hang it on the top of the wheelchair backrest.
    B. Place it on the patient's feet and ask the patient to hold it.
    C. Hang it on the same pole as the patient's IV.
    D. Place it in the patient's lap.

12. The nurse notes vigorous bubbling in the water-seal chamber of a chest-drainage system. Which of the following actions should the nurse take to correct the bubbling?
    A. Examine the entire system and tubing for air leaks.
    B. Lower the level of suction.
    C. Nothing; vigorous bubbling is expected.
    D. Ask the patient to cough forcefully.

13. How can the nurse help monitor effectiveness of therapy for the patient with a pneumothorax and a chest-drainage system?
    A. Palpate for crepitus.
    B. Auscultate lung sounds.
    C. Document color and amount of sputum.
    D. Monitor suction level.

14. Which of the following risk factors presents the greatest threat for respiratory disease?
    A. Smoking
    B. High-fat diet
    C. Exposure to radiation
    D. Alcohol consumption

Unit Seven

Understanding the Gastrointestinal (GI) System

Checklist for Learning Success

Review of Anatomy and Physiology	Major Disorders	Nursing Assessment	Diagnostic Tests	Interventions	Common Medications

☐ Gastrointestinal:
  ☐ Oral cavity/
    pharynx
  ☐ Esophagus
  ☐ Stomach
  ☐ Small intestine
  ☐ Large intestine
  ☐ Aging
	☐ Eating disorders
	☐ Oral/esophageal
	  cancer
	☐ Gastroesophageal
	  reflux disease
	  (GERD)
	☐ Gastritis
	☐ Peptic ulcer disease
	☐ Gastric bleeding
	☐ Gastric cancer
	☐ Constipation/
	  diarrhea
	☐ Appendicitis
	☐ Peritonitis
	☐ Diverticulosis
	☐ Inflammatory bowel
	  disease
	☐ Absorption disorders
	☐ Intestinal
	  obstructions
	☐ Lower
	  gastrointestinal (GI)
	  bleeding
	☐ Colon cancer
		☐ Medical history
		☐ Physical
		  assessment
			☐ Laboratory tests
			☐ Flat plate of abdomen
			☐ Upper GI series
			☐ Lower GI series
			☐ Esophagogastro-
			  duodenoscopy
			  (EGD)
			☐ Colonoscopy
			☐ Gastric analysis
			☐ Stool studies
			☐ IgG antibody test
				☐ GI intubation
				☐ Tube feedings
				☐ Total parenteral
				  nutrition
				  (TPN)/peripheral
				  parenteral
				  nutrition (PPN)
				☐ GI decompression
				☐ Gastric surgeries/
				  complications
				☐ Nursing care after
				  gastric surgery
				☐ Ostomy
				  management
					☐ Antacids
					☐ Antidiarrheal
					☐ Antiemetics
					☐ Bulk-forming
					  agents
					☐ H_2 receptor
					  antagonists
					☐ Laxatives
					☐ Proton pump
					  inhibitors
					☐ Stool
					  softeners
					☐ Sulfasalazine
					  (Azulfidine)
					☐ Vitamin B_{12}

29

GASTROINTESTINAL SYSTEM FUNCTION, ASSESSMENT, AND THERAPEUTIC MEASURES

▶ FUNCTIONS OF THE GASTROINTESTINAL SYSTEM

Fill in the blanks with the appropriate part of the gastrointestinal system.

1. The _LOWER ESOPHAGEAL_ sphincter prevents backup of stomach contents into the esophagus.

2. The _Illeocecal_ valve prevents backup of fecal material from the large intestine into the small intestine.

3. The _CARDIAC_ sphincter prevents backup of duodenal contents into the stomach.

4. The absorption of most of the end products of digestion occurs in the _LARGE_ intestine.

5. The digestion of protein begins in the _Stomach_ .

6. Water and the vitamins produced by the normal flora are absorbed in the _small_ intestine.

7. The _Small_ intestine is the site of action of bile and pancreatic enzymes.

8. The passageway for food into the stomach from the mouth is the _esophagus_ .

9. Voluntary control of defecation is provided by the _external anal_ sphincter.

10. The watery secretion that permits taste and swallowing is produced by the _Salivary_ glands.

11. The process of mechanical digestion is produced by the _teeth_ and _tongue_ in the mouth.

12. The structures in the small intestine that contain capillaries and lacteals for absorption are the _Villi_ .

13. The part of the colon that contracts in the defecation reflex is the _rectum_ .

▶ STRUCTURES OF THE GASTROINTESTINAL SYSTEM

Label the following structures.

▶ VOCABULARY

Unscramble the letters to identify the word described by the definition.

1. Flexible or rigid device consisting of a tube and optical system for observing the inside of a hollow organ or cavity

   Endoscope dontsceped

2. Gurgling and clicking heard over the abdomen caused by air and fluid movement from peristaltic action normally occurring every 5 to 15 seconds at a rate of 5 to 35 per minute

   Bowel _Sounds_ wlebo onudss

3. Examination of the upper portion of the rectum with an endoscope

   laryngoscope locnooscypo

4. Feeding via a tube placed in the stomach

   _____ gvaaeg

5. Immovable accumulation of feces in the bowels

   Impaction mipcaitno

6. Resin obtained from trees to test for occult blood in feces

   guiac gaiuca

7. Device consisting of a fluorescent screen that makes the shadows of objects interposed between the tube and the screen visible

   Fluroscopy ulfroocspeo

8. Fatty stools

   Steatorrhea estaotrhrae

9. A test performed to measure secretions of hydrochloric acid and pepsin in the stomach

   _____ stgairc naayliss

10. Examination of the stomach and abdominal cavity by use of an endoscope

    _____ stgarsopcoy

▶ LABORATORY TESTS

Match the test with its definition.

1. __E__ Stool for lipids
2. __D__ Stool cultures
3. __B__ Stool for occult blood
4. __A__ Carcinoembryonic antigen (CEA)
5. __C__ Stool for ova and parasites

A. Levels may indicate colorectal or other cancer
B. Testing stool for blood that is not visible to the eye
C. Testing stool for intestinal infections caused by parasites
D. Testing stool for the presence of pathogenic organisms in the GI tract
E. Testing stool for excessive amounts of fat

▶ BOWEL PREPARATION

Circle the eight errors in the following paragraph, and insert the correct information.

A stomach preparation is required for several procedures that visualize the lower bowel. This preparation is important for effective test results. An incomplete bowel preparation may prevent the test from being done or cause the need for it to be repeated. This can result in the patient's early discharge and cost savings. The patient usually receives a soft diet 24 hours before the test, and a cool tap-water enema or Fleet enema is given once. Elderly or debilitated patients should be carefully assessed during the administration of multiple enemas, which can fatigue the patient and improve electrolytes. In patients with bleeding or constipation, the bowel preparation may not be ordered by the physician.

► CRITICAL THINKING

Read the following case study, and answer the questions.

Mrs. Davis is a 41-year-old schoolteacher who is admitted to your unit with recurrent lung cancer. She is debilitated and her physician orders total parenteral nutrition (TPN) to be started.

1. Why is the TPN rate started slowly at first? _____

_____

2. Why are serum glucose levels monitored on Mrs. Davis during TPN administration? _____

_____

3. Names types of veins in which TPN may be administered with (a) dextrose of 12 percent or less; (b) dextrose greater than

12 percent. _____

_____

_____

4. Why is it necessary to use an infusion control pump for TPN? _____

_____

_____

5. Why should a TPN rate never be increased to get it back on schedule if the TPN falls behind schedule? _____

_____

_____

6. When TPN is discontinued, why is the infusion slowly weaned off? _____

_____

7. When TPN is ordered to be stopped, why should the patient be fed first if it is not contraindicated? _____

_____

8. Identify one nursing diagnosis and outcome with interventions for the patient on TPN. _____

_____

_____

REVIEW QUESTIONS

Choose the best answer.

1. Which of the following structures are connected by the ileocecal valve?
   A. Duodenum to the stomach
   B. Colon to the small intestine
   C. Stomach to the esophagus
   D. Ileum to the jejunum

2. Mechanical digestion in the stomach is accomplished by which of the following structures?
   A. Mucosa
   B. Smooth muscle layers
   C. Striated muscle layers
   D. Gastric glands

3. Gastric juice contributes to the digestion of which of the following types of nutrients?
   A. Proteins
   B. Fats
   C. Starch

4. The enzymes of the small intestine contribute to the digestion of which of the following types of nutrients?
   A. Proteins
   B. Fats
   C. Disaccharides

5. Bowel sounds heard as soft clicks and gurgles at a rate of four per minute would be documented by the nurse as which of the following types of findings?
   A. Absent
   B. Hyperactive
   C. Hypoactive
   D. Normal

6. To be considered absent, the nurse understands that bowel sounds must be auscultated in each quadrant for which one of the following time intervals?
   A. 2 min
   B. 3 min
   C. 5 min
   D. 15 min

7. Which of the following diagnostic procedures on stool specimens must the nurse collect using sterile technique?
   A. Stool for ova and parasites
   B. Stool for occult blood
   C. Stool culture
   D. Stool for lipids

8. Which of the following diagnostic procedures does the nurse understand does not require the patient to be nil per os (NPO)?
   A. Upper GI series (barium swallow)
   B. Flat plate of the abdomen
   C. Magnetic resonance imaging (MRI)
   D. EGD

9. Which of the following nursing diagnoses would be most appropriate to include in the patient's plan of care following a barium swallow?
   A. Risk for constipation
   B. Risk for pain
   C. Imbalanced nutrition, more than body requirements
   D. Risk for diarrhea

10. Which of the following colors would the nurse expect the patient's stool to be immediately after a barium swallow?
    A. Brown
    B. Black
    C. White
    D. Green

11. Which of the following does the nurse understand is the primary reason a patient is NPO until the gag reflex returns after an EGD procedure?
    A. To rest the vocal cords
    B. To prevent aspiration
    C. To keep the throat dry
    D. To prevent vomiting

12. Which of the following positions would the nurse be correct in using for nasogastric (NG) tube insertion?
    A. Trendelenburg's position
    B. Prone
    C. Sims' position
    D. High Fowler's position

13. A patient who has an NG tube and an intravenous (IV) line states, "I'm so embarrassed to have my family here I have tubes coming out of me everywhere." Which of the following would be an appropriate nursing diagnosis?
    A. Impaired adjustment
    B. Defensive coping
    C. Disturbed body image
    D. Anxiety

14. When inserting a NG tube, it is recommended to have the patient do which of the following to make the insertion easier?
    A. Cough
    B. Swallow
    C. Hold his or her breath
    D. Exhale

30

NURSING CARE OF PATIENTS WITH UPPER GASTROINTESTINAL DISORDERS

▶ VOCABULARY

Unscramble the letters to identify a word described by the definition.

1. Most common cause of peptic ulcers; its recent discovery has revolutionized treatment and cure of most peptic ulcers.

   _____ _____ lehicbocatre ypoilr

2. Loss of appetite

   _____ noraxeai

3. Inflammation of the stomach

   _____ sagrtisti

4. Small, white, painful ulcers that appear on the inner cheeks, lips, gums, tongue, palate, and pharynx

   _____ _____ hpatouhs tsoamtisti

5. Recurrent episodes of binge eating and self-induced vomiting

   _____ _____ lubiami ernvsoa

6. Rapid entry of food into the jejunum causing dizziness, tachycardia, fainting, sweating, nausea, diarrhea, and abdominal cramping

   _____ _____ umdpnig nysdomre

7. Surgical removal of the stomach

   _____ gtrasetcmyo

8. 20 to 30 percent over average weight for age, sex, and height

   _____ boesiyt

9. Condition in which the stomach may protrude above the diaphragm

   _____ _____ ihaatl erhian

10. Following surgical removal of part of the stomach, reanastomosis of the remaining portion to the proximal jejunum

    _____ satgorjujeonsotym

▶ GASTRITIS

Match the description with the type of gastritis associated with it.

1. _____ Heartburn or indigestion

2. _____ Autoimmune gastritis

3. _____ Often caused by overeating

4. _____ Associated with the bacteria *Helicobacter pylori*

5. _____ Associated with difficulty in absorbing vitamin B_{12}

6. _____ Can lead to peritonitis

7. _____ Can be treated with antibiotics

8. _____ Treatment includes a bland diet

A. Acute gastritis
B. Chronic gastritis type A
C. Chronic gastritis type B

▶ PEPTIC ULCER DISEASE

Circle the seven errors in the following paragraph and write the correct information.

Most peptic ulcers are caused by stress. Peptic ulcers are commonly found in the sigmoid colon. Symptoms of peptic ulcers include burning and a gnawing pain in the chest. There is pain and discomfort with a full stomach, which may be relieved by avoiding food. Peptic ulcers cannot be cured. Medication treatment for most peptic ulcers should include anticoagulants as indicated.

▶ GASTRECTOMY

Label the structures as they appear following various types of gastric surgery.

► CRITICAL THINKING

Read the following case study and answer the questions.

Mrs. Sheffield has just returned from surgery. She had a Billroth I procedure. She has a nasogastric tube, a 1000-mL intravenous (IV) of lactated Ringer's solution infusing at 100 mL/h, and a Foley catheter. She is nil per os (NPO). Her vital signs are stable: blood pressure 118/90, pulse 80, respirations 16, and temperature 98° F (36.6° C). Her abdominal dressing is clean, dry, and intact. She is drowsy but easily aroused. After getting Mrs. Sheffield settled in the bed, you connect her nasogastric tube to intermittent low wall suction as ordered by her physician and add another blanket to warm her. Mrs. Sheffield requests something for pain. You administer morphine 5 mg intramuscularly and allow her to rest. An hour later, the nurse's aid tells you that Mrs. Sheffield is vomiting bright red blood. You go to her room and find her lying on her side propped up on one arm vomiting into an emesis basin. Her nasogastric suction catheter contains 250 mL of bright red drainage. Her dressing remains clean and dry. She is diaphoretic and complaining of nausea.

1. What is your first response? _____

   _____

2. What is your next action? _____

   _____

3. Vital signs are now blood pressure 86/60, pulse 96, respirations 24, and temperature 97.6° F (36.4° C). What is your assessment of the new data, and what is your next step? _____

   _____

   _____

4. As you lightly palpate her abdomen, it feels slightly distended, and you suspect that she may be bleeding into her peritoneum. What is your next step? _____

   _____

   _____

5. What do you need to tell the physician? _____

   _____

6. The physician orders a hematocrit and hemoglobin, electrolytes, and oxygen at 2 L via nasal cannula. The physician also tells you to get Mrs. Sheffield ready to return to surgery. What is your priority nursing action? _____

   _____

REVIEW QUESTIONS

Choose the best answer.

1. A patient has a duodenal peptic ulcer and is taking cimetidine (Tagamet). Which of the following side effects related to cimetidine should be included in the teaching plan?
   A. Confusion
   B. Hypertension
   C. Blurred vision
   D. Dry mouth

2. A patient is admitted with chronic gastritis type B. Which of the following signs and symptoms is the nurse likely to find on assessment?
   A. Anorexia
   B. Dysphagia
   C. Diarrhea
   D. Feeling of fullness

3. Which of the following surgical procedures is the most likely treatment for a patient with gastric cancer?
   A. Gastroplasty
   B. Gastrorrhaphy
   C. Gastric stapling
   D. Gastrectomy

4. An asymptomatic patient is admitted with gastric bleeding. For which of the following signs or symptoms of severe gastric bleeding should the nurse monitor?
   A. Hypertension
   B. Diaphoresis
   C. Bounding pulse
   D. Edema

5. A patient had a gastrectomy 2 months ago. The patient comes to the clinic complaining of greasy stools and frequent bowel movements. After the patient's surgical recovery and current eating habits are assessed, which of the following types of diet would be most appropriate for the nurse to teach the patient to use?
   A. Bland diet
   B. High-carbohydrate diet
   C. Low-fat diet
   D. Pureed diet

6. A patient visits her gynecologist and reports that she is very unhappy with her weight, which is 310 lb on her 5-foot 7-inch frame. When planning her care, the nurse knows that the initial treatment for obesity includes which of the following?
   A. Gastroplasty
   B. Billroth I procedure
   C. Billroth II procedure
   D. Diet management

7. A patient has been diagnosed with a hiatal hernia. The patient complains of heartburn and occasional regurgitation. Which of the following interventions should the nurse teach the patient to reduce the symptoms?
   A. Eat small, frequent meals.
   B. Recline for 1 hour after meals.
   C. Sleep flat without a pillow.
   D. Eat a bedtime snack.

8. A patient is having an acute episode of gastric bleeding. The physician orders an IV of 1000 mL of 0.9-percent normal saline, a complete blood cell (CBC) count, a nasogastric tube to low-wall suction, and oxygen by nasal cannula. Which of the following orders should the nurse perform first?
   A. Administer the IV of 1000 mL of 0.9-percent normal saline.
   B. Draw the blood for the CBC cell.
   C. Insert the nasogastric tube.
   D. Apply oxygen by nasal cannula.

9. Which of the following does the nurse understand is a sign or symptom of oral cancer?
   A. Painless ulcer
   B. White painful ulcers
   C. Feeling of fullness
   D. Heartburn

10. Which of the following procedures does the nurse understand is done palliatively for the dysphagia that occurs in inoperable esophageal cancer?
    A. Gastrectomy
    B. Esophageal dilation
    C. Radical neck dissection
    D. Modified neck dissection

11. Which of the following statements by the patient would the nurse evaluate as indicating understanding by the patient of preventive measures for gastroesophageal reflux disease?
    A. I need to eat large meals.
    B. I will sleep without pillows.
    C. I need to lie down for 2 hours after each meal.
    D. I will identify foods that cause discomfort.

31

NURSING CARE OF PATIENTS WITH LOWER GASTROINTESTINAL DISORDERS

▶ VOCABULARY

Match the vocabulary word to the correct definition.

1. _____ Appendicitis

2. _____ Colectomy

3. _____ Colitis

4. _____ Colostomy

5. _____ Diverticulosis

6. _____ Fistula

7. _____ Hernia

8. _____ Ileostomy

9. _____ Intussusception

10. _____ Melena

11. _____ Peritonitis

12. _____ Volvulus

A. Outpouchings in colon
B. Inflammation of colon
C. Telescoping of the bowel
D. Tunnel connection between bowel and another organ
E. Blood in stool
F. Twisting of bowel
G. Inflammation or infection of peritoneum
H. Bulging of abdominal contents through abdominal wall
I. Diversion of small bowel through abdominal wall
J. Removal of large bowel
K. Diversion of large bowel through abdominal wall
L. Inflamed appendix

▶ OSTOMIES

Circle the errors in the following paragraphs and insert the correct information.

1. Michelle Braun is a 16-year-old with ulcerative colitis. She is taking cortisone and amoxicillin (Amoxil). She is on a high-residue diet. She is now admitted to the hospital for a colectomy and elective loop ostomy. You monitor her intake and output (I&O), daily weights, and electrolytes. You also assess for signs of inflammation in her joints, skin, and other parts of her body. You teach her to restrict fluids following surgery to limit the number of stools she has daily.

2. James Key is a 46-year-old with a new sigmoid colostomy. Following surgery you assess his stoma every shift for 3 days to ensure that it remains gray and moist. You explain that the stool will be semiformed and that he will have to irrigate his ostomy every 1 to 2 days to have bowel movements. You contact the dietitian to provide a list of the high-fiber foods that he should avoid.

▶ CRITICAL THINKING

Read the case study and answer the questions.

Mrs. Millie Hendricks is a 90-year-old resident in the nursing home where you work as a practical nurse. She has a history of severe osteoarthritis and has no teeth, but otherwise she is quite healthy. She normally has a bowel movement every other day but has occasional constipation, which she takes care of herself by requesting a dose of Milk of Magnesia. Today when you take Mrs. Hendricks' medications to her, she says, "I think I need a second dose of that Milk of Magnesia; my bowels haven't moved in three days." You look at her medication administration record and find as needed (prn) orders for Milk of Magnesia, psyllium (Metamucil), Senna (Sennakot), or a tap water enema.

1. What should you do before you administer more medication? _____

_____

_____

_____

2. What factors most likely led to Mrs. Hendricks' constipation? _____

_____

_____

_____

3. What will happen if Mrs. Hendricks' bowels do not move today? _____

_____

_____

_____

4. What non-drug interventions will help Mrs. Hendricks' move her bowels? _____

_____

_____

_____

5. After Mrs. Hendricks' bowels have moved, what measures can you institute to prevent constipation next time? _____

_____

_____

_____

REVIEW QUESTIONS

Choose the best answer.

1. A patient visits his physician with complaints of chronic diarrhea that is sometimes bloody. Ulcerative colitis is diagnosed. How should the nurse explain the patient's diagnosis to him?
   A. "You have inflamed sacs throughout your colon."
   B. "Your colon and rectum are inflamed and ulcerated."
   C. "You have ulcerations and fistulas in your small bowel."
   D. "Your colon is spastic and hypertonic."

2. Which of the following laboratory studies does the nurse understand helps monitor ulcerative colitis?
   A. Aspartate aminotransferase (AST)
   B. Creatine phosphokinase (CPK) isoenzymes
   C. Amylase and lipase
   D. Complete blood count (CBC) and electrolytes

3. Which of the following diet instructions should be included in the plan of care to help a patient control ulcerative colitis symptoms?
   A. Drink milk or eat a milk product at least six times daily.
   B. Include four servings daily of whole grain breads or cereals.
   C. Limit coffee to six cups daily.
   D. Avoid fresh fruits and vegetables.

4. A patient who has ulcerative colitis is taken to the emergency department with severe rectal bleeding. Which of the following is the best option for maintaining nutritional status for this patient with ulcerative colitis who must be nil per os (NPO) for an extended period of time?
   A. Nasogastric (NG) tube feedings
   B. Percutaneous endoscopic gastrostomy (PEG) tube feedings
   C. Total parenteral nutrition (TPN)
   D. Intravenous (IV) 5 percent dextrose and water

5. A patient is diagnosed with acute diverticulitis. Which of the following may have placed the patient at risk for developing diverticulitis?
   A. Eating a low-fiber diet
   B. Chronic diarrhea
   C. History of nonsteroidal antiinflammatory drug (NSAID) use
   D. Family history of colon cancer

6. Which of the following foods might a patient with diverticulitis be instructed to avoid in his plan of care?
   A. Peanuts and raspberries
   B. Apples and pears
   C. Red meat and dairy products
   D. Bran and whole grains

7. Which of the following nursing diagnoses is most appropriate to include in the plan of care for a patient with symptoms of a bowel obstruction?
   A. Risk for impaired swallowing related to NPO status
   B. Risk for urinary retention related to fluid volume depletion
   C. Risk for deficient fluid volume related to nausea and vomiting
   D. Risk for impaired coping related to prolonged hospitalization

8. Which of the following explanations by the nurse to reinforce the patient's preoperative education for a loop ostomy would be correct?
   A. "You will have a stoma in the middle of your abdomen that will constantly drain liquid stool."
   B. "You will have a looped bag system to collect stool from your stoma."
   C. "You will have a loop of bowel on your abdomen, but it will not drain stool."
   D. "You will have a loop of bowel on your abdomen that can be put back in after your bowel has healed."

9. Which of the following dietary instructions is most important to include in the plan of care to prevent complications for a patient with an ileostomy?
   A. "Drink lots of fluids to prevent dehydration."
   B. "Avoid fruits and vegetables to prevent diarrhea."
   C. "Avoid milk products to prevent gas."
   D. "Eat plenty of fiber to prevent constipation."

10. A patient is concerned about odor from her ileostomy. Which of the following responses by the nurse would be best?
    A. "A teaspoon of baking soda in your pouch will absorb all the odor."
    B. "The plastic your pouch is made of is odor proof. You shouldn't have to worry about odor as long as you don't have a leak."
    C. "Effluent from an ileostomy has no odor. It's colostomies that can smell bad from time to time."
    D. "Changing your pouch and face plate daily will help prevent odor."

UNIT EIGHT

UNDERSTANDING THE LIVER, GALLBLADDER, AND PANCREAS

CHECKLIST FOR LEARNING SUCCESS

Review of Anatomy and Physiology	Major Disorders	Nursing Assessment	Diagnostic Tests	Interventions	Common Medications
☐ Liver structure and function	☐ Hepatitis	☐ Pain	☐ Alanine aminotransferase, aspartate aminotransferase	☐ Transjugular intrahepatic portosystemic shunt	☐ Diuretics
☐ Gallbladder structure and function	☐ Liver failure	☐ Alcohol history	☐ Albumin	☐ Tamponade	☐ Analgesics
☐ Pancreas structure and function	☐ Acute	☐ Medication history	☐ Amylase	☐ Transplant	☐ Histamine antagonists
☐ Aging changes	☐ Chronic	☐ Gastrointestinal S & S	☐ Ammonia	☐ Cholecystectomy	☐ Lactulose
	☐ Pancreatitis	☐ Skin	☐ Bilirubin	☐ Nutrition	☐ Neomycin
	☐ Cholecystitis	☐ Abdomen	☐ Prothrombin time	☐ Extracorporeal shock wave lithotripsy (ESWL)	
	☐ Cholelithiasis	☐ Mental status	☐ Occult blood	☐ Pain control	
	☐ Cancer		☐ Upper gastrointestinal and lower gastrointestinal series		
			☐ Cholecystogram		
			☐ Liver scan		
			☐ Esophagogastroduodenoscopy		
			☐ Endoscopic retrograde cholangiopancreatography		
			☐ Liver biopsy		

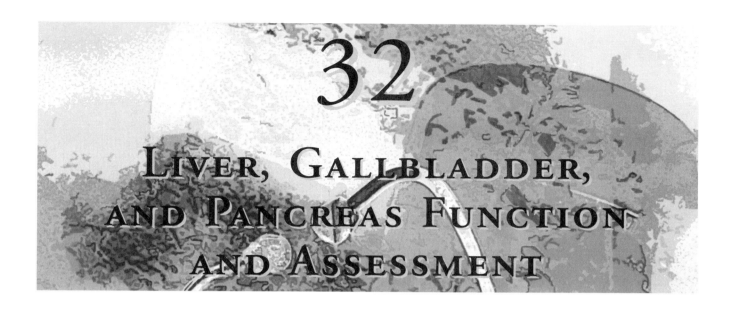

32

LIVER, GALLBLADDER, AND PANCREAS FUNCTION AND ASSESSMENT

▶ VOCABULARY

Match the term or abbreviation with the correct definition.

1. _____ ALT

2. _____ AST

3. _____ Prothrombin time

4. _____ Bilirubin

5. _____ Bile

6. _____ Caput medusae

7. _____ Esophagogastroduodenoscopy

8. _____ Endoscopic retrograde

   cholangiopancreatography

9. _____ Spider angioma

10. _____ Striae

A. Light, silvery lines on the abdomen
B. Bluish-purple vein pattern around umbilicus
C. Endoscopic examination of the esophagus, stomach, and duodenum
D. Substance made by the liver and stored in the gallbladder
E. Endoscopic examination of the common bile duct and pancreatic duct
F. Alanine aminotransferase
G. Thin, reddish-purple vein lines
H. Aspartate aminotransferase
I. Assesses adequacy of blood clotting
J. Substance made by hepatocytes in the liver

▶ PANCREAS

Name the pancreatic enzyme with each function.

1. Digests polypeptides to short chains of amino acids: _____

2. Digests emulsified fats to fatty acids and glycerol: _____

3. Digests starch to maltose: _____

► LIVER

Match each of the following with the proper descriptive statement.

1. _____ Glycogen

2. _____ Beta-oxidation

3. _____ Albumin

4. _____ Bilirubin

5. _____ Lipoproteins

6. _____ Iron and copper

7. _____ Cholesterol

8. _____ Clotting factors

9. _____ Kupffer cells

10. _____ A, D, E, K

A. The vitamins stored by the liver
B. The minerals stored by the liver
C. The form in which excess glucose is stored
D. Helps maintain blood volume
E. Transport fats in the blood
F. The macrophages of the liver
G. Include prothrombin and fibrinogen
H. The process by which fatty acids may be used for energy
I. Formed from old red blood cells and eliminated in feces
J. A steroid synthesized by the liver; excess is excreted in bile

► ANATOMY

Label the structures of the liver, gallbladder, and pancreas.

▶ CRITICAL THINKING

Read the case study and answer the following questions.

Mrs. Margery White, age 54, has come into the clinic "to see why I am always so tired." During the first few minutes with Mrs. White, the nurse notes that Mrs. White's skin appears to be yellow.

1. What other indicators of liver, gallbladder, or pancreas disease might the nurse observe in the first few minutes with Mrs. White? _____

_____

_____

2. What complaints might Mrs. White have? _____

_____

_____

3. What types of information would be important for the nurse to gather regarding Mrs. White's family and social history? __

_____

_____

4. What diagnostic blood work should the nurse anticipate that the physician will order for Mrs. White? _____

_____

_____

5. The physician suspects that Mrs. White has an obstruction in the common bile duct. An ultrasonogram is ordered. Mrs. White is apprehensive. What should the nurse explain about the procedure? _____

_____

_____

R E V I E W   Q U E S T I O N S

Choose the best answer.

1. Which of the following substances is not synthesized by the liver?
   A. Fibrinogen
   B. Albumin
   C. Hemoglobin
   D. Lipoproteins

2. Which of the following structures carries bile and pancreatic juices to the duodenum?
   A. Pancreatic duct
   B. Cystic duct
   C. Hepatic duct
   D. Common bile duct

3. Where does bicarbonate pancreatic juice neutralize hydrochloric acid?
   A. Duodenum
   B. Pancreas
   C. Stomach
   D. Esophagus

4. Bile salts emulsify fats, which means they do which of the following?
   A. Digest them to fatty acids.
   B. Use them for energy.
   C. Break them into smaller pieces.
   D. Digest them to glycerol.

5. Which of the following statements explains why a patient with jaundice is at risk of impaired skin integrity?
   A. Jaundice is associated with thinning of the skin.
   B. Jaundice causes the blood supply to the skin to decrease.
   C. Jaundice is caused by impaired break down of bilirubin, which causes itching.
   D. Jaundice causes the kidneys to produce more uric acid, which causes skin breakdown.

6. The nurse notes that the serum bilirubin level is less today than yesterday in a patient with liver disease. The nurse interprets this to mean what?
   A. Red blood cell destruction is diminishing.
   B. Liver function is probably improving.
   C. Kupffer cell damage is continuing.
   D. The kidneys are compensating for liver dysfunction.

7. When monitoring laboratory results on a patient with pancreatic disease, the nurse should pay particular attention to which of the following laboratory test results?
   A. Serum amylase
   B. Serum bilirubin
   C. Lactic dehydrogenase
   D. Serum cholesterol

8. The nurse auscultates the abdomen of a patient suspected of having gallbladder disease. The normal frequency of bowel sounds is every
   A. 5 to 15 seconds
   B. 15 to 30 seconds
   C. 30 to 60 seconds
   D. 5 to 7 minutes

9. When observing the abdomen of a patient with liver disease, the nurse notes thin, reddish-purple vein lines at various locations on the patient's abdomen. The nurse should note that the patient has which assessment finding?
   A. Striae
   B. Spider angiomas
   C. Caput medusae
   D. Ascites

10. The nurse should question the patient about to take radiopaque tablets in preparation for a gallbladder series about allergies to which of the following?
    A. Bee stings
    B. Adhesive tape
    C. Citrus fruits
    D. Shellfish

33

NURSING CARE OF PATIENTS WITH LIVER, GALLBLADDER, AND PANCREATIC DISORDERS

▶ VOCABULARY

Match the following terms with the appropriate description.

1. _____ Ascites
2. _____ Asterixis
3. _____ Cirrhosis
4. _____ Encephalopathy
5. _____ Fetor hepaticus
6. _____ Hepatorenal syndrome
7. _____ Hepatitis
8. _____ Jaundice
9. _____ Portal hypertension
10. _____ Pruritis
11. _____ Steatorrhea
12. _____ Varices

A. Yellowing of the sclera and skin from excess bilirubin
B. Itching
C. Liver flap
D. Fluid in the abdomen from decreased albumin
E. Neurologic changes from excess ammonia
F. Weakened, swollen veins in the esophagus
G. Foul breath
H. Fatty, foul-smelling stools
I. Increased blood pressure in the portal circulation
J. Scarring and hardening of the liver from inflammation
K. Oliguria and sodium retention without kidney defects
L. Inflammation of the liver cells

▶ LIVER

Fill in the crossword with terms related to the liver.

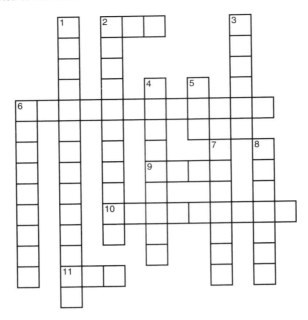

ACROSS

2. Abbreviation for serum hepatitis
6. Snake's head
9. Liver shunt
10. Liver flap
11. Abbreviation for infectious hepatitis

DOWN

1. Confusion and coma are symptoms
2. This complication causes anuria
3. Abdomen circulation
4. Liver inflammation
5. Abbreviation for liver location
6. Liver failure
7. Collection of fluid in peritoneal cavity
8. Dilated esophageal veins

▶ GALLBLADDER

Match the following terms with the appropriate description.

1. _____ Cholecystitis

2. _____ Cholesterol stones

3. _____ Flatulence

4. _____ Murphy's sign

5. _____ Bilirubin

6. _____ Extracorporeal shock wave lithotripsy (ESWL)

7. _____ T-tube

8. _____ Laparoscopic cholecystectomy

9. _____ Chenodeoxycholic acid

10. _____ Cholecystomy

A. Pigment from the breakdown of red blood cells
B. Dissolves cholesterol gallstones
C. An incision into the gallbladder
D. Inflammation of the gallbladder
E. Inability to take a deep breath when fingers are pressed under liver margin
F. Gallstones composed mostly of cholesterol and other fatty acids
G. Intestinal gas expelled via the rectum
H. A procedure that shatters gallstones using sound waves
I. A surgical drain used to ensure that bile freely drains from the gallbladder after surgery
J. Removal of the gallbladder through a small abdominal incision

▶ PANCREAS

In the space on the left, write N or A to indicate whether the assessment finding is normal or abnormal. If the finding is abnormal, indicate the possible cause for the finding in the space on the right.

1. Serum glucose > 150 mg percent _____

2. Serum amylase > 500 IU/L _____

3. Serum lipase = 15 U/L _____

4. Pleural effusion _____

5. Blood pressure and pulse within 15 percent of patient baseline _____

6. Serum albumin < 3.2 g/dL _____

7. Positive Cullen's sign _____

8. Urinary output < 30 mL/hr _____

9. Positive Chvostek's sign _____

10. Foul-smelling, fatty stools _____

▶ CRITICAL THINKING

Read the case study and answer the questions.

Ms. Betty Smith has been diagnosed with hepatic encephalopathy secondary to Laënnec's cirrhosis or chronic liver failure. During the admission process, the nurse notes the following findings: abdomen grossly distended, yellow sclera and skin, multiple bruises, and 2+ pitting edema of the lower extremities. Ms. Smith is noted to be irritable and to have difficulty answering questions and appears to doze off frequently during the interview. The nurse also notes that Ms. Smith scratches her arms and legs frequently. Her laboratory data indicate that her serum bilirubin, ammonia, and prothrombin time are elevated and that her serum albumin, total protein, and potassium are below normal.

1. What data support the diagnosis of Laënnec's cirrhosis? _____

_____

_____

2. What data suggest that Ms. Smith has hepatic encephalopathy? What other evidence might the nurse observe? _____

_____

_____

3. Why are the 2+ pitting edema and abdominal distention of concern? _____

_____

_____

4. What medical treatments can the nurse expect the physician to order for the hepatic encephalopathy? _____

_____

Two days after Ms. Smith was admitted, the nurse notes bright red blood in Ms. Smith's emesis. Ms. Smith also complains of feeling cold, and her pulse is 115 and thready. The nurse calls for help and places Ms. Smith in a semi-Fowler's position.

5. What further treatment can the nurse anticipate for Ms. Smith? _____

_____

6. For what complications of treatment for esophageal varices does the nurse observe? _____

_____

7. What observations does the nurse make to detect bleeding from lack of clotting factors? _____

_____

8. What nursing measures are taken to help Ms. Smith maintain her fluid balance? _____

_____

9. What should Ms. Smith be told about taking acetaminophen (Tylenol)? Why? _____

_____

REVIEW QUESTIONS

Choose the best answer.

1. A patient with ascites is placed on a low-sodium diet. The nurse knows that diet teaching has been successful if the patient selects which of the following meals?
   A. Bologna sandwich with tomato juice
   B. Frankfurter on a bun with pickle relish and skim milk
   C. Baked chicken, white rice, and apple juice
   D. Peanut butter and jelly sandwich with tomato soup

2. Which of the following nursing interventions related to esophageal tamponade with a Senstaken-Blakemore tube is *inappropriate?*
   A. Keeping a pair of scissors at the bedside
   B. Having oral suction available
   C. Maintaining traction on the tube, if ordered
   D. Deflating the gastric balloon periodically

3. Which of the following instructions should be given to the patient with portal hypertension?
   A. Eat spicy, rich foods.
   B. Avoid straining to have a bowel movement.
   C. Increase fluid intake.
   D. Expect urine to be tea colored.

4. Which of the following precautions will protect the nurse who is caring for the patient with hepatitis B?
   A. Reverse isolation
   B. Standard precautions
   C. Respiratory precautions
   D. Enteric precautions

5. Fulminant liver failure is most often caused by which of the following?
   A. Antibiotic use
   B. Vitamin use
   C. Alcohol use
   D. Hepatitis B virus (HBV)

6. A patient with chronic liver failure has asterixis and fetor hepaticas and is confused. The nurse recognizes these as symptoms of which complication?
   A. Hepatic encephalopathy
   B. Hepatorenal syndrome
   C. Portal hypertension
   D. Ascites

7. After treatment of esophageal varices by tamponade, the nurse must closely and carefully observe the patient because bleeding recurs in about _____ percent of patients.
   A. 10
   B. 35
   C. 65
   D. 90

8. Which of the following is not a risk factor for gallbladder disease?
   A. Male
   B. Obese
   C. Multiple pregnancies
   D. Age 40 or older

9. The nurse can expect which of the following pain medications to be ordered for the patient with biliary colic?
   A. Codeine
   B. Morphine
   C. Apomorphine
   D. Meperidine

10. Which of the following is a nonsurgical intervention for the management of biliary colic?
    A. Encouraging a high-fat diet
    B. Giving vitamin K
    C. Giving chenodeoxycholic acid (Chenodiol)
    D. Giving probantheline (Pro-Banthine)

11. Patients with a history of pancreatic disease commonly have a history of which of the following?
    A. High-protein diet
    B. Very-low-fat diet
    C. Excessive alcohol consumption
    D. Excessive intake of vitamin C

12. Patients with acute pancreatitis frequently describe their pain as
    A. Dull, boring, beginning in the mid epigastrium and radiating to the back
    B. Knifelike, centered in the left lower quadrant
    C. Burning, focused over the left flank and radiating to the shoulder
    D. Sharp, severe pain that begins in the right upper quadrant

UNIT NINE

UNDERSTANDING THE RENAL AND URINARY SYSTEM

Review of Renal/Urinary Anatomy and Physiology	Major Renal/ Urinary Disorders	Nursing Assessment	Diagnostic Tests	Interventions	Common Medications
☐ Kidneys	☐ Incontinence	☐ Medical history	☐ Urinalysis	☐ Urinary catheters	☐ Diuretics
☐ Urine	☐ Urinary retention	☐ Medications	☐ Urine culture	☐ Lithotripsy	☐ Kayexalate
☐ Elimination of urine	☐ Urinary tract infections	☐ Vital signs	☐ Blood urea nitrogen	☐ Hemodialysis	☐ Phosphate binders
☐ Aging effects	☐ Urological obstructions	☐ Physical assessment	☐ Creatinine	☐ Peritoneal dialysis	
	☐ Tumors	☐ Intake and output	☐ Creatinine clearance	☐ Continuous renal replacement therapy	
	☐ Polycystic kidney disease	☐ Daily weights	☐ Kidneys-ureter-bladder	☐ Urinary diversion	
	☐ Chronic renal diseases		☐ Intravenous pyelogram		
	☐ Acute/chronic renal failure		☐ Cystoscopy and pyelogram		
	☐ Kidney transplantation				

34

Urinary System Function, Assessment, and Therapeutic Measures

► VOCABULARY

Match the term for an abnormality of the urine or urination with the correct description.

1. _____ Hematuria

2. _____ Dysuria

3. _____ Nocturia

4. _____ Oliguria

5. _____ Enuresis

6. _____ Anuria

7. _____ Polyuria

8. _____ Pyuria

A. Painful urination
B. Decreased urine output (<400 mL per 24 hours)
C. Blood in the urine
D. Voiding during the night
E. Excessive urination (>2000 mL per 24 hours)
F. Absence of urination
G. Presence of pus in the urine
H. Bedwetting

▶ SAMPLE URINALYSIS RESULTS

Review the urinalysis results of the following three patients and determine the most likely cause of the abnormal results.

	Patient A	Patient B	Patient C
Color	Yellow	Dark amber	Yellow-green
Character	Cloudy	Concentrated	Clear
Glucose	Negative	Negative	Negative
Bilirubin	Negative	Negative	2+
Ketones	Small	Negative	Negative
Specific gravity (1.010–1.025)	1.024	1.035	1.025
Hemoglobin	Small	Negative	Negative
pH (5.0–9.0)	6.0	5.2	5.5
Protein	100	Negative	Negative
Urobilinogen (0.2–1.0)	0.2	0.2	0.2
Nitrite	Positive	Negative	Negative
Urine microscopic casts	White blood cell, Red blood cell	Negative	Negative
White blood cells (0–4 HPF)	400	4	1
Red blood cells (0–4 HPF)	90	2	2
Crystals	Negative	2	Negative
Amorphous	Negative	Negative	Negative
Epithelial cells (negative)	3	Negative	2
Bacteria (negative)	4+	Negative	Negative
Yeast (negative)	Negative	Negative	Negative

Patient A: _____

Patient B: _____

Patient C: _____

▶ RENAL DIAGNOSTIC TESTS

Indicate whether each statement is true or false.

1. _____ An x-ray of the renal structures after injection of a radiopaque dye into the venous system is called a renal ultrasound.

2. _____ A diagnostic test in which sound waves are used to outline the structure of the kidney is an intravenous pyelogram.

3. _____ A urine sample that is cultured to determine the kind of bacteria it contains is called a creatinine clearance urine test.

4. _____ A diagnostic test in which the inside of the bladder is visualized is called a cystoscopy.

5. _____ The radiopaque dye used when doing diagnostic tests of the renal system is harmless.

▶ CRITICAL THINKING

Read the case studies and answer the following questions.

Mrs. Bohke is a 54-year-old female patient admitted to the hospital with a diagnosis of pneumonia. During her stay, she tells you she has trouble getting to the bathroom on time and often dribbles before she can get to the bathroom.

1. What type of urinary incontinence does she have? _____

_____

2. What teaching could be done to help her decrease her incontinence? _____

_____

Mrs. Simmon is a 79-year-old woman with a fractured hip and a previous cerebrovascular accident (CVA). She has poor vision but is alert mentally. You find her lying in bed in a puddle of urine, crying. She explains that she was unable to find her call light. You find it lying on the floor out of her reach.

3. What kind of incontinence did Mrs. Simmon experience? _____

_____

_____

4. What actions should the nurse take to ensure that this does not happen again? _____

_____

_____

5. When caring for a patient with incontinence, is it helpful to decrease fluid intake? Why or why not? _____

_____

_____

Choose the best answer.

1. Which of the following is secreted when the blood level of oxygen decreases?
   A. Erythropoietin
   B. Renin
   C. Angiotensin II
   D. Vitamin D

2. Urea is a nitrogenous waste product from the metabolism of which of the following?
   A. Nucleic acids
   B. Amino acids
   C. Muscle tissue
   D. Carbohydrates

3. The kidneys are located behind which of the following structures?
   A. Spinal column
   B. Diaphragm
   C. Peritoneum
   D. Inferior vena cava

4. The renal pyramids make up which kidney structure?
   A. Renal cortex
   B. Renal medulla
   C. Renal pelvis
   D. Renal fascia

5. The process of tubular resorption takes place in which of the following parts of the kidney?
   A. From the glomerulus to Bowman's capsule
   B. From the afferent arteriole to the efferent arteriole
   C. From the peritubular capillaries to the glomerulus
   D. From the renal tubule to the peritubular capillaries

6. When collecting a urine specimen on a newly admitted patient, the nurse should take which of the following actions?
   A. Direct the patient to wash her perineum before collecting the urine specimen.
   B. Have the patient void, throw that urine away, and then collect another specimen at least 2 hours later.
   C. Obtain the first voided urine of the day.
   D. Direct the patient to drink at least three glasses of water.

7. A patient's urinalysis results show the following findings: urine dark amber, bacteria—small amount, nitrite negative, specific gravity 1.035. Which of the following is the best explanation for these results?
   A. Dehydration
   B. Urinary tract infection
   C. Contamination of the specimen from bacteria on the perineum
   D. Contamination from menstruation

8. Which of the following diagnostic test results would the nurse evaluate as being related to renal failure?
   A. Hematocrit 39 percent (38 to 47 percent)
   B. Potassium 4.0 mEq/L (3.6 to 5.0 mEq/L)
   C. Uric acid 2 ng/dL (2.5 to 5.5 ng/dL)
   D. Blood urea nitrogen 10 mg/100 mL (8 to 25 mg/100 mL)

9. A patient is scheduled for an intravenous pyelogram. When giving care, the nurse should recognize that restriction of which of the following is part of the preparation for an intravenous pyelogram?
   A. Salt intake
   B. Fluid intake
   C. Use of tobacco
   D. Physical activities

10. The patient is scheduled for a cystoscopy with basket extraction. Which of the following is the most important nursing care after this kind of surgery?
    A. Measuring urine output
    B. Monitoring daily weights
    C. Observing for symptoms of acute renal failure
    D. Limiting fluid intake

11. A patient, age 48, has urge incontinence. When assessing the patient, the nurse would expect to find which of the following symptoms?
    A. Patient unable to reach the bathroom in time and ends up urinating in underwear
    B. Patient incontinent of small amounts of urine when coughs, sneezes, or bears down
    C. Patient incontinent of urine when has many responsibilities and becomes overloaded
    D. Patient incontinent because unable to tell when needs to urinate and unable to control urination

12. Which of the following actions should the nurse take to prevent development of a urinary tract infection for a patient who has a Foley catheter inserted?
    A. Limit fluid intake to 2000 mL per 24 hours to decrease the flow of urine, which can result in increased contamination.
    B. Wash the perineum with an antibacterial soap three times per 24 hours.
    C. Keep catheter securely taped to the patient, preventing back-and-forth motion of the catheter.
    D. Empty the Foley catheter bag only when needed to prevent contamination of the exit spout.

13. Which of the following actions should the nurse take for a patient who has total urinary incontinence?
    A. Give patient cranberry juice to keep the urine acidic.
    B. Ensure that patient has ready access to the urinal.
    C. Teach patient how to do Kegel exercises to increase perineal tone.
    D. Apply an adult incontinence brief to catch urine and change when necessary.

35

NURSING CARE OF PATIENTS WITH DISORDERS OF THE URINARY TRACT

▶ VOCABULARY
Fill in the blank with the correct term.

1. _____ is inflammation of the urethra.

2. _____ is inflammation of the bladder.

3. _____ is inflammation of the kidney.

4. Surgical repair of the urethra is called _____ .

5. Kidney stones are also called _____ .

6. _____ is surgical incision into the kidney to remove a stone.

7. Unrelieved obstruction of the urinary tract can lead to _____ .

8. A _____ tube may be inserted directly into the kidney pelvis to drain urine.

9. Surgical removal of a kidney is called a _____ .

10. Thickening and hardening of the renal blood vessels is called _____ .

▶ URINARY TRACT INFECTIONS
Answer the following questions.

1. What is the usual cause of urinary tract infections (UTIs) in women? _____

_____

2. What is the usual cause of UTIs in men? _____

_____

3. What advice regarding fluids should be given to patients who are susceptible to UTIs? _____

_____

4. What is the single most important thing a patient with a history of UTIs should be taught? _____

_____

5. Compare cystitis (bladder infection) versus pyelonephritis (kidney infection) by filling out the following chart.

	Cystitis	Pyelonephritis
Symptoms	_____	_____
Urinalysis results	_____	_____
Prognosis	_____	_____

► URINARY TRACT OBSTRUCTIONS
Answer the following questions.

1. What is the most common symptom of cancer of the bladder? _____

2. What is the most common risk factor for cancer of the bladder? _____

3. What is the most common symptom of cancer of the kidney? _____

4. What does the urine look like when a patient has an ileal conduit? _____

5. What nursing care should be provided for a patient with an ileal conduit? _____

6. What is the most important care that should be given a patient with a kidney stone? _____

7. What teaching should be done for the patient to prevent further stone formation if the stone is composed of calcium oxalate? Uric acid? _____

► CRITICAL THINKING
Read the case study and answer the questions.

Mrs. Zins is a 47-year-old woman who has had type 1 diabetes mellitus for over 20 years. Recently she has begun having incidents of hypoglycemia, she is edematous, and her blood pressure has elevated. She is admitted to the hospital for diagnosis and treatment of probable renal failure.

Subjective Data

States that she has been exhausted lately and her skin is itchy
States that she has been very irritable and her husband says she is hard to live with

Objective Data

BP 194/104, P 98, R 22, T 98.4° F (36.9° C)
Jugular vein distention present at 45 degrees
3+ pitting edema of feet and ankles, generalized edema throughout body, including periorbital edema
Weight gain of 20 pounds in 2 months
Skin very dry, flaky

Diagnostic Tests

Fasting blood sugar 56 mg/100 liters
Serum creatinine 5.4 mg/100 liters
Uric acid 8.2 ng/dL

Serum sodium 145 meq/liter
Serum potassium 5.9 meq/liter
Hemoglobin (Hgb) 7.2 g/100ml, Hematocrit (Hct) 22 percent

1. Mrs. Zins has been having incidents of hypoglycemia. Why is this happening? _____

   _____

2. With Mrs. Zins present blood sugar of 56, what kind of juice should the nurse give her? _____

   _____

3. How does diabetes cause chronic renal failure? _____

   _____

4. Is there anything Mrs. Zins could have done to decrease the possibility of developing renal failure? _____

   _____

5. Identify two nursing diagnoses that would be appropriate for Mrs. Zins based on her assessment. _____

   _____

6. What diagnostic test was most indicative of renal failure for Mrs. Zins? _____

   _____

7. Why is Mrs. Zins anemic? _____

   _____

8. What would be the three most important nursing assessments for Mrs. Zins related to her chronic renal failure? _____

   _____

9. What kind of diet will Mrs. Zins most likely receive? _____

   _____

▶ RENAL FAILURE

Fill in the symptoms of renal failure on the figure below.

Neurological system

Oral cavity

Cardiovascular system

Respiratory system

Gastrointestinal system

Renal system

Reproductive system

Skin

Musculoskeletal system

Fluid volume

Choose the best answer.

1. A 72-year-old patient had a cystoscopy, which revealed a bladder cancer. He is admitted to the hospital for a cystectomy and formation of an ileal conduit. The nurse should assess for the most common symptom of cancer of the bladder, which is which of the following?
    A. Nocturia
    B. Dysuria
    C. Urinary retention
    D. Hematuria

2. Postoperatively, the nurse notes the presence of mucus in the urinary drainage. Which of the following actions should the nurse take?
    A. Notify the physician.
    B. Collect a urine specimen for culture and sensitivity.
    C. Measure the specific gravity of the urine.
    D. Recognize that this is a normal occurrence.

3. A patient is admitted to intensive care in hypovolemic shock caused by gastrointestinal bleeding. It is determined that the patient is in acute renal failure. Which of the following is the most significant sign of acute renal failure that the nurse should observe for as part of the nursing assessment?
    A. A rise in blood pressure
    B. An elevation in body temperature
    C. A decrease in urine output
    D. An increase in urine specific gravity

4. When assessing the patient, the nurse notes the following diagnostic tests on the patient's chart. Which of the following diagnostic tests results is most indicative of acute renal failure?
    A. BUN 80 mg/100 mL (8-25) mg/100 L
    B. 24-hour creatinine clearance of 5 mL/min (100 mL/min)
    C. Uric acid 8 ng/dL (2.5-5.5 ng/dL)
    D. Serum creatinine 1.7 mg/100 L (0.5-1.5 mg/100 L)

5. Which of the following snacks is most appropriate for the nurse to serve a patient with acute renal failure to control potassium levels?
    A. Dried peanuts
    B. An orange
    C. Yogurt
    D. A gelatin dessert

6. A patient with severe right flank pain, general weakness, and fever is hospitalized. He has a history of recurrent urinary tract infection, and renal calculi are suspected. On the second hospital day, the patient's urine output drops to 300 mL/24 hr, and he has distention and pain in the suprapubic area. The nurse would evaluate which of the following to be the most likely cause for this sudden change?
    A. Sudden decreased renal perfusion
    B. Inadequate fluid intake
    C. Interstitial fluid shift
    D. Urinary tract obstruction

7. When doing patient teaching, which of the following foods should the patient be taught to avoid for a kidney stone composed of calcium oxalate?
    A. Bread
    B. Beer
    C. Beef
    D. Beans

8. Which of the following is appropriate patient teaching to obtain a midstream urine specimen for culture and sensitivity?
    A. A second-voided specimen is preferred.
    B. The specimen should be collected early in the morning.
    C. The patient should begin voiding, collect the specimen, and then finish voiding in the toilet.
    D. A 24-hour urine specimen is needed; the first void should be discarded.

9. A patient is admitted in chronic renal failure. The patient has a potassium level of 6.4 meq/L. He is put on a cardiac monitor and given Kayexalate by retention enema. When doing the nursing assessment, which of the following is the most significant symptom that the nurse should observe for?
    A. Diarrhea
    B. Irregular heart rhythm
    C. Increased blood pressure
    D. Increased respiratory rate

10. The patient in renal failure has the following symptoms: neck vein distention, periorbital edema, and crackles in the lungs. The nursing diagnosis of excess fluid volume is made. Which of the following nursing assessments is most important for this patient based on the symptoms?
    A. Intake and output
    B. Vital signs
    C. Daily weight
    D. Skin turgor

11. A patient with newly diagnosed chronic renal failure has elevated sodium, potassium, and serum creatinine levels. When the breakfast tray is served, there is a glass of orange juice on it. Which of the following actions should the nurse take first?
    A. Encourage the patient to drink the orange juice for vitamin C to help fight the infection.
    B. Take the orange juice off the tray because it is high in potassium.
    C. Give the patient a smaller glass of orange juice because the patient is on a fluid restriction.
    D. Check the kind of diet the patient is on to determine any restrictions.

12. A patient goes to surgery for a graft insertion for dialysis. The patient asks why it needs to be done. Which of the following is the best explanation by the nurse on the advantages of a graft over a two-tailed subclavian catheter?
    A. "There is a larger blood flow, and dialysis is more efficient."
    B. "There is less risk of clotting with the graft."
    C. "It is easier to access the graft than the two-tailed subclavian."
    D. "It is less likely to be damaged by trauma."

13. After hemodialysis, which of the following nursing interventions is imperative for the nurse to carry out?
    A. Measure stool output.
    B. Weigh the patient.
    C. Check for neck vein distention.
    D. Administer any insulin held previously.

14. The patient has a permanent peritoneal catheter inserted and is begun on CAPD. The patient asks how it works. Which of the following would be the best explanation of how this type of dialysis works?
    A. The peritoneum allows solutes in the dialysate to pass into the intravascular system.
    B. The peritoneum acts as a semipermeable membrane through which solutes move by diffusion and osmosis.
    C. The presence of excess metabolites causes increased permeability of the peritoneum and allows excess fluid to drain.
    D. The peritoneum permits diffusion of metabolites from the intravascular to the interstitial space.

15. A patient on dialysis has a severe cerebrovascular accident and is now semicomatose. His family decides that dialysis should be stopped. He is sent home with his daughter to die. As part of discharge planning, his daughter should be taught to expect which of the following symptoms of untreated end-stage renal failure?
    A. Polyuria, pruritis, and extreme irritability
    B. Dehydration with sunken eyeballs and oliguria
    C. Edema, possible convulsions, then coma
    D. Decreased respiratory rate and cyanosis

16. A patient is admitted who was involved in a motor vehicle accident resulting in trauma to the abdomen and back. He has a ruptured spleen and probable trauma to his kidneys. For which of the following changes in the patient's urine should the nurse observe?
    A. Dysuria
    B. Pyuria
    C. Polyuria
    D. Hematuria

17. A patient is admitted with symptoms of a recent weight gain, 3+ pitting edema of his feet, distended neck veins, and crackles in his lungs. Which of the following nursing diagnoses is most appropriate for this patient's plan of care?
    A. Deficient fluid volume
    B. Excess fluid volume
    C. Imbalanced nutrition, more than body requirements
    D. Noncompliance

UNIT TEN

UNDERSTANDING THE ENDOCRINE SYSTEM

CHECKLIST FOR LEARNING SUCCESS

Review of Anatomy of Physiology	Major Disorders	Nursing Assessment	Diagnostic Tests	Interventions	Common Medications
☐ Antidiuretic hormone	☐ Diabetes insipidus	☐ Fluid balance	☐ 24-hour urine	☐ Monitoring of symptoms	☐ Hormone replacement
☐ Growth hormone	☐ Syndrome of inappropriate secretion of antidiuretic hormone	☐ Mood, affect	☐ T_3 and T_4	☐ Prethyroidectomy and postthyroidectomy care	☐ Calcium
☐ Thyroid-stimulating hormone		☐ Exophthalmos	☐ Thyroid-stimulating hormone		☐ Calcitonin
☐ Adrenocorticotropic hormone		☐ Tremor		☐ Teaching r/t self-care	☐ Thyroid hormone
☐ T_3 and T_4	☐ Acromegaly	☐ Polyuria, polydipsia, polyphagia	☐ Stimulation tests	☐ Diabetes education	☐ Insulin
☐ Calcitonin	☐ Hypothyroidism		☐ Suppression tests		☐ Oral hypogly-cemics
☐ Parathyroid hormone	☐ Hyperthyroidism	☐ Self-monitoring of blood glucose (SMBG)	☐ Thyroid scan		
☐ Glucagon	☐ Goiter		☐ Blood glucose		
☐ Insulin	☐ Hypoparathyroidism	☐ Knowledge of self-care	☐ Glycohemoglobin		
☐ Norepinephrine	☐ Hyperparathyroidism		☐ Glucose tolerance test		
☐ Epinephrine	☐ Pheochromocytoma				
☐ Aldosterone	☐ Addison's disease				
☐ Cortisol	☐ Cushing's syndrome				
☐ Aging changes	☐ Diabetes mellitus				

36
ENDOCRINE SYSTEM FUNCTION AND ASSESSMENT

► VOCABULARY
Complete the following sentences with the appropriate words.

1. Glucose is converted to _____ for storage.

2. High blood glucose is called _____.

3. Emotional tone is called _____.

4. Bulging eyes, or _____, is a symptom of hyperthyroidism.

5. Hormone secretion is regulated through a _____ system.

► HORMONES
Match each hormone with its function. Use each letter only once.

1. _____ Antidiuretic hormone (ADH)

2. _____ Oxytocin

3. _____ Thyroid-stimulating hormone

4. _____ Adrenocorticotropic

5. _____ Growth hormone (GH)

6. _____ Prolactin

7. _____ Follicle-stimulating hormone

8. _____ Luteinizing hormone

9. _____ Thyroxine

10. _____ Calcitonin

11. _____ Parathyroid hormone (PTH)

12. _____ Epinephrine

13. _____ Norepinephrine

14. _____ Cortisol

15. _____ Aldosterone

16. _____ Insulin

17. _____ Glucagon

A. Stimulates growth and secretions of the thyroid gland
B. Increases glucose intake by cells and glycogen storage in the liver
C. Decreases the resorption of calcium from bones; hormone lowers blood calcium level
D. Increases the use of fats and amino acids for energy and has an anti-inflammatory effect
E. Stimulates mitosis and protein synthesis
F. Increases heart rate and force of contraction
G. Causes vasoconstriction throughout the body
H. Increases secretion of cortisol by the adrenal cortex
I. Increases energy production for a normal metabolic rate
J. Directly increases water resorption by the kidneys
K. In men, stimulates secretion of testosterone
L. Increases the conversion of glycogen to glucose in the liver between meals
M. Initiates milk production in the mammary glands
N. Increases the resorption of calcium from bones; raises blood calcium level
O. Increases the resorption of sodium by the kidneys
P. In women, initiates development of ova in ovaries
Q. Causes contraction of the myometrium during labor

▶ ENDOCRINE GLANDS AND HORMONES

Label the figure with the glands of the endocrine system. List the hormone(s) secreted by each gland.

Choose the best answer.

1. Which two hormones help regulate the blood calcium level?
    A. Insulin and glucagon
    B. Calcitonin and PTH
    C. Thyroxine and epinephrine
    D. Cortisol and aldosterone

2. Which hormone is most important for day-to-day regulation of metabolic rate?
    A. Insulin
    B. Epinephrine
    C. GH
    D. Thyroxine

3. What happens when aldosterone increases the resorption of sodium ions by the kidneys?
    A. Water is also reabsorbed back to the blood.
    B. Bicarbonate ions are excreted in urine.
    C. More water is excreted in urine.
    D. Potassium ions are also reabsorbed back to the blood.

4. Which two hormones help maintain blood volume and blood pressure?
    A. Thyroxine and epinephrine
    B. Glucagon and insulin
    C. Aldosterone and ADH
    D. Cortisol and norepinephrine

5. Which of the following hormones has an anti-inflammatory effect?
    A. Epinephrine
    B. Cortisol
    C. Aldosterone
    D. Thyroxine

6. A patient is completing a 24-hour urine test. What should the nurse do to complete the test?
    A. Have the patient void exactly 24 hours after the test was begun and discard the specimen.
    B. Save the last specimen and send it in a separate container.
    C. Have the patient void exactly 24 hours after the test was begun, and add this urine to the remainder of the specimen.
    D. Send only the specimen voided at 24 hours.

7. A 36-year-old female is admitted with hyperthyroidism. How do you assess her thyroid gland function?
    A. Ask her questions about symptoms of hyperthyroidism.
    B. Palpate her thyroid gland for enlargement.
    C. Do a finger stick for a blood glucose level.
    D. Observe for a "buffalo hump" on Mrs. Jenks' back.

8. A patient asks her nurse, "My doctor told me my thyroid scan showed a 'cold spot.' What does that mean?" Which of the following responses by the nurse is best?
    A. "That means you have cancer of the thyroid gland."
    B. "Cold spots are areas that have no living tissue."
    C. "A cold spot is an area that did not pick up the radioactive material they injected."
    D. "Nothing. A cold spot is just part of your thyroid gland."

37

NURSING CARE OF PATIENTS WITH ENDOCRINE DISORDERS

▶ VOCABULARY

Use the following terms to fill in the blanks:

Polydipsia	Euthyroid	Polyuria
Ectopic	Nocturia	Pheochromocytoma
Amenorrhea	Goiter	Dysphagia
Myxedema		

1. A normally functioning thyroid gland produces a _____ state.

2. Enlargement of the thyroid gland is called a _____ .

3. Excessive thirst is called _____ .

4. Excessive urination is called _____ .

5. A _____ is a tumor of the adrenal medulla.

6. Difficulty swallowing is called _____ .

7. Untreated hypothyroidism can lead to _____ coma.

8. _____ is the word for getting up to void during the night.

9. Absence of menses is called _____ .

10. Sometimes hormones are produced outside the endocrine gland in a/an _____ site.

▶ HORMONES

Match the disorder in column one to a hormone imbalance in column two and signs and symptoms in column three.

Disorder	Hormone Problem	Major Signs and Symptoms
Diabetes insipidus	Antidiuretic hormone (ADH) deficiency	Polyuria
Syndrome of Inappropriate ADH Secretion (SIADH)	Growth hormone (GH) deficiency	Growing feet
Cushing's syndrome	High calcium	Moon face
Addison's disease	ADH excess	Labile hypertension
Grave's disease	Steroid excess	Tetany
Hypothyroidism	Deficient steroids	Muscle weakness
Pheochromocytoma	Epinephrine excess	Short stature
Hyperparathyroidism	GH excess	Water retention
Dwarfism	Low T_3 and T_4	Weight gain
Acromegaly	Low calcium	Exophthalmos
Hypoparathyroidism	High T_3 and T_4	Hypotension

▶ CRITICAL THINKING

Read the case study and answer the following questions.

Sam is diagnosed with SIADH related to lung cancer. He enters the hospital for treatment of symptoms.

1. What (fluid-related) nursing diagnosis would be most appropriate for Sam? _____

_____

2. How will you monitor Sam's fluid balance? _____

_____

_____

3. Why is Sam at risk for seizures? _____

_____

_____

4. How will you reduce his risk for injury from seizures? _____

_____

_____

5. What do you expect Sam's urine to look like? _____

_____

6. How will Sam's urine look after treatment is begun? _____

_____

Judy is hospitalized following a motor vehicle accident in which she sustained a head injury. She develops diabetes insipidus (DI).

7. Why does head injury place one at risk for DI? _____

_____

_____

8. What symptoms do diabetes insipidus and diabetes mellitus have in common? _____

_____

_____

9. Will Judy's urine specific gravity be high or low? _____

_____

10. Will Judy's serum osmolality be high or low? _____

_____

11. For which (fluid-related) nursing diagnosis is Judy at risk? _____

_____

12. Judy begins treatment with DDAVP. To what signs of overdose should she be alert? _____

_____

_____

► THYROID DISORDERS

Label each symptom with an R if it suggests hyperthyroidism or an O if it suggests hypothyroidism.

1. _____ Bradycardia

2. _____ Lethargy

3. _____ Restlessness

4. _____ Frequent stools

5. _____ Hypercholesterolemia

6. _____ Dry hair

7. _____ Tremor

8. _____ Insomnia

9. _____ Mental dullness, confusion

10. _____ Warm, diaphoretic skin

11. _____ Weight loss

12. _____ Decreased appetite

REVIEW QUESTIONS

Choose the best answer.

1. A 42-year-old woman enters an outpatient clinic with symptoms of weight gain and fatigue. Laboratory studies are done, and she is diagnosed with primary hypothyroidism. She asks why her thyroid-stimulating hormone (TSH) level is elevated. Which of the following is the best response by the nurse?
   A. "The thyroid makes more TSH to take the place of the deficient T_3 and T_4."
   B. "The TSH will more directly raise the metabolic rate."
   C. "The pituitary makes more TSH to try to stimulate the underactive thyroid."
   D. "The extra fat cells from your weight gain make excess TSH."

2. Which of the following nursing diagnoses would be most appropriate for a patient with weight gain and fatigue related to hypothyroidism?
   A. Imbalanced nutrition, more than body requirements, related to overeating
   B. Impaired gas exchange related to weight gain
   C. Activity intolerance related to fatigue
   D. Ineffective coping related to depression

3. A patient with hypothyroidism is started on levothyroxine (Synthroid), a synthetic thyroid hormone. You know that she understands the side effects of this medication when she makes the following statement:
   A. "I know I should call my doctor if my heart races."
   B. "I understand that I may develop a moon-shaped face."
   C. "The sleepiness I experience when I start this medication will subside within 2 weeks."
   D. "I'll have to watch my diet to avoid further weight gain while on this medication."

4. A 26-year-old female patient is hospitalized for radioactive iodine treatment for hyperthyroidism. Which of the following precautions by the nurse is appropriate?
   A. Talk with the patient only over the intercom system.
   B. Wear gloves when emptying her bedside commode.
   C. Maintain reverse isolation for 3 months.
   D. No precautions are necessary because the dose is small.

5. Following surgery for thyroidectomy, the nurse watches carefully for which of the following signs and symptoms of tetany?
   A. Numb fingers, muscle cramps
   B. Weakness, muscle fatigue
   C. Hallucinations, delusions
   D. Dyspnea and tachycardia

6. Assessment of which of the following will best assist the nurse to detect the onset of thyrotoxicosis?
   A. Peripheral pulses
   B. Serum sodium
   C. Vital signs
   D. Incision site

7. Which of the following dietary recommendations will reduce the risk of kidney stones in the patient with hyperparathyroidism?
   A. Limit meat products
   B. Limit bread products
   C. Increase fluids
   D. Increase citrus fruits

8. The nurse develops the nursing diagnosis of pain related to bone demineralization for a patient with hypoparathyroidism. Which of the following goals is most appropriate?
   A. Serum calcium level will be <20 mg/dL
   B. Patient will state correct dietary restrictions
   C. Patient will perform activities of daily living (ADL) without injury
   D. Patient will verbalize acceptable pain level

9. An excess of which hormone is responsible for acromegaly?
   A. TSH
   B. Insulin
   C. Growth hormone
   D. Adrenocorticotropic hormone (ACTH)

10. A patient enters a clinic with possible Cushing's syndrome. Which of the following assessment findings support this diagnosis?
    A. Weight loss, pale skin
    B. Buffalo hump, easy bruising
    C. Nausea, vomiting
    D. Polyuria, polydipsia

11. Which assessment activity by the nurse is most important for the patient with a pheochromocytoma?
    A. Vital signs
    B. Daily weights
    C. Peripheral pulses
    D. Bowel sounds

12. Which of the following nursing diagnoses is most appropriate for the patient admitted in addisonian crisis?
    A. Imbalanced nutrition: more than body requirements
    B. Disturbed body image
    C. Deficient fluid volume
    D. Acute pain

38

NURSING CARE OF PATIENTS WITH DISORDERS OF THE ENDOCRINE PANCREAS

▶ VOCABULARY

Fill in the blanks.

1. Glucose in the urine is called _____.

2. _____ is too much sugar in the blood.

3. _____ is too little sugar in the blood.

4. Deep, sighing respirations from diabetic acidosis are called _____ respirations.

5. Excessive hunger is called _____.

6. Excessive thirst is called _____.

7. The patient who gets up to urinate at night has _____.

8. The time when insulin is working its hardest after injection is called its _____ action time.

9. The length of time insulin works is called its _____.

10. The Diabetes Control and Complications Trial (DCCT) says that individuals who maintain _____ control of their diabetes will have fewer long-term complications.

▶ HYPOGLYCEMIA AND HYPERGLYCEMIA

Place an R in front of each symptom of hyperglycemia and an O in front of each symptom of hypoglycemia.

1. _____ Tremor

2. _____ Polydipsia

3. _____ Polyuria

4. _____ Lethargy

5. _____ Irritability

6. _____ Fruity breath

7. _____ Sweating

8. _____ Abdominal pain

▶ LONG-TERM COMPLICATIONS OF DIABETES

Match the complication with its signs and symptoms.

1. _____ Retinopathy

2. _____ Neuropathy

3. _____ Hyperosmolar, hyperglycemic, nonketotic syndrome

4. _____ Diabetic ketoacidosis (DKA)

5. _____ Nephropathy

6. _____ Gastroparesis

7. _____ Infection

A. Ketones in the blood and urine
B. Burning pain in legs and feet
C. Fever
D. Profound hyperglycemia without ketonemia
E. Impaired vision
F. Food intolerance
G. Microalbuminuria

▶ CRITICAL THINKING

Read the case study and answer the following questions.

Jennie is a 56-year-old overweight woman admitted to your medical unit with type cellulitis of the left leg. She has a history of diabetes; her blood sugar level is 436. She tells you that she takes human N insulin 38 units every morning and human R insulin 10 units with each meal and at bedtime.

1. Chart the action of Jennie's insulin over the course of 24 hours.

Insulin action (y-axis)

Time   0600   1200   1800   2400   0600

2. Jennie tells you that her physician wants her to keep her blood sugar level between 100 and 150 mg/dL. You know that a normal blood sugar level is 60 to 115. Why the discrepancy? _____

_____

_____

3. When you enter Jennie's room to check her 4 P.M. vital signs, she says she has a headache. By the time you finish taking her blood pressure, she has developed a cold sweat. What is happening? What should you do? Why did it occur at 4 P.M.?

_____

_____

4. At 5 P.M., you check Jennie's blood sugar level and find that it is 80 mg/dL. What is your next step? _____

_____

_____

5. List three things that may have caused Jennie's blood sugar level to drop. _____

_____

_____

6. You explain to Jennie the importance of eating three meals a day on a regular schedule. She asks why. How do you explain this to her? _____

_____

7. Jennie is discharged and follows her diet, exercise, and insulin regimen carefully. She even loses 50 lb. One year after her first admission, she is brought into the emergency department with a blood sugar level of 32. Why has her blood sugar level dropped? _____

_____

_____

8. Jennie's physician discontinues her insulin and starts her on glipizide (Glucotrol) 5 mg twice a day. What are two ways this oral hypoglycemic works? _____

_____

_____

9. You teach Jennie to take her glipizide (Glucotrol) at what times each day? Why? _____

_____

_____

10. Does Jennie have type 1 or type 2 diabetes? How do you know? _____

_____

_____

REVIEW QUESTIONS

Choose the best answer.

1. A 56-year-old gentleman visits his physician with symptoms of diabetes mellitus. He is placed on an exercise and diet plan. Which type of diabetes does he have?
   A. Type 1
   B. Type 2
   C. Insulin-dependent diabetes mellitus
   D. Gestational

2. In addition to stimulating insulin production, glyburide (Micronase) has which of the following effects?
   A. Stimulate gluconeogenesis
   B. Promote fat breakdown
   C. Increase tissue sensitivity to insulin
   D. Enhance appetite

3. Which of the following symptoms do you expect if a patient with diabetes forgets to take a dose of glyburide (Micronase)?
   A. Cold, clammy sweat
   B. Tachycardia, nervousness, hunger
   C. Chest pain, shortness of breath
   D. Fatigue, thirst, blurred vision

4. What is an acceptable blood sugar range for a patient with diabetes?
   A. 46 to 98 mg/dL
   B. 100 to 140 mg/dL
   C. 180 to 250 mg/dL
   D. 350 to 600 mg/dL

5. Insulin is usually given by which route?
   A. Oral
   B. Intramuscular
   C. Intravenous
   D. Subcutaneous

6. Before giving insulin, the nurse always checks which of the following?
   A. Recent potassium level
   B. Blood sugar level
   C. Urine ketones
   D. White blood cell count

7. Your patient is taking NPH insulin every morning. At which of the following times should the patient observe for signs and symptoms of low blood sugar level?
   A. 1 hour after administration of insulin
   B. 6 to 12 hours after administration of insulin
   C. 24 to 36 hours after administration of insulin
   D. NPH insulin does not cause low blood sugar level

8. Some patients take regular insulin four times a day, before meals and at bedtime. The peak action of regular insulin is how long?
   A. 30 to 60 minutes
   B. 1 to 2 hours
   C. 2 to 5 hours
   D. 8 to 12 hours

9. Which of the following are symptoms of low blood sugar level?
    A. Nausea and vomiting
    B. Glycosuria
    C. Cold sweat and tremor
    D. Pruritic rash

10. Which of the following is an appropriate treatment for hypoglycemia?
    A. Raisins
    B. Cheese
    C. Tylenol
    D. Beef jerky

11. Some patients use subcutaneous glucagon for emergency episodes of which of the following conditions?
    A. Hyperglycemia
    B. Ketonuria
    C. Diabetic ketoacidosis
    D. Hypoglycemia

12. Which of the following is a major risk factor of type 2 diabetes?
    A. Obesity
    B. Viral infection
    C. Binge eating
    D. Hypertension

13. A patient on an American Diabetes Association diet receives a breakfast tray and does not care for the oatmeal. Which of the following foods can substitute for a half a cup of oatmeal?
    A. 4 oz of orange juice
    B. Two strips of bacon
    C. 1 oz of cheese
    D. A slice of wheat toast

UNIT ELEVEN

UNDERSTANDING THE GENITOURINARY AND REPRODUCTIVE SYSTEM

Review of Anatomy and Physiology	Major Disorders	Nursing Assessment	Diagnostic Tests	Interventions	Common Medications
☐ Female reproductive system	☐ Breast cancer	☐ History	☐ Mammogram	☐ Breast surgeries	☐ Antibiotics
☐ Female hormones	☐ Menstrual disorders	☐ Breast assessment	☐ Biopsy	☐ Hysterectomy	☐ Hormone replacement therapy
☐ The menstrual cycle	☐ Infections	☐ Breast self-examination (BSE)	☐ Hormone tests	☐ Contraception	☐ Oral contraceptives
☐ Male reproductive system	☐ Displacement disorders	☐ Sexual function	☐ Pelvic examination	☐ Prostatectomy	
☐ Male hormones	☐ Fertility disorders	☐ Testicular self-examination (TSE)	☐ Papanicolaou (Pap) smear	☐ Transurethral resection of the prostate (TURP)	
☐ Aging changes	☐ Tumors of the cervix, uterus, and ovaries		☐ Endoscopic examinations	☐ Teaching	
	☐ Prostatitis		☐ Cystourethroscopy		
	☐ Benign prostatic hypertrophy (BPH)		☐ Digital rectal examination (DRE)		
	☐ Prostate cancer		☐ Prostate specific antigen (PSA)		
	☐ Penile disorders		☐ Fertility testing		
	☐ Testicular disorders				
	☐ Erectile dysfunction				
	☐ Sexually transmitted diseases (STDs)				

39

GENITOURINARY AND REPRODUCTIVE SYSTEM FUNCTION AND ASSESSMENT

► VOCABULARY

Complete the following sentences with the correct term from the chapter.

1. A _____ may be done to view the inside of the uterus with an endoscope.

2. During some diagnostic procedures, a body cavity is filled with carbon dioxide to make it easier for the physician to view structures. This is called _____ .

3. A male patient should have a yearly _____ _____ _____ to detect prostate cancer.

4. Some men have excessive breast tissue, or _____ .

5. If the urethral opening is on the underside of the penis, it is called _____ .

6. Fluid in the scrotum is called a _____.

7. If the scrotum feels like a bag of worms when palpated, it is called a _____ .

8. Another word for sexual desire is _____ .

9. The beginning of menstruation in the female is called _____ .

10. X-ray examination of the breasts is called _____ .

▶ ANATOMY AND PHYSIOLOGY

Label the structures of the male and female reproductive systems.

► FEMALE REPRODUCTIVE STRUCTURES

Match the female reproductive structures with the correct descriptive statement.

1. _____ Fallopian tube
2. _____ Myometrium
3. _____ Bartholin's glands
4. _____ Vestibule
5. _____ Endometrium
6. _____ Ovarian follicle
7. _____ Corpus luteum

A. Site of development of an ovum
B. Becomes the maternal placenta
C. Contains the urethral and vaginal openings
D. Secretes progesterone and estrogen after ovulation
E. The usual site of fertilization
F. Secrete mucus at the vaginal orifice
G. Contracts for labor and delivery

► MALE REPRODUCTIVE SYSTEM

Number the following in proper sequence with respect to the pathway sperm travel from the testes.

_____ Ejaculatory duct

_____ Epididymis

_____ Urethra

_____ Seminiferous tubules

_____ Ductus deferens

► DIAGNOSTIC TESTS

Match the following tests with their descriptions.

1. _____ Cytology
2. _____ Colposcopy
3. _____ Sonography
4. _____ Computed tomography (CT) scan
5. _____ Magnetic resonance imaging
6. _____ TSE

A. Scope examination of the vagina
B. Examination of cells using a microscope
C. Mapping of tissues according to their densities using sound waves
D. Mapping of tissue by using radio frequency radiation and magnetic fields
E. Self-examination of the male testicles
F. Computer-assisted recording of very precise x-ray pictures of layers of tissue

► CRITICAL THINKING

Read the case studies and answer the following questions.

1. Mr. White comes to see his physician for a yearly checkup. As you are taking his blood pressure, he says, "I don't need that rectal examination, do I? I had prostate surgery last year." How do you respond? _____

_____

_____

2. Mrs. Bitner has just returned from having an endoscopic examination. She says, "Something went wrong, I just know it. Look at my belly. I look like I'm 9 months pregnant." How do you respond? _____

_____

_____

3. Ms. Wilson comes to the clinic with complaints of excessive vaginal discharge. While asking her some initial questions, you learn that she has multiple sex partners. How do you respond? _____

_____

_____

4. Mr. Brown is being admitted to the hospital for complications of diabetes. While collecting initial data, you learn that although he is married, he is no longer sexually active. How do you respond? _____

_____

_____

REVIEW QUESTIONS

Choose the best answer.

1. Which of the following male reproductive structures carries semen through the penis to the exterior?
   A. Urethra
   B. Epididymis
   C. Ductus deferens
   D. Ejaculatory duct

2. Which layer of the uterus will become the maternal portion of the placenta?
   A. Myometrium
   B. Endometrium
   C. Epimetrium
   D. Serosa

3. Which of the following descriptions best describes the position of the uterus?
   A. Superior to the bladder with the fundus most anterior
   B. Anterior to the bladder with the cervix most inferior
   C. Inferior to the bladder with the cervix most superior
   D. Posterior to the bladder with the fundus most inferior

4. Which of the following hormones stimulates the mammary glands to produce milk after pregnancy?
   A. Progesterone
   B. Estrogen
   C. Oxytocin
   D. Prolactin

5. Strong contractions of the smooth muscle of the uterus for labor and delivery are brought about by which of the following hormones?
   A. Progesterone
   B. Follicle-stimulating hormone (FSH)
   C. Oxytocin
   D. Luteinizing hormone (LH)

6. According to the American Cancer Society, how often should breast self-examination be done?
   A. Weekly
   B. Monthly
   C. Yearly
   D. Semiannually

7. When should men over age 40 have digital rectal examinations?
   A. Weekly
   B. Monthly
   C. Every other month
   D. During yearly physician visit

8. A patient being prepared for cystourethrography asks what is going to be done to him. Which is the best reply by the nurse?
   A. "The doctor will put an endoscope into your bladder."
   B. "You will have a catheter put in, then a dye will be injected and x-rays will be taken."
   C. "You will have a small needle inserted through your lower abdomen and into your bladder."
   D. "You will have an intravenous injection of dye, then x-rays will be taken as it travels through your kidneys."

9. How should the nurse prepare a patient for a routine Pap smear?
   A. Give her an enema.
   B. Ask her to empty her bladder.
   C. Ask her to give blood for a test.
   D. Set out a suture tray and local anesthetic.

10. Which of the following positions is advised for doing a portion of the breast self-examination?
   A. Supine
   B. Simm's
   C. Kneeling
   D. Fowler's

11. Which supplies should the nurse set out when assisting with collecting gonorrhea bacteria for culture?
   A. Clear swab
   B. Chlamydia kit
   C. Charcoal swab
   D. Viral collection kit

12. Why are additional tests used to verify mammography findings?
   A. The mammogram needs no other verification.
   B. Mammograms are unable to show lesions in breast tissue.
   C. The mammogram is the most expensive test, and therefore is best.
   D. Many things can cause shadows on a mammogram besides cancer.

13. What danger does magnetic resonance imaging pose?
   A. It gives the body radiation poisoning.
   B. It bombards the body with too much sound.
   C. It will heat any metal in the body to a high temperature.
   D. It poisons the body with the chemicals that must be injected to outline the cavities.

14. Which of the following describes a wet mount?
   A. Pap smears
   B. Cultures of bacteria from vaginal discharge
   C. Combinations of sodium chloride and potassium hydroxide in a bottle
   D. Smears of discharge on slides, which must be taken to the microscope immediately after they are obtained

40

NURSING CARE OF WOMEN WITH REPRODUCTIVE SYSTEM DISORDERS

▶ VOCABULARY

Match the term with its definition.

1. __C__ Imperforate
2. __D__ Colporrhaphy
3. __B__ Dysmenorrhea
4. __I__ Cryotherapy
5. __E__ Agenesis
6. __G__ Dyspareunia
7. __A__ Cystocele
8. __F__ Rectocele
9. __H__ Anteversion
10. __I__ Salpingo-oophorectomy

A. Bladder sags into vaginal space
B. Painful menstruation
C. Not having expected openings
D. Surgical repair of a part of the vagina
E. Undeveloped
F. Rectum sags into the vagina
G. Painful intercourse
H. Forward turning
I. Removal of fallopian tubes and ovaries
J. Freezing of tissue

▶ BREAST SURGERIES

Match the following breast surgery terms with their descriptions.

1. __E__ Mastopexy
2. __A__ Mastectomy
3. __C__ Reduction mammoplasty
4. __B__ Augmentation mammoplasty
5. __D__ Reconstructive mammoplasty

A. Surgery to remove a breast
B. Surgery to increase the size of the breasts
C. Surgery to decrease the size of the breasts
D. Surgery to rebuild a breast after mastectomy
E. Surgery to change the position of the breasts

► MENSTRUAL DISORDERS

Match the following menstrual disorders with their description.

1. _E_ Amenorrhea
2. _C_ Menorrhagia
3. _A_ Dysmenorrhea
4. _B_ Polymenorrhea
5. _D_ Hypomenorrhea

A. Difficult or painful menstruation
B. Menses more often than every 21 days
C. Passing more than 80 mL of blood per menses
D. Less than expected amount of menstrual bleeding
E. Absence of menstrual periods for 6 months or three previous cycle lengths once cycles have been established

► MASTECTOMY CARE

Circle the errors in the following scenario and write the correct information in the space provided.

You are assigned to care for Mrs. Joseph, who is 1 day postoperative following a right radical mastectomy. You know that she is not anxious, because she had a left mastectomy a year ago and knows everything to expect. You listen to her breath sounds and find them clear, so it is not necessary to have her cough and deep breathe. You encourage her to lie on her right side to prevent bleeding. You use her right arm for blood pressures, because both arms are affected and the right one is more convenient. You also encourage her to avoid use of her right arm to prevent injury to the surgical site. You provide a balanced diet and plenty of fluids to aid in her recovery.

_____

_____

_____

_____

► CRITICAL THINKING

Read the case study and answer the following questions.

A 21-year-old female college student attends the physician's office where you work and comments with evident frustration that she has a yeast infection again. She has type 1 diabetes mellitus and takes her insulin routinely. However, she seldom tests her blood glucose level, because, she says, "I don't have time to mess with that stuff as often as I should." She comments that every time she goes home on weekends to visit her parents (a 3-hour bus trip), she develops a very uncomfortable vaginal yeast infection.

1. What factors may be contributing to her frequent yeast overgrowths? _____

_____

_____

2. What suggestions can you give her to help prevent this problem? _____

_____

_____

Choose the best answer.

1. What is a disadvantage of using a condom with spermicide for contraception?
   - A. Relatively expensive
   - B. Many systemic drug side effects
   - C. Very low success rate
   - D. Cannot be initiated by the woman without male agreement

2. Which pH concentration describes the normal vaginal environment?
   - A. Basic
   - B. Acidic
   - C. Neutral

3. How will a douche affect a vaginal examination to determine the type of pathogen present?
   - A. Helps clear the area for better visualization.
   - B. Does not affect the outcome negatively or positively.
   - C. May wash away evidence of the pathogen, making diagnosis difficult.
   - D. Baking soda douche must be done before the examination to neutralize the pH.

4. Which of the following is a danger associated with receiving estrogen without progestins?
   - A. Cancer
   - B. Heart disease
   - C. Osteoporosis
   - D. Atrophic vaginitis

5. After a radical mastectomy with lymph node removal, which of the following nursing interventions will help prevent swelling?
   - A. Restricting all movement of the affected arm
   - B. Raising the affected arm above the heart on pillows
   - C. Applying warm moist heat to the arm
   - D. Holding the arm close to the body with a sling

6. Cervical cancer is very treatable if diagnosed early. Which of the following is a known risk factor for cervical cancer?
   - A. Tight underwear
   - B. Frequent Papanicolaou smears
   - C. Multiple sexual partners
   - D. Beginning sexual activity late in life

7. A patient had a pan hysterectomy 4 days ago for endometrial cancer. She found out yesterday that she has metastases to her lungs. When asked about her plans after discharge, she answered sharply that she "cannot plan for any future, because there isn't going to be any!" She then started to cry. Which of the following nursing diagnoses best fits this situation?
   - A. Anticipatory grieving
   - B. Body image disturbance
   - C. Sleep pattern disturbance
   - D. Noncompliance

8. Which of the following is a risk factor for development of breast cancer?
   - A. Late menarche
   - B. No pregnancies
   - C. Early menopause
   - D. Early first pregnancy

9. A patient with breast cancer is being treated with tamoxifen citrate, which deprives cancer cells of the estrogen that makes them grow. This is an example of which mode of therapy?
   - A. Hormonal therapy
   - B. Radiation therapy
   - C. Cytotoxic chemotherapy
   - D. Biological response modifier therapy

10. If a patient is taking cytotoxic chemotherapy drugs to fight cervical cancer, maintaining adequate nutrition is often a problem because of nausea and mouth sores. Which of the following nursing actions will best help increase the patient's food intake?
    - A. Provide very hot or cold foods.
    - B. Provide a bland diet.
    - C. Avoid fresh fruits and vegetables.
    - D. Administer antiemetic medications before meals.

11. A 38-year-old patient had a reduction mammoplasty 4 days ago. When changing her dressing the nurse notes redness, swelling, and some thick yellow drainage escaping from areas of the incision line around her left nipple. Which of the following nursing interventions is appropriate?
    - A. Give it another day or two to heal before getting concerned.
    - B. Tell the patient that this is the way all breast reductions look until they are healed.
    - C. Tell the patient that you have never seen such poor healing of a breast reduction.
    - D. Promptly report the situation to the registered nurse and document it in the patient's chart.

12. Which of the following lifestyle modification measures is most likely to increase premenstrual syndrome symptoms?
    - A. Restricting alcohol intake
    - B. Avoiding smoking
    - C. Drinking strong hot coffee
    - D. Eating a low-salt diet

41

NURSING CARE OF MALE PATIENTS WITH GENITOURINARY DISORDERS

▶ VOCABULARY

Fill in the blanks in the following sentences with words from the chapter.

1. A ___Cystoscopy___ is a test that uses an endoscope to view the bladder.

2. Surgery to remove the prostate gland is called a ___TURP___ .

3. When semen goes into the bladder during intercourse, it is called ___retrograde ejaculation___

4. An erection that lasts too long is called ___priaprism___ .

5. ___Phimosis___ is the term used to describe uncircumcised foreskin that cannot be extended over the head of the penis.

6. ___Smegma___ is a cottage cheese-like secretion made by the gland of the foreskin.

7. Surgical removal of the foreskin is called ___Circumcision___ .

8. ___Cryptorchid___ is a birth condition in which one or both of the testicles have not descended into the scrotum.

9. The male reproductive gland where sperm is made is the ___testicle___ .

10. The skin sac behind the penis that holds the testicles is the ___Scrotum___ .

11. The hollow tube along the back side of the testicle that stores sperm is the ___epididimus___ .

12. Inflammation or infection of a testicle is called ___Orchititis___ .

13. The correct term for male impotence is ___erectile dysfunction___

14. A ___Varicocele___ is varicose veins of the scrotum.

15. Surgical cutting of the vas deferens as a method of birth control is called a ___vasectomy___ .

DISORDERS OF THE MALE REPRODUCTIVE SYSTEM
Match the disorder with its definition.

1. _____ Benign prostatic hypertrophy (BPH)
2. _E_ Hydronephrosis
3. _A_ Hematuria
4. _B_ Peyronie's disease
5. _J_ Priapism
6. _G_ Epididymitis
7. _D_ Infertility
8. _F_ Orchitis
9. _H_ Dysuria
10. _I_ Reflux

A. Blood in the urine
B. Curved penis
C. Noncancerous overgrowth of prostate tissue
D. Inability to reproduce
E. Distention of kidney with retained urine
F. Inflammation of the testicles
G. Inflammation or infection of the tube where sperm matures
H. Painful or difficult urination
I. Backward flow of urine
J. Prolonged erection

ERECTILE DYSFUNCTION
Unscramble the causes of erectile dysfunction.

aeiioctdmn _____

sssrte _____

eeiophysnnntr _____

PRUT _____

threa flraeiu _____

tiellpum lersssoic _____

CRITICAL THINKING
Read the case study and answer the following questions.

Mr. Washington is a 62-year-old retired teacher who comes to the urgent care center complaining that he "can't pass water."

1. What initial questions do you ask to further assess Mr. Washington's problem? _____

2. What do you think is happening? _____

3. What care do you anticipate as the physician examines him? _____

4. What can result if the problem continues untreated? _____

Mr. Washington is transferred to the local hospital where BPH is confirmed. He is scheduled for a transurethral resection of the prostate (TURP). He asks the nurse, "What's a TURP?"

5. How would you explain a TURP to Mr. Washington? _____

_____

6. Following surgery, Mr. Washington has a three-way Foley catheter. What is the purpose of this type of catheter? How does the nurse total intake and output (I&O) at the end of the shift? _____

_____

_____

7. Bladder spasms are common after TURP. How will you know if this is happening? What interventions will help? _____

_____

_____

8. Mr. Washington is discharged. The next day he calls the nursing unit and says in a panicky voice, "I just wet my pants! I can't hold my urine! This is worse than not being able to go at all!" How do you respond? What can he do? _____

_____

_____

REVIEW QUESTIONS

Choose the best answer.

1. The nurse completes a nursing history on a patient admitted for a TURP. Which of the following symptoms is typically seen with BPH?
   A. A feeling of incomplete bladder emptying after voiding
   B. Difficulty maintaining an erection
   C. Grossly bloody urine
   D. Pain in the lower back that radiates to the hips during urination

2. A patient tells his nurse that he has delayed having a TURP because he is afraid it will affect his sexual function. Which response by the nurse is most appropriate?
   A. "Don't worry about sterility; sperm production is not affected by this surgery."
   B. "Would you like some information about implants used for impotence?"
   C. "This type of surgery rarely affects the ability to have an erection or ejaculation."
   D. "There are many methods of sexual expression that are alternatives to sexual intercourse."

3. A patient returns from surgery following a TURP with a three-way Foley catheter and continuous bladder irrigation. Postop orders include meperidine (Demerol) 75 mg IM q3h as needed for pain, belladonna and opium (B & O) suppository q4h as needed, and strict I&O. The patient complains of painful bladder spasms, and the nurse observes blood-tinged urine on the sheets. Which action should the nurse take?
   A. Give the Demerol.
   B. Give the B&O suppository.
   C. Warm the irrigation solution to body temperature.
   D. Notify the physician STAT.

4. A patient who has just had a TURP asks his nurse to explain why he has to have the bladder irrigation because it seems to increase his pain. Which of the following explanations by the nurse is best?
   A. "The bladder irrigation is needed to stop the bleeding in the bladder."
   B. "Antibiotics are being administered into the bladder to prevent infection."
   C. "The irrigation is needed to keep the catheter from becoming occluded by blood clots."
   D. "Normal production of urine is maintained with the irrigations until healing can occur."

5. A post-TURP patient experiences dribbling following removal of his catheter. Which action should the nurse take?
   A. Have him restrict fluid intake to 1,000 mL/day.
   B. Teach him to perform Kegel's exercises 10 to 20 times per hour.
   C. Reinsert the Foley catheter until he regains urinary control.
   D. Reassure him that incontinence never lasts more than a few days.

6. A 36-year-old gentleman is scheduled for a unilateral orchiectomy for treatment of testicular cancer. He is withdrawn and does not interact with the nurse. Which action is most appropriate?
   A. Identify the problem with a nursing diagnosis of impaired communication related to the diagnosis of cancer.
   B. Set a patient outcome that the patient will verbalize his concerns about his diagnosis.
   C. Ask the patient whether he is worried about future sexual functioning.
   D. Assess the patient's concerns related to his diagnosis and treatment.

7. A 28-year-old man is diagnosed with acute epididymitis. Which of the following symptoms supports this diagnosis?
   A. Burning and pain on urination
   B. Severe tenderness and swelling in the scrotum
   C. Foul-smelling ejaculate and severe scrotal swelling
   D. Foul-smelling urine and pain on urination

8. Which of the following interventions is inappropriate for the patient with epididymitis?
   A. Maintaining bed rest
   B. Elevating the testes
   C. Increasing fluid intake
   D. Applying hot packs to the scrotum

9. Which of the following nursing actions is most appropriate when doing perineal care on an uncircumcised male patient?
   A. Leave the foreskin retracted so air can keep the area dry.
   B. Do not retract the foreskin during washing.
   C. Replace the foreskin over the head of the penis after washing.
   D. Use alcohol and a cotton swab to clean under the foreskin.

10. What is the best way to detect testicular cancer early?
    A. Monthly testicular self-examination (TSE)
    B. Yearly digital rectal examination (DRE)
    C. Annual physician examination
    D. Annual ultrasonography

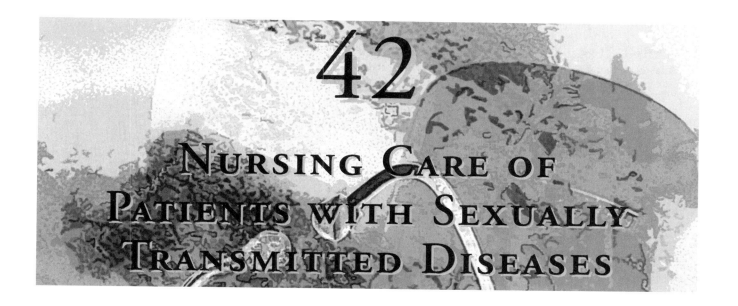

42

NURSING CARE OF PATIENTS WITH SEXUALLY TRANSMITTED DISEASES

▶ VOCABULARY

Match the term with its definition.

1. _____ Condylomatous

2. _____ Gumma

3. _____ Chancre

4. _____ Cytotoxic

5. _____ Herpetic

6. _____ Puerperal

A. Relating to herpes
B. Rubbery tumor
C. Red ulcer from syphilis
D. Wartlike
E. Poison to cells
F. Time following childbirth

▶ INFLAMMATORY DISORDERS

Match the following inflammation words with their definitions.

1. _____ Proctitis

2. _____ Urethritis

3. _____ Cervicitis

4. _____ Endometritis

5. _____ Conjunctivitis

A. Inflammation of the rectum and anus
B. Inflammation of the cervix
C. Inflammation of the urethra
D. Inflammation of parts of the eye
E. Inflammation of the lining of the uterus

▶ TRANSMISSION OF SEXUALLY TRANSMITTED DISEASES

Match the number of the sexually transmitted disease (STD) in the mother with the letter for the potential disease of the baby.

1. _____ Herpes

2. _____ Hepatitis

3. _____ Gonorrhea

4. _____ Genital warts

A. Ophthalmia neonatorum
B. Becoming a chronic carrier of hepatitis B virus
C. Disseminated herpes infection of skin, membranes, and nerves
D. Development of similar lesions on the baby and possible increased cancer risk

▶ BARRIER METHODS FOR SAFER SEX

List the teaching that should accompany each of the following barriers against STDs.

1. Male condoms

_____

_____

_____

2. Female condoms

_____

_____

_____

3. Diaphragms _____

_____

_____

_____

4. Rubber gloves _____

_____

_____

_____

5. Double condoms _____

_____

_____

_____

▶ CRITICAL THINKING

Read the case study and answer the following questions.

James Edwards, an old friend of yours from high school, enters the physician's office where you work. He is accompanied by a beautiful, exotic-looking lady. He seats her and then motions to one side of the room as if he wishes to speak to you there. When you arrive there, he whispers, "What do you think; isn't she a beauty? We all have to settle down sometime and I figure that face over the breakfast table certainly won't spoil my appetite!" You compliment him on his choice of an attractive partner and ask what you can do for him today. You find out that he has met this woman through an international dating agency and that she has come to marry him. He wants you to just give him the paperwork for both of them to get the blood test for STDs—just to make sure they don't have anything contagious. He is in a hurry and figures that they can give the blood first and then he would come right back and see the doctor and find out the results for both of them.

1. What misunderstandings does James have about STD diagnosis? _____

_____

_____

2. Legally and ethically, does James have a right to be told his fiancee's test results? _____

_____

_____

3. What procedures should occur before any testing is done? _____

_____

_____

4. Is James likely to get his answer about whether he has a contagious STD today? _____

_____

_____

REVIEW QUESTIONS

Choose the best answer.

1. Syphilis has how many stages?
    A. One
    B. Two
    C. Three
    D. Four

2. Which of the following actions by a nurse would be *least* likely to result in patient comfort when attending an STD clinic?
    A. Addressing the patient by name
    B. Standing with your arms crossed as you talk with the patient
    C. Making eye contact appropriate for the patient's culture
    D. Asking the nature of the problem in an area that maintains privacy

3. Chemical treatments to destroy genital wart tissue are cytotoxic, which means that they do which of the following?
    A. They poison wart cells.
    B. They cause wart cells to grow.
    C. They increase blood flow to the wart cells.
    D. They cause wart cells to have more oxygen.

4. A 36-year-old woman comes into the hospital in active labor for her fourth child. When asked about her prenatal care, she states that she certainly knows by now how things should go and felt healthy, so she did not bother to go to a doctor. She has vesicles evident on her perineum. Which of the following is the *least* appropriate action to take?
    A. Maintain universal precautions.
    B. Politely reprimand her for putting her baby at risk of herpes.
    C. Prepare for the possibility that she may be delivered by cesarean section.
    D. Document and notify the registered nurse about the vesicles as soon as possible.

5. A 23-year-old woman is deciding whether to engage in sexual activity with a man she is just getting to know. She wonders whether he might have an STD. Which of the following statements about transmission of STDs is a groundless myth?
    A. Not everyone who can transmit a disease shows symptoms.
    B. Most people who have STDs have poor hygiene.
    C. You may not know about the person's past sexual contacts or the contacts of their contacts.
    D. By the time you get around to inspecting a partner for symptoms, emotions may cloud your judgment.

6. Which of the following actions is the most effective STD risk-reduction strategy?
    A. Taking oral contraceptive pills
    B. Lifelong monogamy of both partners
    C. Using a male condom with spermicide
    D. Using a female condom with spermicide

7. Diagnosis of chlamydia requires what special equipment?
    A. Chlamydia slide
    B. Chlamydia swab
    C. Chlamydia wet mount
    D. Chlamydia collection kit

8. A Venereal Disease Research Laboratory slide test (VDRL) and a rapid plasma reagin are both blood tests to diagnose which disorder?
    A. Herpes
    B. Syphilis
    C. Gonorrhea
    D. Chlamydia

9. Which of the following is the treatment of choice for a nonpregnant patient who has *Trichomonas?*
    A. Bed rest
    B. Penicillin
    C. Frequent bathing
    D. Baking soda douches

10. A psychological "herpes syndrome" has been documented in the medical and popular literature. Which of the following reactions is common in a patient who is experiencing herpes syndrome?
    A. Vesicles over most of the body
    B. Feelings of shame
    C. Fever and night sweats
    D. Psychotic behavior

11. Which virus causes genital warts?
    A. Cytomegalovirus
    B. Herpes simplex virus type II
    C. Human papillomavirus
    D. Human immunodeficiency virus

12. Papanicolaou smears can diagnose all types of STDs.
    A. True
    B. False

13. Having an STD gives immunity to developing that STD in the future.
    A. True
    B. False

14. What should nurses teach about STD risk reduction?
    A. As long as there is a condom, there is no risk.
    B. There is always risk involved in anything worthwhile.
    C. Barrier protection with spermicide reduces risk but does not eliminate it.
    D. Worrying about risks makes a person more susceptible to developing an STD.

15. Which statement correctly describes the symptoms of urethritis syndrome in men?
    A. Constipated stool and inadequate urination
    B. Chancres, gummas, and vesicles on the urethra
    C. Difficult, painful, and frequent urination and a urethral discharge
    D. Infrequent, inadequate urination with yellow urine and pain in the legs

UNIT TWELVE

UNDERSTANDING THE MUSCULOSKELETAL SYSTEM

Review of Anatomy and Physiology	Major Musculoskeletal Disorders	Nursing Assessment	Diagnostic Tests	Interventions	Common Medications
☐ Skeletal system	☐ Osteoarthritis	☐ Medical history	☐ Alkaline Phosphatase	☐ Amputation	☐ Allopurinol (Zyloprim)
☐ Muscular system	☐ Rheumatoid arthritis	☐ Medications	☐ Erythrocyte sedimentation rate	☐ Prosthesis	☐ Analgesics
☐ Aging effects	☐ Gout	☐ Vital signs	☐ Serum calcium/ phosphorus/uric acid	☐ Casts	☐ Anticoagulant
	☐ Systemic lupus erythematosus	☐ Physical assessment	☐ Muscle enzymes	☐ Closed reduction	☐ Antirheumatic drugs
	☐ Muscular dystrophy	☐ Deformities/limb length	☐ Rheumatoid factor	☐ Continuous passive motion machine	☐ Biophosphonates
	☐ Carpal tunnel syndrome	☐ Crepitation	☐ Arthrocentesis	☐ Diet therapy	☐ Calcitonin (Calcimar)
	☐ Fractures	☐ Swelling	☐ Arthrography	☐ External fixation	☐ Corticosteroid
	☐ Complications of fractures	☐ Range of motion	☐ Arthroscopy	☐ Heat and cold	☐ Cox II selective inhibitors
	☐ Osteomyelitis	☐ Muscle strength	☐ Bone scan	☐ Hip protectors	☐ Muscle relaxants
	☐ Osteoporosis	☐ Pain	☐ Electromyography (EMG)	☐ Open reduction/ internal fixation	☐ Nonsteroidal antiinflammatory drugs (NSAIDs)
	☐ Paget's disease	☐ Neurovascular checks	☐ Magnetic resonance imaging (MRI)	☐ Rest, ice, compression, elevation	☐ Raloxifene (Evista)
	☐ Bone cancer		☐ Myelogram	☐ Total joint replacement	
			☐ X-rays	☐ Traction	

43

MUSCULOSKELETAL FUNCTION AND ASSESSMENT

▶ STRUCTURE OF NEUROMUSCULAR JUNCTION AND SARCOMERES

Label the structures from the following word list.

Acetylcholine   Axon terminal   Sarcomere
Acetylcholine receptors Myosin filament   Synaptic cleft
Actin filament   Sarcolemma   Vesicle of acetylcholine

187

► NEUROMUSCULAR JUNCTION
Match each part of the neuromuscular junction with the proper descriptions. Each part will have two correct answers.

1. _____ _____ Synapse

2. _____ _____ Axon terminal

3. _____ _____ Sarcolemma

A. Contains the transmitter acetylcholine
B. The cell membrane of the muscle fiber
C. The space between the muscle fiber and the motor neuron
D. Has receptors for acetylcholine
E. An impulse is transmitted by the diffusion of acetylcholine
F. The end of the motor neuron

► SYNOVIAL JOINTS
Match each part of a synovial joint with the correct description.

1. _____ Articular cartilage

2. _____ Joint capsule

3. _____ Synovial membrane

4. _____ Synovial fluid

5. _____ Bursae

A. Lines the joint capsule and secretes synovial
B. Prevents friction within the joint cavity
C. Encloses the joint similar to a sleeve
D. Permit tendons to slide easily across a joint
E. Provides a smooth surface on the joint surfaces of bones

► VOCABULARY
Match the word with its definition.

1. __C__ Symphysis

2. __A__ Ball and socket

3. __D__ Hinge

4. __E__ Condyloid

5. __B__ Pivot

6. __F__ Gliding

7. __H__ Saddle

8. __G__ Bursa

9. __J__ Crepitation

10. __I__ Synovitis

A. Movement in all planes
B. Rotation
C. Disk of fibrous cartilage between bones
D. Movement in one plane
E. Hinge with some lateral movement
F. Side-to-side movement
G. Small sacs of synovial fluid between joints and tendons
H. Movement in several planes
I. Swollen synovial tissue within the joint
J. Grating sound as joint or bone moves

► DIAGNOSTIC TESTS
Match the diagnostic tests to the appropriate description.

1. _____ X-ray

2. _____ Arthrogram

3. _____ MRI

4. _____ Arthroscopy

5. _____ Arthrocentesis

6. _____ Bone scan

7. _____ Alkaline phosphatase

8. _____ Calcium

9. _____ Phosphorus

10. _____ Erythrocyte sedimentation rate

11. _____ Uric acid

A. Dye required to view joint structures: tendons, ligaments, cartilage
B. Radio waves and magnetic field view of soft tissue
C. Bones show up as white areas
D. Insertion of a needle into a joint space to remove fluid, obtain a specimen, or instill medication
E. An endoscopy of joints with local or general anesthesia
F. Serum level of enzyme that is made by osteoblasts to mineralize bone
G. After being injected, the radioisotope Napertechnate is taken up by bone and 2 hours later a camera scans the body front and back
H. Serum level of substance stored in bone that makes bone rigid
I. Serum test for inflammation
J. Serum level of substance that mineralizes bones and teeth
K. Serum level for end product of purine metabolism

▶ CRITICAL THINKING

Read the case study and answer the questions.

Mr. John Allen, 45, was in an automobile accident and comes to the emergency department with a fractured femur.

1. What information should the nurse include in Mr. Allen's history? _____

_____

2. What areas should Mr. Allen's physical assessment focus on first? _____

_____

3. What tests can the nurse anticipate will be done on Mr. Allen? _____

_____

4. What types of teaching should the nurse do? _____

_____

REVIEW QUESTIONS

Choose the best answer.

1. Absorbing shock between adjacent vertebrae is the function of disks made of
   - A. Smooth muscle
   - B. Synovial fluid
   - C. Fibrous cartilage
   - D. Adipose tissue

2. Which of the following is the transmitter at neuromuscular junctions?
   - A. Sodium ions
   - B. Acetylcholine
   - C. A nerve impulse
   - D. Cholinesterase

3. Muscles are attached to bones by which of the following?
   - A. Tendons
   - B. Ligaments
   - C. Fascia
   - D. Other muscles

4. Which of the following is the part of the brain that initiates muscle contraction?
   - A. Parietal lobe
   - B. Cerebellum
   - C. Frontal lobe
   - D. Temporal lobe

5. Which of the following organ systems is not considered directly necessary for muscle contraction?
   - A. Circulatory system
   - B. Digestive system
   - C. Respiratory system
   - D. Nervous system

6. The nurse is inspecting the knee of a patient who reports pain and stiffness in it. As the patient moves the knee the nurse hears a grating sound. The nurse documents the grating sound as which of the following?
   - A. Friction rub
   - B. Crepitation
   - C. Effusion
   - D. Subcutaneous emphysema

7. When the nurse observes a joint that has a grating sound with movement, which of the following actions should the nurse take next?
   - A. Adduct the extremity.
   - B. Flex the joint.
   - C. Avoid joint movement.
   - D. Abduct the extremity.

8. The nurse is gathering functional data on a patient with rheumatoid arthritis. Which of the following areas would the nurse include in the assessment?
   - A. Response to treatment
   - B. Ability to prepare food
   - C. Appearance of joints
   - D. Lung sounds

9. Following a patient's bone biopsy, the nurse inspects the biopsy site. The nurse is assessing for which of the following complications that may occur immediately following a biopsy?
   - A. Joint dislocation
   - B. Crackles
   - C. Infection
   - D. Hematoma formation

10. The nurse understands that increased pain that is unresponsive to analgesic medication in a patient who has had a biopsy may indicate which of the following biopsy complications?
   A. Bleeding in soft tissue
   B. A low pain tolerance
   C. An allergic reaction
   D. Inadequate analgesic dose

11. A patient, age 66, has rheumatoid arthritis. Which of the following symptoms would the nurse most likely be told was the first symptom that caused the patient to seek health care?
   A. Cold intolerance
   B. Stiff, sore joints
   C. Shortness of breath
   D. Crepitation

12. The nurse is admitting a patient scheduled at 9:00 AM for an arthroscopy of the knee. Which of the following would be included in nursing preoperative care for this patient?
   A. A soft breakfast
   B. No food after midnight
   C. Explaining the surgical procedure
   D. Explaining the anesthetic agents

44

NURSING CARE OF PATIENTS WITH MUSCULOSKELETAL AND CONNECTIVE TISSUE DISORDERS

► VOCABULARY

Fill in the blank for the word that is formed by the word building.

1. _____ arthron—joint + itis—inflammation

2. _____ arthro—joint + plasty—creation of

3. _____ synovia—synovial fluid or tissue + itis—inflammation

4. _____ arthro—joint + centesis—puncture of a cavity

5. _____ hyper—excessive + uric—uric acid + emia—in blood

6. _____ sclero—hardening + derma—skin

7. _____ vascul—blood vessel + itis—inflammation

8. _____ poly—many + myo—muscle + itis—inflammation

9. _____ a—without + vascular—blood + necrosis—death

10. _____ re—again + plant—to plant + tion—process

11. _____ hemi—half + pelv—pelvis + ectomy—removal of

12. _____ fascia—fibrous tissue + otomy—opening into

13. _____ osteo—bone + myel—bone marrow + itis—inflammation

14. _____ osteo—bone + sarco—flesh + oma—tumor

▶ FRACTURES

Match the type of fracture with its definition.

1. _____ More than two fragments that appear to float
2. _____ Fragment overrides the other fragment
3. _____ Splintered and bent, occurring mainly in children
4. _____ More than two fragments driven into each other
5. _____ Extends into articular surface
6. _____ Runs along axis of bone
7. _____ Oblique fracture line
8. _____ Spontaneous fracture from bone disease
9. _____ Fracture spirals around shaft of bone
10. _____ From repeated stress (jogging)
11. _____ At right angle to bone

A. Transverse
B. Stress
C. Spiral
D. Pathological
E. Oblique
F. Longitudinal
G. Interarticular
H. Impacted
I. Greenstick
J. Displaced
K. Comminuted

▶ PROSTHESIS CARE EDUCATION

Indicate whether the statement is true or false, and correct false statements.

1. _____ Have a wooden prosthesis refinished at least every 3 months.
2. _____ Clean the prosthesis socket with alcohol and water, and dry it completely.
3. _____ Replace worn inserts and liners when they become too soiled to clean adequately.
4. _____ Check all mechanical parts such as bolts periodically for unusual sounds or movement.
5. _____ Oil the mechanical parts as instructed by the physician.
6. _____ Use garters to keep socks or stockings in place.
7. _____ Replace shoes when they wear out with new ones of a different height and type.

▶ HEALTH PROMOTION FOR PATIENTS WITH GOUT

Fill in the blanks.

1. Avoid high _____ foods, such as organ meats, shellfish, and oily fish such as _____.

2. _____ alcohol.

3. Drink plenty of _____, especially water.

4. Avoid all forms of _____ and drugs containing _____.

5. _____ diuretics.

6. Avoid excessive physical or emotional _____.

▶ PROGRESSIVE SYSTEMIC SCLEROSIS

Find the eight errors and insert the correct information.

Progressive systemic sclerosis (PSS), called systemic scleroderma, is similar to systemic lupus erythematosus in that it can affect one body organ and other connective tissues. PSS is as common as lupus but has a higher mortality rate.

PSS is characterized by pain that develops into fibrosis (scarring), then sclerosis (softening) of tissues. Autoimmunity is the likely cause. Like some of the other systemic connective tissue diseases, abnormal antibodies damage abnormal tissue.

PSS affects men more than women, usually between 30 and 50 years of age. The disease tends to progress slowly and does not respond well to treatment. Spontaneous remissions and exacerbations occur.

▶ CRITICAL THINKING

Complete the nursing diagnosis of impaired physical mobility for a patient with a hip replacement.

IMPAIRED PHYSICAL MOBILITY RELATED TO HIP PRECAUTIONS AND SURGICAL

Intervention	Rationale	Evaluation
_____ _____ Place overhead frame and trapeze on bed; teach patient how to use it. Assess the patient for and take measures to prevent complications of immobility: _____ _____ _____ _____ _____	Activity is restricted due to hip precautions and weight-bearing limitations. _____ _____ _____ _____	_____ _____ Does patient use overbed frame and trapeze for movement? Does patient experience complications of immobility?

REVIEW QUESTIONS

Choose the best answer.

1. A patient is in skin traction using a foam boot with Velcro fasteners for a fractured hip. The nurse would document this type of skin traction as which of the following?
   A. Gardner tongs
   B. Buck's traction
   C. Crutchfield tongs
   D. Steinmann pin

2. A patient sustains a closed fracture of his right tibia and is placed in a long-leg plaster cast, which is still damp. Which of the following methods should the nurse use to move the cast without causing complications?
   A. Have the patient move own leg.
   B. Palm the cast to move it.
   C. Use fingertips to grasp cast.
   D. Avoid moving the cast until it is dry.

3. A patient is being treated with gold therapy for rheumatoid arthritis. Which of the following interventions is essential when gold therapy is started?
   A. Removing all metal objects patient is wearing
   B. Assessing allergies to iodine
   C. Giving a test dose of gold
   D. Planning a biweekly dosing schedule

4. A patient asks why he must receive a test dose of gold therapy. Which of the following is the most appropriate response by the nurse?
   A. To avoid waste of expensive gold
   B. To determine the necessary dose
   C. To determine the therapeutic response
   D. To assess for an allergic reaction

5. The nurse is caring for a patient who has a fractured ankle that is in a cast. The patient has morphine 10 to 15 mg intramuscularly ordered every 3 to 4 hours. The patient received morphine 10 mg 2 hours and 45 minutes ago and is rating the pain at 10+ and moans that leg hurts. The patient has good capillary refill. Which of the following actions is most appropriate for the nurse to take next?
   A. Apply ice to the cast.
   B. Notify the physician immediately.
   C. Remove the pillow under the cast.
   D. Prepare morphine 15 mg for administration.

6. The nurse turns a 2-day postoperative patient with a right total hip replacement using three pillows between the legs. The nurse later returns and finds the patient lying supine with legs crossed. Which of the following should the nurse assess to determine whether a complication has developed?
   A. The right knee for crepitation
   B. The left leg for internal rotation
   C. The left leg for loss of function
   D. The right leg for shortening

7. Discharge teaching for patients who have gout includes diet teaching. The patients will require additional teaching if they say they will be eating which one of the following?
   A. Cod
   B. Chicken
   C. Eggs
   D. Liver

8. Which of the following medications should a patient with gout be encouraged to avoid to prevent a gout attack?
   A. Aspirin
   B. Tylenol
   C. Nonsteroidal anti-inflammatory drugs
   D. Narcotics

9. The nurse is reviewing a erythrocyte sedimentation rate (ESR) for a patient. Which of the following does the nurse understand is the purpose of an ESR test?
   A. To identify the number of red blood cells the patient has
   B. To determine sedimentation found in red blood cells
   C. To identify the presence of systemic inflammation
   D. To diagnose various types of arthritis

10. Which of the following is a common nursing diagnosis that the nurse will include in the plan of care for a patient with lupus?
    A. Fatigue
    B. Impaired mobility
    C. Impaired swallowing
    D. Impaired tissue perfusion

11. Which of the following is the recommended protocol for caring for a severed body part that may be replanted?
    A. Cover it with a warm dry towel.
    B. Wrap it in a cool moist cloth.
    C. Place it on dry ice.
    D. Wrap it in a dry sterile dressing.

Unit Thirteen

Understanding the Neurological System

CHECKLIST FOR LEARNING SUCCESS

Review of Anatomy and Physiology	Major disorders	Nursing Assessment	Diagnostic Tests	Interventions	Common Medications
□ Central nervous system (CNS) □ Brain □ Spinal cord □ Peripheral nervous system (PNS) □ Cranial nerves □ Spinal nerves □ Sympathetic □ Para-sympathetic □ Aging changes	□ CNS infections □ Headaches □ Transient ischemic attack (TIA) □ Brain attack □ Aneuryms □ Seizures □ Traumatic brain injury (TBI) □ Hematomas □ Brain tumors □ Herniated disk □ Spinal cord injury □ Parkinson's disease □ Alzheimer's disease □ Multiple sclerosis □ Myasthenia gravis □ Amyotrophic lateral sclerosis (ALS) □ Guillain-Barré □ Cranial nerve disorders	□ Level of consciousness (LOC) (Glasgow coma scale) □ Pupils □ Muscle function □ Cranial nerves □ Intracranial pressure (ICP) monitoring	□ Lumbar puncture □ Computed tomography (CT) scan □ Magnetic resonance imaging (MRI) □ Angiogram □ Myelogram □ Electroencephalogram (EEG)	□ Positioning □ Nutrition □ Interventions for swallowing □ Activities of daily living (ADLs) □ Communication □ Rehabilitation □ ICP monitoring □ Intracranial surgery	□ Anticoagulants □ Thrombolytics □ Corticosteroids □ Platelet aggregation inhibitors □ Diuretics □ Anticonvulsants

45

NEUROLOGICAL FUNCTION AND ASSESSMENT

▶ VOCABULARY

Fill in the blank with the correct term.

1. Difficulty swallowing is called __Dysphagia__ .

2. _____ is a disorder of the spinal nerve root that causes pain along the nerve path.

3. A patient might say his leg feels like it is asleep to describe a _____ .

4. Abnormal flexion posturing when eliciting best motor response is called __decortical__ posturing.

5. Abnormal extension posturing when eliciting best motor response is called __decebrink__ posturing.

6. _____ is the term that describes unequal pupils.

7. Involuntary eye movement is called __nystigmus__ .

8. Permanent muscle contractions are called _____ .

9. Difficulty speaking because of muscle dysfunction is called __APHASIA__ .

10. Patients who have difficulty speaking after a stroke are experiencing _____ .

▶ DIAGNOSTIC TESTS

Describe the procedure, and preprocedure and postprocedure care, for each of the following diagnostic tests.

1. Myelogram

_____

_____

_____

2. EEG

_____

_____

_____

3. Lumbar puncture

_____

_____

_____

4. MRI

_____

_____

_____

5. CT scan

_____

_____

_____

▶ **ANATOMY**
Label the parts of the sensory and motor neurons.

Label the parts of the brain.

ANATOMY
Match the part of the brain with the function it controls.

1. _____ Cerebrum

2. _____ Medulla oblongata

3. _____ Occipital lobe

4. _____ Cerebellum

5. _____ Temporal lobe

A. Vision center
B. Speech
C. Equilibrium and coordination
D. Respiratory center
E. Information storage

ASSESSMENT OF CRANIAL NERVES
Match the following assessment tools with the nerve to be tested.

1. __C__ Cotton ball

2. __D__ Snellen chart

3. __e__ Use hands to check neck/shoulder strength

4. __A__ Tuning fork or whisper

5. __C__ Tongue blade and cotton swab

A. Acoustic (VIII)
B. Spinal accessory (XI)
C. Trigeminal (V)
D. Optic (II)
E. Vagus (X)

CRITICAL THINKING
Read the case study and answer the following questions.

Mrs. Pickett is admitted to the nursing home where you work as a nurse (LPN/LVN). She had a stroke 2 weeks ago and is not strong enough to go to a rehabilitation facility. She has left-sided weakness. You collect admitting data to help determine her plan of care.

1. Mrs. Pickett tells you she needs to get up to go to the bathroom. What are some things you can do to determine if she is

able to do this? _____

_____

_____

2. Mrs. Pickett's first meal is served. What do you do to assess her ability to eat safely? _____

_____

_____

3. Mrs. Pickett says, "Will you go to the kitchen and get me one of those cookies I like?" How do you assess whether she is confused? _____

_____

_____

4. Mrs. Pickett is weak on her left side. Why do you think her blood pressure will be more accurate in her right arm? _____

_____

_____

REVIEW QUESTIONS

Choose the best answer.

1. Which of the following parts of a neuron transmits impulses away from the cell body?
   A. Dendrite
   B. Axon
   C. Neurolemma
   D. Synapse

2. Which type of neuron transmits impulses from the central nervous system to the muscles and glands?
   A. Afferent
   B. Efferent

3. Which part of the body is supplied by nerves from the thoracic cord?
   A. Head
   B. Trunk
   C. Hips
   D. Coccyx

4. Which part of the brain controls breathing?
   A. Medulla
   B. Cerebellum
   C. Cerebrum
   D. Thalamus

5. When a neurologist asks a patient to smile, which cranial nerve is being tested?
   A. II optic
   B. VII facial
   C. X vagus
   D. XI accessory

6. The neurologist tests the fourth (trochlear) and sixth (abducens) cranial nerves together by having a patient do which of the following?
   A. Turn his head to the right and left.
   B. Identify whispering in his ears.
   C. Say "ahhh."
   D. Follow his finger with his eyes.

7. Which of the following responses indicates sympathetic nervous system function?
   A. Tachycardia, dilated pupils
   B. Increased peristalsis, abdominal cramping
   C. Hypoglycemia, headache
   D. Pupil constriction, bronchoconstriction

8. Which neurotransmitter mediates the sympathetic response?
   A. Norepinephrine
   B. Acetylcholine
   C. Prostaglandin
   D. Serotonin

9. Which of the following nursing actions prepares a patient for a lumbar puncture?
   A. Administering enemas until clear
   B. Removing all metal jewelry
   C. Positioning the patient on his or her side
   D. Removing the patient's dentures

10. Which of the following nursing interventions is appropriate after a lumbar puncture?
    A. Have the patient lie flat for 6 to 8 hours.
    B. Keep the patient from eating or drinking for 4 hours.
    C. Monitor the patient's pedal pulses q4h.
    D. Keep the head of the bed elevated 30 degrees for 24 hours.

11. A patient is scheduled for an MRI and asks what to expect. Which of the following responses by the nurse is best?
    A. "It is the measurement of muscle contraction after stimulation by tiny needle electrodes."
    B. "Electrodes will be placed on your scalp to measure activity of the brain."
    C. "A scan of the brain will be done after injection of a radioisotope."
    D. "It is a noninvasive test that uses magnetic energy to visualize internal parts."

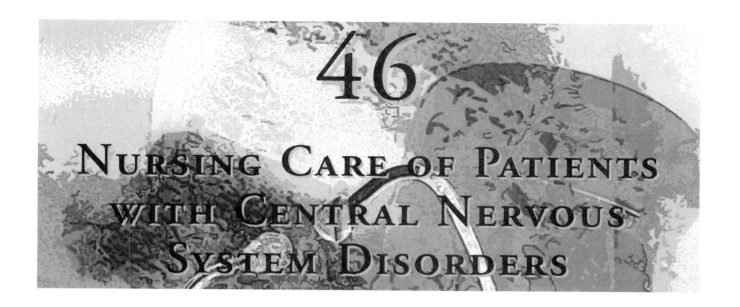

46

Nursing Care of Patients with Central Nervous System Disorders

▶ VOCABULARY

Match the term with the correct definition.

1. _____ Contralateral hemiparesis

2. _____ Ipsilateral hemiplegia

3. _____ Quadriplegia

4. _____ Paraplegia

5. _____ Photophobia

6. _____ Thrombotic

7. _____ Aphasia

8. _____ Dysphagia

9. _____ Hemianopsia

10. _____ Flaccid

A. All four extremities paralyzed
B. Sensitive to light
C. Difficulty swallowing
D. Caused by a clot
E. Inability to speak or understand language
F. Paralyzed on same side
G. Paralyzed lower extremities
H. Vision lost in half of visual field
I. Weak on opposite side
J. Without muscle tone

▶ DRUGS USED FOR CENTRAL NERVOUS SYSTEM DISORDERS

Match the drug with its action.

1. _____ Mannitol

2. _____ Heparin

3. _____ Ticlid

4. _____ Decadron

5. _____ Tissue plasminogen activator

A. Anticoagulant
B. Osmotic diuretic
C. Platelet aggregation inhibitor
D. Thrombolytic
E. Corticosteroid

▶ ALZHEIMER'S DISEASE

Match the stage of disease with its primary symptom.

1. _____ Stage 1

2. _____ Stage 2

3. _____ Stage 3

4. _____ Stage 4

A. Terminal
B. Confused
C. Forgetful
D. Ambulatory dementia

▶ CENTRAL NERVOUS SYSTEM DISORDERS

Match the signs and symptoms with the correct disorders.

1. _____ Unconscious at accident scene

2. _____ Flaccid right side

3. _____ Hypotension, loss of sympathetic function

4. _____ Nuchal rigidity

5. _____ High blood pressure, bradycardia, diaphoresis

6. _____ Brief period of staring

7. _____ Automatic repetitive movement such as picking or lip smacking

8. _____ Status epilepticus

9. _____ Rising weakness

10. _____ Numbness, weakness, spasticity

A. Spinal shock
B. Absence seizure
C. Multiple sclerosis
D. Guillain-Barré syndrome
E. Meningitis
F. Brain attack
G. Autonomic dysreflexia
H. Complex partial seizure
I. Epidural bleed
J. Continuous seizure

▶ SPINAL DISORDERS

Determine whether each of the following symptoms is associated with lumbar spine or cervical spine dysfunction.

_____ Radiating pain to the ankle

_____ Deltoid weakness

_____ Diminished triceps reflex

_____ Footdrop

_____ Inability to walk on the toes

▶ CRITICAL THINKING

Brain Attack

Read the case studies and answer the questions.

   Mrs. Saunders is a 70-year-old retired secretary admitted to your unit from the emergency department with a diagnosis of brain attack (stroke). She has a history of hypertension and atherosclerosis, and she had a carotid endarterectomy 6 years ago. She is 40 percent over her ideal body weight and has a 20 pack-year smoking history. Her daughter says her mother has been having short episodes of confusion and memory loss for the past few weeks. This morning she found her mother slumped to the right in her recliner, unable to speak.

1. Explain the pathophysiology of a cerebrovascular accident. Which type of stroke is most likely the cause of Mrs. Saunders'

   symptoms? _____

   _____

   _____

2. Mrs. Saunders is flaccid on her right side. What is the term used to describe this? _____

   _____

3. Which hemisphere of Mrs. Saunders' brain is damaged? _____

4. List four risk factors for stroke evident in Mrs. Saunders' history. _____

_____

_____

5. Mrs. Saunders appears to understand when you speak to her but is only able to speak in garbled words. What is the term for this? _____

_____

_____

6. Neurological checks are ordered every 2 hours for 24 hours, then every 4 hours. When you enter her room and call her name, she opens her eyes. She is able to squeeze your hand with her left hand when you ask her to but is only able to make incomprehensible sounds. What is her score on the Glasgow Coma Scale? List seven symptoms of rising intracranial pressure (ICP) that you will watch for. _____

_____

_____

7. List two medications that the physician may order. Why might they be used? _____

_____

_____

8. Identify a nursing diagnosis related to Mrs. Saunders' right-sided paralysis. List three interventions to prevent complications. _____

_____

_____

9. How will you protect Mrs. Saunders' skin? List at least three interventions. _____

_____

_____

10. As you enter Mrs. Saunders' room on her third day on your unit, you find her agitated, trying to speak, and trying to get out of bed. List at least three ways you might find out what she wants. _____

_____

_____

11. Before feeding Mrs. Saunders for the first time, what reflex do you check? How do you do this? _____

_____

_____

12. Mrs. Saunders has some difficulty swallowing and pockets her food in her right cheek. List three interventions you might try. _____

_____

_____

_____

13. Mrs. Saunders begins to move her right hand slightly and is able to say her daughter's name when she enters the room. She is prepared for discharge to a rehabilitation facility. List three ways you might prepare her family for her move and her eventual discharge home. _____

_____

_____

14. What class of drugs might be ordered for Mrs. Saunders to prevent another stroke? _____

_____

_____

Spinal Cord Injury

Mr. Granger is a 23-year-old admitted to your unit with a C5-6 spinal cord injury following an auto accident. You collect the following subjective data:

Pain in cervical spine

You also collect the following objective data:

No sensation or movement below the level of the injury
Blood pressure 80/60
Pulse 45
Respirations shallow
Temperature 97° F

1. Explain Mr. Granger's hypotension, hypothermia, and bradycardia. _____

_____

_____

2. Why are Mr. Granger's respirations shallow? _____

_____

_____

3. Explain the purpose of each of the following therapies. How will they benefit Mr. Granger? _____

_____

Cervical traction: _____

_____

Vasopressor administration: _____

_____

Insertion of a urinary catheter: _____

_____

4. Mr. Granger suddenly becomes anxious and dyspneic. He is using his accessory muscles with each breath. Explain what is happening. _____

_____

_____

5. What treatment would you expect, and why will it be beneficial to Mr. Granger? _____

_____

_____

6. List two priority nursing diagnoses and goals for Mr. Granger's acute stage. _____
_____
_____

7. What are two health learning needs Mr. Granger faces in his acute stage? _____
_____
_____

REVIEW QUESTIONS

Choose the best answer.

1. A patient reports severe back pain that radiates from the back to the left knee. Which of the following is the most likely cause of the pain?
    A. Muscular injury
    B. Herniated lumbar disk
    C. Impaired peripheral circulation
    D. A tumor of the femur

2. A patient asks the nurse what side effects to expect from the antispasmodic medication the patient is taking. Which of the following side effects is most common with antispasmodics?
    A. Hypoglycemia
    B. Hypotension
    C. Drowsiness
    D. Dyspnea

3. Which of the following treatments would be least likely to be prescribed for acute back pain?
    A. Physical therapy
    B. Vigorous exercise
    C. Analgesics
    D. Anti-inflammatory medications

4. Which of the following problems during the immediate postoperative course following microdiskectomy should be reported to the physician immediately?
    A. Incisional pain
    B. Decreased range of motion
    C. Inability to move the left leg
    D. Muscle spasm

5. A 46-year-old woman is admitted to the rehabilitation unit with left-sided hemiparesis resulting from a subarachnoid hemorrhage. She is not oriented to her surroundings or situation, but she does recognize her family. On admission, she tells her nurse that she can walk to the bathroom without assistance. Which of the following responses by the nurse is best?
    A. Allow her to ambulate unassisted, to encourage positive self-esteem.
    B. Ask her to demonstrate her ability to ambulate.
    C. Leave her alone while the nurse checks the transfer sheet for orders.
    D. Ask another staff member to help the nurse ambulate the patient.

6. A brain-injured patient becomes easily frustrated when unable to complete a task. Which of the following responses by the nurse will best help the patient get the task done?
    A. Perform the task for the patient.
    B. Tell the patient not to worry about it.
    C. Break the task down into simple steps.
    D. Have another patient demonstrate how to perform the task.

7. The nurse is assessing a patient who has had a subarachnoid hemorrhage and finds the patient lethargic and irritable. Within minutes of awakening, the patient vomits. Which of these is the most likely cause of these symptoms?
    A. Hydrocephalus
    B. The flu
    C. Food poisoning
    D. Brainstem herniation

8. Which of the following is a common long-term result of subarachnoid hemorrhage?
    A. Bowel dysfunction
    B. Memory impairment
    C. Pneumonia
    D. Neck pain

9. The primary reason for starting antibiotics immediately after the lumbar puncture for a patient suspected of having meningitis is what?
    A. To determine whether the patient will have an allergic reaction
    B. To increase the likelihood of successfully treating the meningitis
    C. To prevent resistant strains of bacteria from developing
    D. To determine whether the antibiotics will compromise auditory function

10. Which of the following signs is least likely after rupture of an arteriovenous malformation?
    A. Seizures
    B. Hemiparesis
    C. Encephalitis
    D. Memory impairment

11. Which of the following settings is most therapeutic for an agitated head-injured patient?
    A. A lively public place
    B. A structured, quiet environment
    C. A family waiting room with lots of visitors
    D. A hallway near the nurse's station

12. Decreasing level of consciousness is a symptom of which of the following physiological phenomena?
    A. Increased ICP
    B. Sympathetic response
    C. Parasympathetic response
    D. Increased cerebral blood flow

13. Which of the following blood pressure changes alerts the nurse to increasing ICP?
    A. Gradual increase
    B. Rapid drop followed by gradual increase
    C. Widening pulse pressure
    D. Rapid fluctuations

14. You are assigned to monitor a patient receiving mannitol for increasing ICP. Which of the following measurements will determine whether the mannitol is effective?
    A. Pulse rate
    B. Blood sugar level
    C. Comfort level
    D. Urine output

15. Which of the following nursing interventions will help prevent a further increase in ICP?
    A. Encourage fluids.
    B. Elevate the head of the bed.
    C. Provide physical therapy.
    D. Reposition the patient frequently.

47

NURSING CARE OF PATIENTS WITH PERIPHERAL NERVOUS SYSTEM DISORDERS

▶ VOCABULARY

Fill in the blanks with the correct terms.

1. Muscles that are not used become wasted, or _____ .

2. Some diseases are characterized by remissions and _____ .

3. Tic douloureux causes nerve pain, or _____ .

4. An early symptom of myasthenia gravis is drooping eyelids, also called _____ .

5. Symptoms of Guillain-Barré syndrome are caused by _____ of axons.

6. Myasthenia gravis is sometimes treated with _____ , which separates blood cells from plasma to remove antibodies.

7. Muscle twitching or _____ occur in amyotrophic lateral sclerosis.

8. The chemical that breaks down acetylcholine is called _____ .

▶ PERIPHERAL DISORDERS

Underline incorrect information in the following case studies. Write the correct information in the space provided.

1. Miss Mary Garvey sees her physician because she has been seeing double off and on for several weeks and has been fatigued. Her physician suspects myasthenia gravis and schedules her for a carotid ultrasound. He confirms his suspicions with a Tensilon test. He explains to Miss Garvey that she has a disease that is characterized by a decrease in the neurotransmitter norepinephrine. He begins her on Mastadon and prednisone. Her nurse teaches her the importance of getting regular exercise and recommends joining a local health and exercise club.

2. Mr. Tom Neura has a history of trigeminal neuralgia. He enters the emergency department with severe pain in his left wrist. The physician orders a narcotic analgesic because Mr. Neura's third cranial nerve is inflamed. Once the acute pain has subsided, Mr. Neura is discharged with instructions to get plenty of fresh air and to take his phenytoin (Dilantin) as ordered.

3. Mrs. Mattie Schultz is admitted with exacerbated multiple sclerosis. Her legs are becoming weaker, causing difficult walking, and she has been having difficulty swallowing. You know that buildup of myelin on her neurons is responsible for her weakness. You assess her for stressors that might have caused her exacerbation, such as a urinary tract infection (UTI) or upper respiratory tract infection (URI). Mattie is started on thyroid stimulating hormone (TSH) to stimulate her thyroid, which will help reduce her symptoms. She is also placed on sulfamethoxazole (Bactrim) for the UTI you identified through your excellent assessment and on diazepam (Valium) for urinary retention.

▶ CRITICAL THINKING

Read the case study and answer the following questions.

Reverend Wilson is a 50-year-old minister who sees his physician when he develops weakness in his arms and legs and has difficulty carrying out his job duties. He is diagnosed with amyotrophic lateral sclerosis (ALS).

1. Mrs. Wilson asks what ALS is. How do you describe it for her? _____

_____

2. Reverend Wilson returns to the physician's office several months after his initial diagnosis because he fell walking to the podium to preach. What is happening? What can he do about it? _____

_____

3. Reverend Wilson is concerned about continuing in his job and asks if his mind is going to be affected. How do you respond?

_____

_____

4. He develops painful muscle spasms. What medications might be ordered to help relieve them? _____

_____

5. Reverend Wilson stabilizes for a while. A year later he is admitted to the hospital with aspiration pneumonia. What probably happened? What nursing diagnosis is appropriate in this situation? List an appropriate goal and two or three interventions. _____

_____

_____

6. Reverend Wilson's condition deteriorates, and he has to retire. He becomes confined to a wheelchair. He has a gastrostomy tube inserted because he is no longer able to swallow. What additional nursing diagnoses are now appropriate? _____

_____

REVIEW QUESTIONS

Choose the best answer.

1. A 32-year-old male patient is admitted to your medical unit with a diagnosis of Guillain-Barré syndrome. His legs are weak, and he is unable to walk without assistance. Which of the following is most likely responsible for this syndrome?
   A. Bacterial infection
   B. Heredity
   C. High-fat diet
   D. Autoimmune reaction

2. Patients with Guillain-Barré syndrome should be closely monitored. Which of the following assessments is most likely to signal acute problems related to this syndrome?
   A. Increasing blood urea nitrogen (BUN) and creatinine
   B. Deteriorating arterial blood gases (ABG)
   C. Drop in Hgb and Hct
   D. Rising serum potassium

3. A woman sees her primary care provider because of extreme fatigue for the past 2 months; she has difficulty lifting even light objects. Her physician suspects myasthenia gravis. Which of the following tests do you anticipate assisting with to confirm this diagnosis?
   A. Mestinon test
   B. Quinine tolerance test
   C. Pulmonary function studies
   D. Tensilon test

4. Which drug class is used to reduce symptoms of muscle weakness from myasthenia gravis?
   A. Anticholinesterase drugs
   B. Anticholinergic drugs
   C. Adrenergic drugs
   D. Beta-blocker drugs

5. A 39-year-old homemaker sees her physician after she falls twice for seemingly no reason. Diagnostic tests are done, and she is diagnosed with multiple sclerosis. Which of the following explanations will help her understand her disease?
   A. "You have a buildup of myelin in your nervous system, causing congestion and muscle weakness."
   B. "You are missing a neurotransmitter that is important to muscle contraction."
   C. "The receptor sites on your muscles are damaged, so they can't contract correctly."
   D. "The insulation on your nerve cells is damaged, which makes the impulses to the muscles slow."

6. Which of the following medications might be ordered to help control symptoms of multiple sclerosis, and possibly induce a remission?
   A. Acyclovir (Zovirax)
   B. Adrenocorticotropic hormone (ACTH)
   C. Thyrotropin
   D. Diphenhydramine (Benadryl)

7. Many neuromuscular disorders can impair respiratory function. What intervention can a home care nurse recommend to help prevent complications in patients with impaired respiratory function?
   A. Antibiotics as needed
   B. Elevate the head of the bed
   C. Bed rest
   D. Suction q4h

8. Which of the following nursing interventions will help prevent complications in the patient with Bell's palsy?
   A. Megavitamin therapy
   B. Elastic bandages
   C. Application of ice to the affected area
   D. Lubricating eyedrops

9. Which of the following assessment actions will help the nurse determine if the patient with Bell's palsy is receiving adequate nutrition?
   A. Monitor meal trays.
   B. Measure intake and output.
   C. Check twice-weekly weights.
   D. Assess swallowing reflex.

10. The nurse admits a 26-year-old Navajo Indian patient to your unit with pneumonia and sepsis. He is unusually small for his age and is sexually underdeveloped. Which of the following medical diagnoses should the nurse suspect?
    A. Navajo neuropathy
    B. Acquired immune deficiency syndrome (AIDS)
    C. Tuberculosis
    D. Cerebral palsy

11. The nurse notes frequent muscle twitching when collecting admission data on a patient admitted for increasing muscle weakness. Which of the following terms should the nurse use to document this?
    A. Fasciculations
    B. Atrophy
    C. Chorea
    D. Neuropathy

12. A 19-year-old nursing student develops trigeminal neuralgia. Which of the following actions will most likely aggravate her pain?
    A. Sleeping
    B. Eating
    C. Reading
    D. Cooking

UNIT FOURTEEN

UNDERSTANDING THE SENSORY SYSTEM

CHECKLIST FOR LEARNING SUCCESS

Review of Sensory Anatomy and Physiology	Major Sensory Disorders	Nursing Assessment	Diagnostic Tests	Interventions	Common Medications
☐ Eye structures	☐ Vision	☐ Medical history	☐ Vision	☐ Corrective eyewear	☐ Cycloplegics
☐ Eye function	☐ Eye infections/ inflammation	☐ Psychosocial history	☐ Amsler grid	☐ Trabeculoplasty	☐ Cholinergics (Miotics)
☐ Ear structures	☐ Refractive errors	☐ Medications	☐ Angiography	☐ Trabeculectomy	☐ Acetazolamide (Diamox)
☐ Ear function	☐ Blindness	☐ Physical assessment	☐ GDx access	☐ Cyclocryotherapy	☐ Timolol (Timoptic)
☐ Aging effects	☐ Diabetic retinopathy	☐ Vision:	☐ Intraocular pressure	☐ Iridotomy/ iridectomy	☐ Cerumenolytics
	☐ Retinal detachment	☐ Pupillary reflexes	☐ Ophthalmoscopy	☐ Scleral buckling	
	☐ Glaucoma	☐ Accommodation	☐ Slit lamp	☐ Supportive services	
	☐ Cataracts	☐ Romberg test	☐ Visual acuity	☐ Postoperative eye care	
	☐ Macular degeneration	☐ Hearing:	☐ Hearing	☐ Irrigation	
	☐ Hearing	☐ Rinne test	☐ Audiometric	☐ Hearing aids	
	☐ Hearing loss	☐ Weber test	☐ Caloric test	☐ Myringotomy	
	☐ External ear		☐ Otoscopic	☐ Stapedectomy	
	☐ Otosclerosis		☐ Tympanometry	☐ Postoperative ear care	
	☐ Ménière's disease				

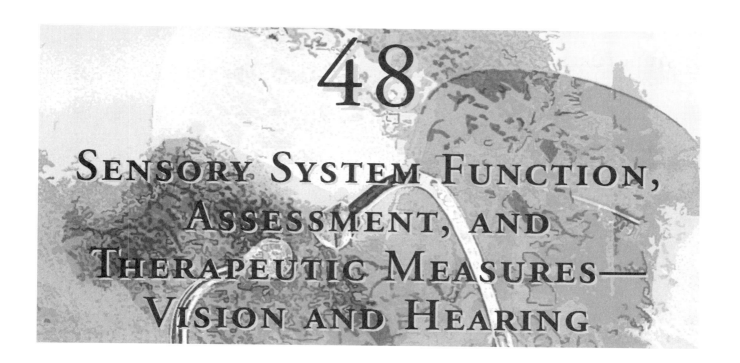

48

SENSORY SYSTEM FUNCTION, ASSESSMENT, AND THERAPEUTIC MEASURES— VISION AND HEARING

▶ STRUCTURES OF THE EYE

Label the following structures.

Anterior chamber
Aqueous humor
Canal of Schlemm
Choroid layer
Ciliary body
Conjunctiva
Cornea

Fovea
Inferior rectus muscle
Iris
Lens
Optic disc
Optic nerve
Posterior chamber

Pupil
Retina
Retinal artery and vein
Sclera
Superior rectus muscle
Suspensory ligaments
Vitreous humor

► STRUCTURES OF THE EAR

Label the following structures.

Auricle   Incus
Cochlea   Malleus
Ear canal   Semicircular canals
Eighth cranial nerve   Stapes
Eustachian tube   Tympanic membrane (eardrum)

► VISION

Number the following in the proper sequence as they are involved in the process of vision.

_____ A. Cornea   _____ E. Occipital lobe

_____ B. Vitreous humor   _____ F. Lens

_____ C. Optic nerve   _____ G. Retina

_____ D. Aqueous humor

► HEARING

Number the following in the order they function in the process of hearing when sound waves enter the ear canal.

_____ A. Eardrum   _____ F. Stapes

_____ B. Oval window   _____ G. Fluid in the cochlea

_____ C. Incus   _____ H. Hair cells in the organ of Corti

_____ D. Eighth cranial nerve _____ I. Temporal lobes

_____ E. Malleus

▶ VOCABULARY

Define the following terms and use them in a sentence.

Nystagmus

    Definition: _____

    Sentence: _____

Tropia

    Definition: _____

    Sentence: _____

Accommodation

    Definition: _____

    Sentence: _____

Ptosis

    Definition: _____

    Sentence: _____

Arcus senilis

    Definition: _____

    Sentence: _____

Ophthalmologist

    Definition: _____

    Sentence: _____

Optometrist

    Definition: _____

    Sentence: _____

Optician

    Definition: _____

    Sentence: _____

▶ DIAGNOSTIC TESTS

Fill in the table.

Assessment Test	Purpose of Test	Normal Test Results
_____ Visual fields	_____ _____	OD 20/20, OS 20/20, OU 20/20 _____
_____	Extraocular movement	_____
Accommodation	_____	Eyes turn inward and pupils constrict when focusing on a near object
_____ Weber	_____	Air conduction more than bone conduction _____
_____	Balance/vestibular function	_____

▶ CRITICAL THINKING

Read the case study and answer the following questions.

Ms. Sally LittleThunder works on a computer as a data processor. She is complaining of recurring eye discomfort about 2 hours after she begins work each day.

1. What do you suspect is wrong with Ms. LittleThunder?

_____

_____

2. For what environmental factors should the nurse assess?

_____

_____

3. To protect Ms. LittleThunder from eyestrain, what safety measures should be implemented in her office?

_____

_____

REVIEW QUESTIONS

Choose the best answer.

1. Which of the following would the nurse explain to the patient is indicated by a Snellen chart finding of 20/80?
    A. The eye can see at 80 feet what the normal eye can see at 20 feet.
    B. The eye can see at 20 feet what the normal eye can see at 80 feet.
    C. The eye can see four times what the normal eye can see.
    D. The eye sees normally.

2. Which of the following would indicate that the patient has a normal corneal light reflex?
    A. The eye focuses the image in the center of the pupil.
    B. The eyes converge to focus on the light.
    C. Constriction of both pupils occurs in response to bright light.
    D. Light is reflected at the same spot in both eyes.

3. The examiner shines a light in the patient's eyes and notes that the pupils are round and constrict from 4 to 2 mm bilaterally. Next, the examiner asks the patient to focus on a far object, then on the examiner's finger as it is brought from 3 feet distance to 5 inches distance. The pupils constrict bilaterally and the eyes turn inward. Which of the following would be the correct documentation of these findings?
    A. Pupils 2 mm
    B. Pupils constricted
    C. PERRLA
    D. Pupils normal

4. When testing visual fields, the nurse is assessing which of the following parts of vision?
    A. Peripheral vision
    B. Near vision
    C. Distance vision
    D. Central vision

5. In planning safe care for the older adult, which of the following conditions would not cause visual problems?
    A. Glaucoma
    B. Cataracts
    C. Macular degeneration
    D. Arcus senilis

6. Which of the following statements does the nurse understand is true concerning air conduction of sound in the ear?
    A. It is caused by the vibration of bones in the skull.
    B. It is less efficient than bone conduction.
    C. It is heard longer than bone conduction.
    D. It is caused by transmission of heat through the air.

7. Which of the following assessment findings could indicate a hearing loss?
    A. Patient converses easily with nurse.
    B. Patient answers questions appropriately.
    C. Patient's face is relaxed during conversation.
    D. Patient speaks in a very loud voice.

8. Which of the following statements would the nurse understand is true when assessing normal auditory acuity using the Rinne test?
   A. The patient perceives sound equally in both ears.
   B. Air conduction is heard longer than bone conduction in both ears.
   C. Bone conduction is heard longer than air conduction in both ears.
   D. The patient's left ear will perceive the sound better than the right ear.

9. Which of the following would indicate to the nurse that a substance is toxic to the ear?
   A. Otoplasty
   B. Otalgia
   C. Ototoxic
   D. Tinnitus

10. Which of the following subjective data questions would assist the nurse in assessing the patient's eye health?
   A. "Have you had any recent upper respiratory infections?"
   B. "Have you ridden in a car recently?"
   C. "Have you been scuba diving lately?"
   D. "Have you seen halos around lights?"

11. When assessing the external ear, the nurse palpates a small protrusion of the helix called a Darwin tubercle. The nurse would document this finding as which of the following?
   A. A normal finding
   B. An abnormal finding
   C. A normal finding only in the older adult
   D. An abnormal finding only in the older adult

12. Which of the following tests would the nurse use as an initial screening test to determine hearing loss?
   A. Romberg test
   B. Otoscopic examination
   C. Caloric test
   D. Whisper voice test

13. Which of the following would the nurse use to document a finding that the patient's ear is draining?
   A. Otorrhea
   B. Otalgia
   C. Ototoxic
   D. Tinnitus

14. Which of the following terms indicates that the patient has a hearing loss caused by aging?
   A. Otoplasty
   B. Otalgia
   C. Presbycusis
   D. Tinnitus

49

NURSING CARE OF PATIENTS WITH SENSORY DISORDERS— VISION AND HEARING

▶ **VOCABULARY**

Match the following terms with the appropriate definition.

1. _____ Carbuncle

2. _____ Cholesteatoma

3. _____ Mastoiditis

4. _____ Barotrauma

5. _____ Labyrinthitis

6. _____ Presbycusis

A. Hearing loss caused by aging
B. Inflammation or infection of the inner ear
C. Complication of otitis media
D. Epithelial cystlike sac filled with skin and sebaceous material
E. Several hair follicles forming an abscess
F. Pressure in the middle ear caused by atmospheric changes

▶ **ERRORS OF REFRACTION**

Draw a picture showing the eye size and focal point differences in a) hyperopia and b) myopia.

► PRESBYOPIA

Circle the seven errors in the following paragraph, and insert the correct information.

Presbyopia is a condition in which the lenses increase their elasticity resulting in a decrease in ability to focus on far objects. The loss of elasticity causes light rays to focus in front of the retina, resulting in hyperopia. This condition usually is associated with aging and generally occurs before age 40. Because accommodation for close vision is accomplished by lens contraction, people with presbyopia exhibit the ability to see objects at close range. They often compensate for blurred close vision by holding objects to be viewed closer. Complaints of eye strain and mild occipital headache are common.

► VISUAL AND HEARING DATA COLLECTION

Describe how you would know that a patient has the following condition based on data collection (include diagnostic tests and examinations).

Macular degeneration (dry type) _____

_____

Cataract _____

_____

Hordeolum _____

_____

Acute angle-closure glaucoma _____

_____

External otitis _____

_____

Impacted cerumen _____

_____

Otitis media _____

_____

Otosclerosis _____

_____

► GLAUCOMA

Circle the seven errors in the following paragraph, and insert the correct information.

Glaucoma is characterized by abnormal pressure outside the eyeball. This pressure causes damage to the cells of the acoustic nerve, the structure responsible for transmitting visual information from the ear to the brain. The damage is evident, progressive, and reversible until the end stages when initially loss of central vision occurs, and then eventually blindness. Once glaucoma occurs, the patient can be cured.

▶ CONDUCTIVE HEARING LOSS
Circle the six errors in the following paragraph, and insert the correct information.

Conductive hearing loss is interference with conduction of light waves through the external auditory canal, the eardrum, or the middle ear. The inner ear is involved in a pure conductive hearing loss. Conductive hearing loss is a neural problem. Causes of conductive hearing loss include cerumen, foreign bodies, infection, perforation of the tympanic membrane, trauma, fluid in the middle ear, cysts, tumor, and otosclerosis. Many causes of conductive hearing loss such as infection, foreign bodies, or impacted cerumen cannot be corrected. Hearing devices may not improve hearing for conditions that cannot be corrected. Hearing devices are most effective with conductive hearing loss when inner ear and nerve damage are present.

▶ OTOSCLEROSIS
Circle the nine errors in the following paragraph, and insert the correct information.

Otosclerosis results from the formation of new bone along the incus. With new bone growth, the incus becomes mobile and causes conductive hearing loss. Hearing loss is most apparent after the sixth decade. Otosclerosis usually occurs less often in women than in men. The disease usually affects one ear. It is thought to be a hereditary disease. The primary symptom of otosclerosis is rapid hearing loss. The patient usually experiences bilateral conductive hearing loss, particularly with soft, high tones. Otoectomy is the treatment of choice.

▶ CRITICAL THINKING
Read the case study and answer the following questions.

Mr. Nyugen, age 70, reports that he has difficulty seeing at night, so much so that he has given up driving. When questioned further, he also states, "I used to be an avid reader, but I guess I'm getting too old to read, the words aren't very clear." The nurse examines his eye and finds that he is sensitive to light, has opacity of both lenses, and denies any pain.

1. What do you suspect is wrong with Mr. Nyugen? _____

_____

2. For which diagnostic tests should you prepare Mr. Nyugen? _____

_____

3. After the physician has made a definitive diagnosis, Mr. Nyugen asks you to explain the surgical procedure and recovery regimen to him. Outline your teaching plan. _____

_____

_____

REVIEW QUESTIONS

Choose the best answer.

1. Which of the following would be a symptom the nurse would expect to find during assessment of a patient with macular degeneration?
   A. Increased ability to distinguish colors
   B. Sudden loss of vision
   C. Loss of far vision
   D. Loss of central vision

2. Which of the following type of eyedrops does the nurse understand is given to constrict the pupil, permitting aqueous humor to flow around the lens?
   A. Osmotic
   B. Myotic
   C. Mydriatic
   D. Cycloplegic

3. Which of the following safety instructions should the nurse give a patient who has temporarily dilated pupils?
    A. Keep eyes closed.
    B. Do not drive for 8 hours.
    C. Wear sunglasses.
    D. Avoid caffeinated beverages.

4. Which of the following procedures does the nurse understand is used to correct otosclerosis?
    A. Myringotomy
    B. Myringoplasty
    C. Mastoidectomy
    D. Stapedectomy

5. The nurse understands that labyrinthitis is treated primarily with which of the following drug categories?
    A. Antihistamines
    B. Antispasmotics
    C. Antiinflammatories
    D. Antiemetics

6. Which of the following types of hearing loss does the nurse understand is most improved with the use of a hearing aid?
    A. Conductive
    B. Sensorineural
    C. Mixed
    D. Central

7. Which of the following would the nurse explain to a patient is the main purpose of a hearing aid?
    A. Amplify background noise.
    B. Occlude the ear.
    C. Amplify musical sounds.
    D. Improve ability to hear.

8. Which of the following would the nurse explain to the patient is the triad of symptoms associated with Meniere's disease?
    A. Hearing loss, vertigo, and tinnitis
    B. Nystagmus, headache, and vomiting
    C. Nausea, vomiting, and pain
    D. Nystagmus, vomiting, and pain

9. Which of the following actions would the nurse include in the plan of care to reduce the symptoms of the patient who has vertigo?
    A. Avoid noises.
    B. Avoid sudden movements.
    C. Encourage fluid intake.
    D. Administer analgesics.

10. A patient is diagnosed with acute bacterial conjunctivitis. In providing patient teaching the nurse would tell the patient that this condition is more commonly known as which of the following?
    A. Glaucoma
    B. Astigmatism
    C. Color blindness
    D. Pinkeye

11. Which of the following is usually the first symptom of a cataract that the nurse would expect a patient to report during assessment?
    A. Dry eyes
    B. Eye pain
    C. Blurring of vision
    D. Loss of peripheral vision

12. Which of the following would the nurse teach the patient is the most common site for ear infections?
    A. Outer ear
    B. Inner ear
    C. Middle ear
    D. Semicircular canal

13. Which of the following nursing interventions would have the highest priority in the plan of care for the postoperative eye patient?
    A. Do not leave the patient unattended at any time.
    B. Teach the patient not to bend over.
    C. Report sudden onset of acute pain.
    D. Apply sandbags to either side of the head.

14. Which of the following descriptions by the nurse would best explain glaucoma to a patient?
    A. "There is an increase in the amount of vitreous humor."
    B. "There is an increase in the intraocular pressure."
    C. "There is a decrease in the amount of aqueous humor."
    D. "There is a decrease in the intraocular pressure."

15. Which of the following is a symptom that the nurse would expect to find during assessment of a patient experiencing acute angle-closure glaucoma?
    A. Flashing lights
    B. Lens opacity
    C. Halos around lights
    D. Vertigo

16. Which of the following activities would the nurse teach a patient to avoid so that intraocular pressure is not increased after eye surgery?
    A. Sitting upright in bed
    B. Coughing
    C. Chewing food vigorously
    D. Reading a book

UNIT FIFTEEN

UNDERSTANDING THE INTEGUMENTARY SYSTEM

CHECKLIST FOR LEARNING SUCCESS

Review of Anatomy and Physiology	Major Disorders	Nursing Assessment	Diagnostic Tests	Interventions	Common Medications
☐ Epidermis	☐ Pressure ulcers	☐ History	☐ Cultures	☐ Dressings	☐ Antibiotics
☐ Dermis	☐ Dermatitis	☐ Color	☐ Biopsy	☐ Balneotherapy	☐ Antivirals
☐ Appendages	☐ Herpes simplex	☐ Lesions	☐ Wood's light	☐ Topical medications	☐ Corticosteroids
☐ Subcutaneous tissue	☐ Herpes zoster	☐ Moisture	☐ Skin tests	☐ Plastic surgery	☐ Analgesics
☐ Aging changes	☐ Fungal infections	☐ Edema			☐ Chemotherapy
	☐ Cellulitis	☐ Vascular markings			
	☐ Acne	☐ Integrity			
	☐ Parasites	☐ Cleanliness			
	☐ Pemphigus				
	☐ Burns				
	☐ Malignant lesions				

50

INTEGUMENTARY FUNCTION, ASSESSMENT, AND THERAPEUTIC MEASURES

▶ INTEGUMENTARY STRUCTURES

Match each integumentary structure with its proper description.

1. _____ Epidermis

2. _____ Dermis

3. _____ Subcutaneous tissue

4. _____ Collagen fibers

5. _____ Eccrine glands

6. _____ Receptors

7. _____ Melanin

8. _____ Stratum corneum

9. _____ Stratum germinativum

A. If unbroken, prevents entry of pathogens
B. Give strength to the dermis
C. Detect changes in the external environment
D. Contains the accessory structures of the skin, such as glands
E. Made of both living and nonliving cells
F. Mitosis takes place to produce new epidermis
G. Stores fat
H. Acts as a barrier to ultraviolet light
I. Stimulated by exercise or heat

▶ VOCABULARY

Match the word with its definition.

1. _____ Absence or loss of hair, especially of the head

2. _____ A bruise of various size; the color may be blue-black, changing to greenish-brown or yellow with time

3. _____ Diffuse redness over the skin

4. _____ Small, purplish, hemorrhagic spots on the skin

5. _____ Resistance of the skin to being grasped between the fingers

A. Ecchymosis
B. Erythema
C. Petechiae
D. Turgor
E. Alopecia

▶ PRIMARY SKIN LESIONS

Match the lesion with its description.

1. _____ Macule
2. _____ Papule
3. _____ Nodule
4. _____ Vesicle
5. _____ Bulla
6. _____ Pustule
7. _____ Wheal
8. _____ Plaque
9. _____ Cyst

A. Solid elevated lesion
B. Vesicle or blister larger than 1 cm
C. Flat, nonpalpable change in skin color
D. Round, transient elevation of the skin caused by dermal edema and surrounding capillary dilation
E. Patch or solid, raised lesion on the skin or mucous membrane that is greater than 1 cm
F. Palpable solid raised lesion
G. Small elevation of skin or vesicle or bulla that contains pus
H. Closed sac or pouch tumor that consists of semisolid, solid, or liquid material
I. Small raised area that contains serous fluid, less than 0.5 cm

▶ DIAGNOSTIC SKIN TESTS

Match the test with its definition.

1. _____ Skin biopsy
2. _____ Wood's light examination
3. _____ Scratch test
4. _____ Patch test

A. Superficial testing with allergen for immediate reaction
B. Excision of small piece of tissue for microscopic assessment
C. Superficial testing with allergen for delayed hypersensitivity reaction
D. Use of ultraviolet rays to detect fluorescent materials in skin and hair

▶ CRITICAL THINKING

Read the case study and answer the questions.

Mr. Carr is admitted to a medical unit after having a hemorrhagic stroke. His vital signs are stable, but he is disoriented except to person. He is on bed rest and is often restless. He responds appropriately to questions intermittently. His left side is flaccid, but he can move his right side. The nurse notes that Mr. Carr rarely moves himself into a different position. He is of thin build. He is receiving an intravenous of dextrose 5 percent/0.9-percent normal saline. He has difficulty swallowing and has not eaten. Mr. Carr is diaphoretic and his linen is damp.

1. Why is Mr. Carr at high risk for developing pressure ulcers? _____

_____

_____

2. How many calories is Mr. Carr receiving? _____

_____

_____

3. What are priority nursing diagnoses and nursing interventions for Mr. Carr related to his skin needs? _____

_____

_____

4. Why would a pressure-relieving device be appropriate for Mr. Carr? _____

_____

_____

REVIEW QUESTIONS

Choose the best answer.

1. Which of the following is the mechanism of heat loss that depends on evaporation?
   A. Sweating
   B. Fat storage
   C. Vasoconstriction in the dermis
   D. Vasodilation in the dermis

2. How do arterioles in the dermis respond to a cold environment?
   A. Dilate to release heat
   B. Constrict to release heat
   C. Dilate to conserve heat
   D. Constrict to conserve heat

3. Which of the following is the tissue that stores fat in subcutaneous tissue?
   A. Fibrous connective tissue
   B. Stratified squamous epithelium
   C. Adipose tissue
   D. Areolar connective tissue

4. When the ultraviolet rays of the sun strike the skin, they stimulate the formation of which of the following?
   A. Vitamin A and keratin
   B. Melanin and vitamin D
   C. Sebum and vitamin A
   D. Keratin and melanin

5. Which of the following is the layer of skin that, if unbroken, prevents the entry of most pathogens?
   A. Stratum corneum
   B. Papillary layer
   C. Stratum germinativum
   D. Dermis

6. White blood cells, which destroy pathogens that enter breaks in the skin, are found in which of the following?
   A. Stratum corneum
   B. Keratinized layer
   C. Subcutaneous tissue
   D. Adipose cells

7. In which of the following developmental age-groups would less elasticity and moisture of the skin be a normal finding?
   A. Adolescent
   B. Young adult
   C. Middle-aged adult
   D. Elderly adult

8. Which of the following terms is used to document a bluish discoloration of the skin?
   A. Cyanosis
   B. Erythema
   C. Jaundice
   D. Pallor

9. The nurse understands that an elderly person may be more sensitive to cold temperatures due to which of the following?
   A. Slower cell division in the epidermis
   B. Deterioration of collagen and elastin fibers
   C. Less fat in the subcutaneous layer
   D. Death of melanocytes in the skin

10. The nurse is caring for a patient with a skin tear. Which of the following dressings is most appropriate for the nurse to apply to a skin tear?
    A. Moist sterile gauze
    B. Hydrocolloid
    C. Paste
    D. Transparent dressing

11. Which of the following actions should the nurse take when new petechiae are observed on the patient's skin?
    A. Cleanse the skin.
    B. Apply warm, moist compresses.
    C. Inform the registered nurse or physician.
    D. Apply heat to the area.

51

NURSING CARE OF PATIENTS WITH SKIN DISORDERS

▶ VOCABULARY

Match the word with its definition.

1. _____ To lose color

2. _____ Inflammation of cellular or connective tissue

3. _____ Skin lesion that occurs in acne vulgaris

4. _____ Inflammation of the skin

5. _____ A fungal infection of the skin

6. _____ Acute or chronic inflammatory skin condition

7. _____ The growth of skin over a wound

8. _____ Hard scab or dry crust from necrotic tissue

9. _____ Removal of a slough or scab formed on skin and underlying tissue of severely burned skin

10. _____ Thickened or hardened from continued irritation

11. _____ Disease of the nails due to fungus

12. _____ Infestation with lice

13. _____ Acute or chronic serious skin disease characterized by the appearance of bullae (blisters) of various sizes on normal skin and mucous membranes

14. _____ Severe itching

15. _____ Chronic inflammatory skin disorder in which epidermal cells proliferate abnormally quickly

16. _____ Describes fluid that contains pus

17. _____ Any acute, inflammatory, purulent bacterial dermatitis

18. _____ Disease of the sebaceous glands marked by increase in the amount, and often alteration of the quality, of sebaceous secretion

19. _____ Describes fluid consisting of serum and blood

A. Serosanguineous
B. Seborrhea
C. Pyoderma
D. Purulent
E. Psoriasis
F. Pruritus
G. Pemphigus
H. Pediculosi
I. Onychomycosis
J. Lichenified
K. Escharotomy
L. Eschar
M. Epithelialization
N. Eczema
O. Dermatophytosis
P. Dermatitis
Q. Comedone
R. Cellulitis
S. Blanch

► BENIGN SKIN LESIONS

Match the lesion with its definition.

1. _____ Cyst
2. _____ Seborrheic keratosis
3. _____ Keloid
4. _____ Pigmented nevi
5. _____ Warts
6. _____ Hemangiomas

A. Small, common growths caused by a virus
B. Vascular tumors of dilated blood vessels
C. Saclike growth with a definite wall
D. Scar formation at site of trauma or surgical incision
E. Light brown to dark brown patches, plaques, or papules that occur mainly in older patients
F. Flesh colored to dark brown macule or papule

► PLASTIC SURGERY PROCEDURES

Fill in the blanks.

1. A _____ is done to correct nasal septal defects.

2. A _____ is referred to as a rhytidoplasty.

3. Removal of bags under the eyes is known as _____ .

► CRITICAL THINKING

Read the case study and answer the questions.

Mrs. Miller, age 59, is admitted for a femoral-popliteal bypass graft. She has non-insulin-dependent diabetes mellitus. After surgery, she is in the intensive care unit (ICU) and is hypotensive for 24 hours. Her leg is painful and she barely moves. During her bath, the nurse notes a dark red-black area 4 inches in diameter and 2 inches deep on her sacral area and a reddened oozing area on the heel of her right foot.

1. Why did these dark red-black and red areas develop? _____

_____

2. To plan Mrs. Miller's care, what stage are these discolored areas? _____

_____

The surgeon is notified of these areas and orders turning every 2 hours, elevation of the right foot, and a sheepskin pad.

3. What is the benefit and effectiveness of each of these ordered interventions? _____

_____

_____

4. Why should the nurse discuss the use of the sheepskin with the surgeon? _____

_____

_____

Choose the best answer.

1. Which of the following activities creates a mechanical force that the nurse understands can lead to the formation of a pressure ulcer?
   A. Massaging nonreddened areas
   B. Whirlpool baths
   C. Pulling a patient up in bed
   D. Range-of-motion exercises

2. The nurse notes a pressure ulcer on the left heel of a bedridden patient. The area is a deep crater with no damage to the muscle or bone. Which of the following defines the stage of this ulcer?
   A. Stage I
   B. Stage II
   C. Stage III
   D. Stage IV

3. Which of the following dressings does the nurse understand should be used on an infected stage III pressure ulcer?
   A. Sterile gauze
   B. Transparent film (Opsite)
   C. Hydrocolloid (DuoDERM)
   D. Occlusive

4. A patient has a wound with moderate blood-tinged fluid draining from it. Which of the following would be an appropriate description of this drainage for the nurse to document?
   A. Purulent drainage
   B. Serosanguineous drainage
   C. Copious drainage
   D. Serous drainage

5. Which of the following would be most appropriate for the nurse to use to clean a noninfected pressure ulcer?
   A. 45 psi pressure flushing
   B. Gentle flushing with a needleless 30-mL syringe.
   C. Gentle scrubbing with gauze and normal saline
   D. Flushing with a 30-mL syringe with an 18-gauge needle

6. The nurse finds the skin on the arms of a burn patient to be white and hard. It is inelastic and insensitive to pressure. Which of the following does the nurse understand this burn would be classified as?
   A. Superficial
   B. Superficial partial thickness
   C. Deep partial thickness
   D. Full thickness

7. A patient with full-thickness burns has surgery for skin grafting. One day postoperatively the area around the graft is red and warm, and there is a foul smell under the dressing. Which of the following actions would be most appropriate by the nurse?
   A. Remove the dressing.
   B. Apply an occlusive dressing.
   C. Apply an antibiotic ointment dressing.
   D. Notify the registered nurse and physician.

8. A 62-year-old woman is admitted to the hospital with a lesion on her face that is a small, pearly papule. It has a rolled, waxy edge with crusting and ulceration. Which of the following types of skin cancer does the nurse suspect?
   A. Basal cell
   B. Squamous cell
   C. Malignant melanoma

9. Which of the following does the nurse understand is the most metastatic type of skin cancer when planning care for a patient with skin cancer?
   A. Basal cell
   B. Squamous cell
   C. Malignant melanoma

10. A 92-year-old woman is admitted from a nursing home to the hospital for a colon resection. Four days postoperatively she reports that her perineum is sore. It is reddened and has whitish discharge. She has been on three intravenous antibiotics. Which of the following problems does the nurse suspect?
    A. Monilial intertrigo
    B. Psoriasis
    C. Herpes zoster
    D. Thrush

UNIT SIXTEEN

UNDERSTANDING THE IMMUNE SYSTEM

Review of Anatomy and Physiology	Major Disorders	Nursing Assessment	Diagnostic Tests	Interventions	Common Medications
☐ Immune:	☐ Immune:	☐ Medical history	☐ Blood studies	☐ Immunotherapy	☐ Antihistamines
☐ Antigens	☐ Allergic rhinitis	☐ Physical assessment	☐ Radiographic tests	☐ Surgical management	☐ Antiretrovirals
☐ Lymphocytes	☐ Atopic dermatitis		☐ Biopsies	☐ New therapies	☐ Corticosteroids
☐ Antibodies	☐ Anaphylaxis		☐ Skin tests		☐ Epinephrine
☐ Mechanisms of immunity	☐ Urticaria		☐ Gene testing		☐ Immunosuppressives
☐ Types of immunity	☐ Angioedema				☐ Immunoglobulin
☐ Aging effects	☐ Hemolytic transfusion reaction				☐ Non-nucleoside analog reverse transcriptase inhibitors
	☐ Serum sickness				☐ Nucleoside analog reverse transcriptase inhibitors
	☐ Contact dermatitis				☐ Nucleotide analogue reverse transcriptase inhibitors
	☐ Transplant rejection				☐ Protease inhibitors
	☐ Pernicious anemia				☐ Ribonucleotide reductase onhibitors
	☐ Idiopathic autoimmune hemolytic anemia				☐ Rho (D) immune globulin (RhoGAM)
	☐ Hashimoto's thyroiditis				☐ Thyroxine
	☐ Ankylosing spondylitis				☐ Vitamin B_{12}
	☐ Hypogamma-globulinemia				
	☐ Human immuno-deficiency virus (HIV)/Acquired immune deficiency syndrome (AIDS)				

52

IMMUNE SYSTEM FUNCTION, ASSESSMENT, AND THERAPEUTIC MEASURES

▶ **STRUCTURES OF THE IMMUNE SYSTEM**

Label the following structures.

▶ IMMUNE SYSTEM CELLS

Match each cell of the immune system with the correct description.

1. _____ Memory cells

2. _____ Helper T cells

3. _____ Cytotoxic T cells

4. _____ Plasma cells

5. _____ Suppressor T cells

6. _____ Macrophages

7. _____ B cells

A. Phagocytize pathogens labeled with antibodies
B. Produce antibodies
C. Limit the immune response once the pathogen has been destroyed
D. Initiate a rapid immune response if the pathogen reenters the body
E. Destroy cells directly by lysing their membranes
F. May become plasma cells or memory cells
G. Participate in antigen recognition and activate B cells

▶ ANTIBODIES

Name the proper class of antibodies for each of these functions.

1. Found on mucous membranes: _____

2. Provides long-term immunity: _____

3. Form the receptors on B cells: _____

4. Important in allergic reactions: _____

5. Cross the placenta to fetal circulation: _____

6. Found in breast milk: _____

7. The first antibody produced in an infection: _____

▶ VOCABULARY

Fill in the blank.

1. _____ are chemical markers that identify cells or molecules.

2. _____ is the ability to destroy pathogens or other foreign material and to prevent further cases of certain infectious diseases.

3. _____, _____, and _____ are the three types of lymphocytes.

4. _____ mature in the thymus gland.

5. Antibodies are also called _____.

6. _____ is the type of immunity that involves only T cells.

7. _____ is the type of immunity in which a person has recovered from a disease and now has antibodies and memory cells specific for that pathogen.

8. The immunoglobulin _____ crosses the placenta and provides long-term immunity following recovery from an illness.

9. Lymph node enlargement with tenderness is usually indicative of _____.

10. The _____ of a white blood cell differential are increased in bacterial and acute infection.

▶ IMMUNE SYSTEM

Match the word with the definition.

1. _____ Allergy shots

2. _____ Tests for antibodies to human immunodeficiency virus (HIV), used as

   a screening test

3. _____ Important in allergic reactions and attaches to mast cells

4. _____ Swelling around the eyes

5. _____ A test done to confirm a diagnosis, determine a prognosis, or evaluate

   effectiveness of treatment

6. _____ Found in secretions of all mucous membranes

7. _____ Itching

8. _____ An abnormal protein found in plasma during an acute inflammatory process

A. Periorbital edema
B. Biopsies
C. Pruritus
D. Enzyme-linked immunosorbent assay
E. IgE
F. C-reactive protein
G. Immunotherapy
H. IgA

▶ NURSING ASSESSMENT—SUBJECTIVE (HISTORY)

Find the 12 errors and correct the information.

Demographic data

The patient's age, gender, race, and ethnic background are important. Systemic lupus erythematosus affects men eight times more frequently than women. The patient's place of birth gives insight to ethnic ties. Where the patient has lived and does live may shed light on the current illness. The patient's occupation such as that of a coal miner may contribute to gastrointestinal symptoms.

Rare signs and symptoms found with immune system disorders include fever, fatigue, joint pain, swollen glands, weight gain, and skin rash.

History

Food, medication, and environmental allergies should include those that the patient experiences and those present in the family history. With a family history, a previous exposure to a substance is required before a severe reaction occurs. Conditions such as allergic rhinitis, systemic lupus erythematosus, ankylosing spondylitis, and asthma are thought to be either familial or have a congenital genetic predisposition. If the patient's thymus gland has been removed (thymectomy), B-cell production may be altered. Corticosteroids and immunosuppressants enhance the immune response. The patient's lifestyle may place the patient at low risk for contracting the HIV. The patient's diet and usage of vitamins give insight into the depletion reserve of the immune system. Stress (environmental, physical, and psychological) can enhance immune system function.

▶ CRITICAL THINKING

Read the case study and answer the following questions.

David Case, age 29, is visiting the physician because he has been extremely fatigued for several months and now has swollen lymph nodes in his neck. On palpation, the area feels enlarged, nontender, hard, and fixed.

1. What categories of data collection should the nurse obtain? _____

   _____

   _____

2. What might the palpation findings indicate? _____

   _____

3. What categories of data collection would be important to explore in detail? _____

_____

_____

Choose the best answer.

1. A baby is born temporarily immune to the diseases to which the mother is immune. The nurse understands that this is an example of which of the following types of immunity?
   A. Naturally acquired passive immunity
   B. Artificially acquired passive immunity
   C. Naturally acquired active immunity
   D. Artificially acquired active immunity

2. Immunity to a disease after recovery is possible because the first exposure to the pathogen has stimulated the formation of which of the following?
   A. Antigens
   B. Memory cells
   C. Complement
   D. Natural killer cells

3. CD4$^+$ T-cell levels can be elevated in patients with which of the following conditions?
   A. An autoimmune disorder
   B. Cancer
   C. Acquired immune deficiency syndrome
   D. Allergies

4. Which of the following is the function of macrophages and neutrophils?
   A. Phagocytosis
   B. Antibody production
   C. Complement fixation
   D. Suppression of autoimmunity

5. The activation of B cells in immoral immunity is assisted by which of the following?
   A. Cytotoxic T cells
   B. Helper T cells
   C. Suppressor T cells
   D. Neutrophils

6. Which of the following are chemical markers that identify cells or molecules?
   A. Antibodies
   B. Antigens
   C. T cells
   D. B lymphocytes

7. The thymus gland role with the immune system is which of the following?
   A. Maturates B cells
   B. Maturates red blood cells
   C. Maturates platelets
   D. Maturates T cells

8. Which of the following types of cells is the immune system's shutoff mechanism?
   A. Plasma cells
   B. Helper T cells
   C. Suppressor T cells
   D. B lymphocytes

9. Which of the following is the humoral immune response?
   A. B cells phagocytize the foreign antigen.
   B. T cells are stimulated by B cells and turn into plasma cells, which produce antibodies or memory cells.
   C. B cells are stimulated by T helper cells or macrophages and turn into plasma cells, which produce antibodies or memory cells.
   D. T cells produce antibodies.

10. Mrs. Miller's children were just diagnosed with chickenpox. Mrs. Miller had chickenpox as a child and is not concerned with contracting the disease when caring for her children. What type of immunity does Mrs. Miller have?
    A. Active natural immunity
    B. Passive natural immunity
    C. Passive artificial immunity
    D. Active artificial immunity

11. Autoimmunity is defined as a phenomenon involving which of the following?
    A. Production of endotoxins that destroy B lymphocytes
    B. Inability to differentiate self from nonself
    C. Overproduction of reagin antibody
    D. Depression of the immune response

12. Antibodies are made of which of the following types of substances?
    A. Fat
    B. Sugar
    C. Protein
    D. Carbohydrate

13. Which of the following immunoglobulins is first produced during an acute infection?
    A. IgG
    B. IgM
    C. IgE
    D. IgD

53

NURSING CARE OF PATIENTS WITH IMMUNE DISORDERS

► VOCABULARY

Match the term with its definition.

1. _____ An anaphylactic-type reaction

2. _____ The type of antibodies that attach to mast cells

3. _____ Elimination of the offending environmental stimuli

4. _____ Very dry, pruritic, edematous skin

5. _____ Sudden, severe reaction characterized by smooth muscle spasms and capillary permeability changes

6. _____ Urticaria

7. _____ Types of drugs used to prevent transplant rejection

8. _____ Painless subcutaneous and dermal erythemic eruptions with diffuse edema

9. _____ Requires lifelong vitamin B_{12} injections

10. _____ Red blood cell (RBC) fragments seen with microscope

11. _____ Infant may be asymptomatic until 6 months old

12. _____ Causes may include heat, cold, pressure, and stress

13. _____ Patient education includes a diet low in iodine and high in bulk, protein, and carbohydrates

14. _____ Patient education includes frequent movement and the use of a hard mattress and no pillow when sleeping

A. Urticaria
B. Angioedema
C. Anaphylaxis
D. Pernicious anemia
E. Hashimoto's thyroiditis
F. Idiopathic autoimmune hemolytic anemia
G. Hypogammaglobulinemia
H. Allergic rhinitis
I. Hives
J. Type I
K. IgE
L. Ankylosing spondylitis
M. Atopic dermatitis
N. Immunosuppressive

▶ IMMUNE DISORDERS

Fill in the blank.

1. The way hypersensitivity reactions are classified include _____ , _____ , _____ , and _____ .

2. When allergic rhinitis occurs seasonally, it is called _____ .

3. Complications of allergic rhinitis are _____ , _____ , _____ , and _____ .

4. _____ is a complication of atopic dermatitis.

5. The first drug of choice for anaphylaxis is _____ .

6. Urticaria is commonly called _____ .

7. Angioedema differs from urticaria in that angioedema _____ , _____ , and _____ .

8. The _____ is used to diagnose a hemolytic transfusion reaction.

9. _____ and _____ are two complications that can occur with a hemolytic transfusion reaction.

10. Today, serum sickness tends to occur when _____ and _____ are administered to patients.

11. _____ and _____ are two food additives that can trigger an anaphylactic reaction.

12. _____ is the most common cause of contact dermatitis.

13. Patients with pernicious anemia are unable to absorb _____ .

14. _____ is a process whereby abnormal RBCs are removed and replaced with normal RBCs.

15. Ankylosing spondylitis is a chronic progressive inflammatory disease of the _____ , _____ , and _____ joints.

REVIEW QUESTIONS

Choose the best answer.

1. A patient has allergic rhinitis. In planning care for the patient, the nurse understands that if he does not remain compliant with his treatment, he is at risk for developing which of the following?
    A. Sinusitis
    B. Anaphylaxis
    C. Lymphadenopathy
    D. Angioedema

2. A patient reports on admission that she was "very sick" with erythromycin in the past. She is to receive erythromycin now. Which of the following actions should the nurse take regarding giving the antibiotic?
    A. Give the antibiotic.
    B. Give half of the dose.
    C. Do not give the antibiotic.
    D. Give the antibiotic as the patient's condition requires it.

3. A patient is given penicillin via intravenous piggyback and develops an anaphylactic reaction. Which of the following should be the nurse's first action?
    A. Call the doctor.
    B. Call for help.
    C. Maintain the antibiotic.
    D. Turn off the antibiotic.

4. As the nurse assesses a patient, which of the following is a symptom that may be found that the patient with anaphylaxis may be experiencing?
    A. Dermatitis
    B. Delirium
    C. Sinusitis
    D. Wheezing

5. Which of the following is the medication of choice for anaphylaxis that the nurse should anticipate would be ordered?
    A. Epinephrine
    B. Theophylline (Theo-Dur)
    C. Digoxin (Lanoxin)
    D. Furosemide (Lasix)

6. A patient is admitted with a 2-month history of fatigue, shortness of breath, pallor, and dizziness. She is diagnosed with idiopathic autoimmune hemolytic anemia. On reviewing her laboratory results, the nurse notes which of the following that confirms this diagnosis?
    A. RBC fragments
    B. Macrocytic, normochromic RBCs
    C. Microcytic, hypochromic RBCs
    D. Hemoglobin molecules

7. A patient, age 45, has had a portion of his stomach removed. He must take vitamin B$_{12}$ injections. If the patient does not take the vitamin B$_{12}$ injections, he will develop which of the following?
    A. Iron deficiency anemia
    B. Pernicious anemia
    C. Sickle cell anemia
    D. Acquired hemolytic anemia

8. A patient is diagnosed with Hashimoto's thyroiditis and asks what causes it. The nurse would respond that the destruction of the thyroid in this condition is due to which of the following?
    A. Antigen-antibody complexes
    B. Autoantibodies
    C. Viral infection
    D. Bacterial infection

9. Which of the following is a disease process characterized by a chronic progressive inflammation of the sacroiliac and costovertebral joints and adjacent soft tissue?
    A. Rheumatoid arthritis
    B. Kyphosis
    C. Scoliosis
    D. Ankylosing spondylitis

10. A patient was walking in the woods when she disturbed a beehive. She asks to be taken to the emergency department immediately because she is allergic to bee stings. Which of the following symptoms would the nurse expect to see upon admission?
    A. Pallor around the sting bites
    B. Numbness and tingling in the extremities
    C. Respiratory stridor
    D. Retinal hemorrhage

11. A 45-year-old patient has a long-standing history of allergies to pollen. Which of the following actions indicates that the patient does not understand how to control this disease?
    A. Staying indoors on dry, windy days
    B. Driving her car with the windows open
    C. Refusing to walk outside in the spring
    D. Working in her garden on sunny days

12. The nurse would evaluate that the patient understands what triggers allergic rhinitis by which of the following patient responses?
    A. "Parenteral medications"
    B. "Topical creams and ointments"
    C. "Ingested food and medications"
    D. "Airborne pollens and molds"

13. The nurse understands that an anaphylactic reaction is considered which of the following types of hypersensitivity reactions?
    A. Type I
    B. Type II
    C. Type III
    D. Type IV

14. As the nurse cares for a patient with angioedema, the nurse understands that angioedema differs from urticaria in that angioedema is characterized by which of the following?
    A. Angioedema is more pruritic.
    B. Angioedema has a deeper and more widespread edema.
    C. Angioedema has small, fluid-filled vesicles that crust.
    D. Angioedema lasts a shorter time.

54

NURSING CARE OF PATIENTS WITH HIV DISEASE/AIDS

► VOCABULARY
Fill in the blank with the correct term.

1. _____ is the final phase of a chronic, progressive immune function disorder caused by the human immunodeficiency virus (HIV).

2. The _____ is an important part of the human immune system and defends the body against very primitive invaders such as fungi, yeast, and other viruses.

3. _____ is a diagnostic test done to detect antibodies to HIV antigen on test plates.

4. _____ are a primary complication of HIV infection and invade the body because of an impaired immune system.

5. _____ occurs in most patients with the acquired immune deficiency syndrome (AIDS) and is characterized by the occurrence of an involuntary baseline body weight loss of more than 10 percent and weakness or fever for more than 30 days or chronic diarrhea of two loose stools daily for more than 30 days.

6. _____ measures the amount of HIV RNA in plasma and is extremely important for determining prognosis and monitoring the response to antiretroviral therapy.

► DIAGNOSTIC TESTS
Describe the procedure, and preprocedure and postprocedure care, for each of the following diagnostic tests.

1. Enzyme-linked immunosorbent assay (ELISA) test _____

   _____

   _____

   _____

2. Viral load _____

   _____

   _____

3. CD4$^+$ cell count _____

   _____

   _____

▶ HIV

a. HIV is transmitted through _____, _____, and _____.

b. HIV may stay latent for _____ years.

c. Fatigue, headache, fever, and generalized lymphadenopathy may be seen during the _____ stages of HIV infection.

d. _____ are increasingly becoming infected with HIV.

▶ HIV AND AIDS

Indicate whether the following are true or false, and correct false statements.

1. If a health care worker is stuck with a needle from a patient with AIDS, exposure to the virus may occur even if gloves were worn. _____

2. HIV is caused by AIDS. _____

3. Individuals who are not men who have sex with men or who are intravenous drug users probably do not need to worry about contracting HIV and developing AIDS. _____

4. If the nurse suctions a patient with a fresh tracheostomy who is diagnosed with HIV and blood-tinged sputum gets in the nurse's eyes, the nurse may contract the virus. _____

5. Once a person is infected with HIV, the diagnosis can be made using laboratory tests within 1 to 2 days.

_____

6. A patient with AIDS should always be put into isolation for the protection of health care workers.

_____

▶ CRITICAL THINKING

Answer the following questions.

1. Jack Swope, age 26, has been diagnosed HIV positive. He asks, "Do I have AIDS and am I going to die?" What should you say to him? _____

_____

_____

2. When is the patient with HIV considered to have AIDS? _____

_____

3. Jack now is diagnosed with AIDS with a CD4$^+$ count of 200. At this time, he is asymptomatic. He is started on Bactrim (Septra). Why? _____

_____

4. (a) Jack is 6 feet tall and weighs 135 lb. He is malnourished. Why? _____

_____

(b) What can you do as a nurse to improve Jack's nutrition? _____

_____

5. Six months after being diagnosed with AIDS, Jack develops dementia. Why? _____

_____

6. How can a nurse contract HIV from a patient? _____
_____

7. How should the home health nurse teach family members of a patient with AIDS to clean the patient's home? _____
_____

Choose the best answer.

1. The nurse understands that a common method of HIV transmission is via which of the following?
   A. Saliva
   B. Tears
   C. Breast milk
   D. Semen

2. Which of the following would the nurse evaluate as laboratory data that support the occurrence of AIDS?
   A. Viral load (HIV RNA) 10,000 copies/mL, 900 CD4+ cells
   B. Viral load (HIV RNA) 12,000 copies/mL, 700 CD4+ cells
   C. Viral load (HIV RNA) 20,000 copies/mL, 500 CD4+ cells
   D. Viral load (HIV RNA) 24,000 copies/mL, 200 CD4+ cells

3. Which of the following diets would the nurse include in the plan of care for a person with AIDS?
   A. A high-protein, high-calorie diet divided into six small meals
   B. A low-fat, soft diet divided into eight small meals
   C. A high-carbohydrate, fat-restricted diet divided into four meals
   D. A high-fat, high-calorie diet divided into three meals

4. Which of the following is an appropriate nursing intervention to prevent infection in patients with AIDS?
   A. Prohibiting patients who are severely immunodeficient from having visitors
   B. Obtaining a low-microbial diet for patient with CD4+ cell count of less than 500
   C. Wearing protective gear such as gown, mask, gloves, and goggles when entering the room
   D. Ensuring protective barrier isolation precautions are in place

5. A patient who is being tested for HIV asks what tests are used. The nurse would be correct in stating that the test used to confirm HIV infection is which of the following?
   A. CD4+ cell count and thymus function
   B. B-cell and T-cell count
   C. ELISA and Western blot
   D. CD4+, viral load, and ELISA

6. The nurse is caring for a patient with HIV who has diarrhea. Which of the following would be most therapeutic to teach the patient to avoid in the diet to reduce diarrhea?
   A. Potassium-rich food
   B. Raw fruits and vegetables
   C. Liquid nutritional supplements
   D. Frozen products

7. The nurse is teaching a patient newly diagnosed with AIDS about complications of the disease. Which of the following is the most common malignancy seen with AIDS?
   A. Kaposi's sarcoma
   B. Liver cancer
   C. Pancreatic cancer
   D. Stomach cancer

8. The nurse is taking vital signs of a pregnant woman during her first prenatal visit. The patient asks the nurse if she has to have an HIV test. Which of the following is the nurse's best response?
   A. "Yes, all pregnant women must have the test."
   B. "If you do not have multiple sex partners or inject drugs, it is not necessary."
   C. "Governmental guidelines require an HIV test for all pregnant woman."
   D. "After voluntary pretest counseling, you decide whether HIV testing should be done."

9. The nurse is caring for a patient with HIV. Which of the following foods would the nurse teach the patient is safe to eat to reduce the risk of infection?
   A. Raw fruits
   B. Cooked vegetables
   C. Raw vegetables
   D. Caesar dressing

10. When caring for a patient with AIDS, which of the following nursing actions would be most appropriate for infection control?
    A. Wear gloves at all times.
    B. Wear gloves for blood/body fluid contact.
    C. Wear gown and mask at all times.
    D. Wear a mask during patient contact times.

UNIT SEVENTEEN

UNDERSTANDING MENTAL HEALTH CARE

Review of Basic Concepts	Major Disorders	Nursing Assessment	Diagnostic Tests	Interventions	Common Medications
☐ Mental health	☐ Anxiety disorders	☐ Appearance and behavior	☐ DSM-IV	☐ Milieu therapy	☐ Antipsychotics
☐ Mental illness	☐ Mood disorders	☐ Reality orientation	☐ Blood tests	☐ Psychoanalysis	☐ Antianxiety agents
☐ Nature vs. nurture	☐ Somatoform disorders	☐ Thinking	☐ Computed tomography (CT) scan	☐ Behavior modification	☐ Antidepressants
☐ Psychoanalytic theory	☐ Schizophrenia	☐ Memory	☐ Positron emission therapy (PET) scan	☐ Cognitive therapies	☐ Stimulants
☐ Psychobiologic theory	☐ Substance abuse disorders	☐ Speech		☐ Person-centered therapy	☐ Antiparkinsonism agents
☐ Coping		☐ Mood and affect		☐ Counseling	
		☐ Judgment		☐ Group therapy	
		☐ Perception		☐ Electroconvulsive therapy (ECT)	
				☐ Relaxation therapy	

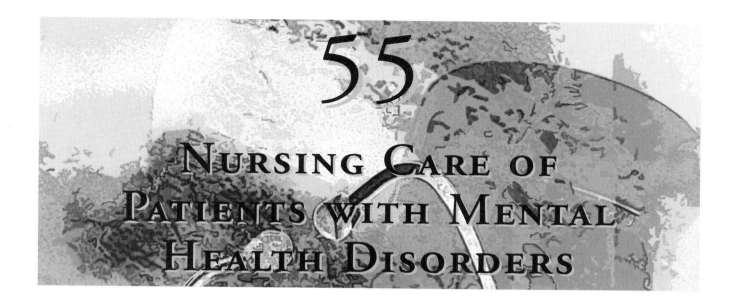

55

NURSING CARE OF PATIENTS WITH MENTAL HEALTH DISORDERS

▶ VOCABULARY

Fill in the blanks with the correct terms.

1. _____ is the way one adapts to a stressor.

2. The ability to think rationally and process thoughts is referred to as _____ ability.

3. _____ is the use of medication to treat psychological disorders.

4. Computerized instruments are used to provide information about behavior in _____ therapy.

5. An irrational fear is called a/an _____ .

6. A repetitive thought or urge is called a/an _____ .

7. Manic-depressive illness is also called _____ depression.

8. Physical symptoms that have no known organic cause may indicate the presence of a/an _____ disorder.

9. People with_____ cannot distinguish between their reality and society's reality.

10. Abrupt withdrawal from alcohol may cause a disorder called _____ _____ .

▶ DEFENSE MECHANISMS

Label the defense mechanism being used in each of the following statements.

1. The patient with cancer says, "I know if I take my vitamins I'll be fine." _____

2. The student who comes unprepared to a clinical says, "I woke up late because my instructor gave us too much work to do and I had to stay up all night, and my kids are sick and the car isn't working." _____

3. The man who always wanted to be a lawyer but was not accepted into law school says, "Lawyers are all crooked. I would never trust one." _____

4. The teen who didn't make the football team says, "I've decided to give up trying to play in sports. I'm much better at piano." _____

5. The woman who was raped says, "Why are you calling me to set up rape counseling? I was not raped and I do not need counseling." _____

6. The man who is passed over for a promotion yells at his son for a minor mistake: "You are so stupid. You never do anything right." _____

7. An adolescent says to his mother, "I got a B on my project because you made me do chores too long." _____

8. The woman who cheated on an examination turns in extra work and states, "Here is some extra work I did. I really want to learn this material." _____

9. A teen tells her date, "I'm sorry I can't go out tonight; I have to wash my hair." _____

10. The student nurse tells the instructor, "I don't think I can do that catheter. I am feeling sick to my stomach. I think I ate some bad food in the cafeteria." _____

▶ CRITICAL THINKING

Read the case study and answer the following questions.

Mrs. Jewel is a 48-year-old woman admitted to your unit with cellulitis of her lower legs and diabetes mellitus. She is disabled because of arthritis and morbid obesity. As you collect some initial data, you notice that her hair is dirty and unkempt, her clothes are dirty, and she has an unpleasant body odor. You also find that she does not appear to have a good understanding of her health or self-care needs. You decide to assess her mental status.

1. What factors related to Mrs. Jewel's appearance provide information about her mental status? How can you find out if this is unusual behavior for her? _____
_____
_____

2. Mrs. Jewel is alert. What questions can you ask to assess orientation? _____
_____
_____

3. How might you determine whether Mrs. Jewel's thought processes are intact? _____
_____
_____

4. What questions can you ask to assess Mrs. Jewel's recent and remote memory? _____
_____
_____

5. How do you assess speech and ability to communicate? _____
_____
_____

6. You determine that Mrs. Jewel's affect is inappropriate. What does this mean? _____
_____
_____

7. How can you assess Mrs. Jewel's judgment? _____
_____
_____

8. How can perception be assessed? _____
_____
_____

REVIEW QUESTIONS

Choose the best answer.

1. Which of the following sources of data will best help the nurse determine if the patient has a threat to his or her mental health?
   A. Intelligence testing
   B. Behavior and its appropriateness to the situation
   C. Opinion of his or her doctor
   D. Opinion of family members

2. Which of the following defense mechanisms is being used by the person who always seems to blame others for his problems?
   A. Denial
   B. Projection
   C. Rationalization
   D. Transference

3. Which of the following nursing actions is necessary for psychotherapy to be effective?
   A. Encourage the patient to repress feelings.
   B. Punish inappropriate behavior.
   C. Establish a therapeutic patient—staff relationship.
   D. Give the patient advice as to how to solve the problem.

4. A patient being treated with haloperidol (Haldol) for organic dementia becomes hard to arouse, then stays sleepy after the next three doses. You know that sedation may occur with this drug. As his nurse, which of the following actions should you take first?
   A. Notify your supervisor or physician according to agency policy.
   B. Realize that tolerance will occur and continue giving the drug.
   C. Discontinue the drug immediately.
   D. Administer an antidote.

5. Which of the following responses to anxiety is a cause for concern?
   A. A student studies late into the night to prepare for a difficult examination.
   B. A woman takes deep breaths before going into the grocery store because shopping makes her nervous.
   C. A pilot has an alcoholic drink before a stressful flight.
   D. A young man gets the opinions of several of his friends before asking a woman out.

6. Which of the following nursing actions is appropriate immediately following electroconvulsive therapy?
   A. Restrain the patient's extremities for 24 hours.
   B. Stay with the patient until he or she is oriented.
   C. Discharge the patient to home with instructions to rest.
   D. Administer oxygen at 6 L per minute.

7. The nurse is collecting admission data on a new patient with a long health history. Which of the following life events is considered a stressor?
   A. Gallbladder surgery at age 46
   B. Divorce at age 50
   C. Loss of job at age 55
   D. Whatever the patient says is stressful

8. A patient calls you into her room and says, "Quick, nurse, there is a dog in the corner. Please get him out. I am terrified of dogs." You see no dog in the corner. Which of the following responses is best?
   A. "You know we don't allow dogs in the hospital."
   B. "We have been through this before. You know full well that there is no dog in the corner."
   C. "I do not see a dog. Let's take a walk down to the snack room."
   D. "What kind of a dog is it? What makes you so scared of dogs?"

9. A patient is starting on lithium for bipolar disorder. Which of the following nutrients should be carefully maintained in his diet?
   A. Potassium
   B. Sodium
   C. Selenium
   D. Tyramine

10. The nurse is making a home visit to a patient with schizophrenia who has been noncompliant with taking medications. Which of the following sources of data is most reliable when determining if the patient has been taking medications as prescribed?
    A. Ask the patient.
    B. Ask the significant other.
    C. Count pills in the bottles.
    D. Check with the pharmacy to see if refills have been picked up.

11. Which of the following is one of the most effective treatments for alcoholism?
    A. Group support, such as Alcoholics Anonymous
    B. Drug therapy
    C. Electroconvulsive therapy
    D. Reducing but not totally eliminating alcohol consumption

12. Which of the following behaviors by the nurse may aggravate the behavior of a patient with schizophrenia?
    A. Providing written instructions on when to take medications
    B. Speaking in short, simple sentences
    C. Maintaining a structured environment
    D. Speaking in low tones to other staff members when the patient is present

1

ANSWERS

► VOCABULARY

Auscultation
Definition: Listening for sounds such as bowel or lung sound, usually with a stethoscope.

Assessment
Definition: Exploring a situation to gather information and data.

Critical thinking
Definition: Use of knowledge and skills to make the best decisions possible that increase the probability of a desirable outcome.

Inspection
Definition: The use of observation skills to systematically gather data that can be seen.

Objective data
Definition: Factual information obtained through physical assessment and diagnostic tests. Objective data are observable or knowable through the health care worker's five senses. Referred to as *signs*.

Palpation
Definition: The use of the fingers or hands to feel something.

Percussion
Definition: Tapping technique used by physicians and advanced practice nurses to determine the consistency of underlying tissues.

Subjective data
Definition: Information that is provided verbally by the patient and referred to as *symptoms*.

► SUBJECTIVE AND OBJECTIVE DATA

1. Subjective (symptom)
2. Subjective (symptom)
3. Objective (sign)
4. Objective (sign)
5. Subjective (symptom)
6. Objective (sign)
7. Subjective (symptom)
8. Objective (sign)
9. Subjective (symptom)
10. Subjective (symptom)
11. Objective (sign)
12. Objective (sign)
13. Subjective (symptom)
14. Objective (sign)
15. Objective (sign)

► INSPECTION, PERCUSSION, PALPATION, AUSCULTATION

1. **(D)**   6. **(C)**
2. **(C)**   7. **(D)**
3. **(C)**   8. **(A)**
4. **(C)**   9. **(C)**
5. **(A)**   10. **(B)**

► CRITICAL THINKING

There are many possible patient need categories for this patient. One category has been completed for feedback. (See the figure on page 249.)

► REVIEW QUESTIONS

The correct answers are in **boldface.**

1. **(c)** is a nursing diagnosis. (a, b, d) are medical diagnoses.
2. **(a)** is a medical diagnosis. (b, c, d) are nursing diagnoses.
3. **(b)** Palpation of the abdomen can alter auscultation findings. (a, c, d) are incorrect.
4. **(c)** Assessment, or collecting data, is the first step in the nursing process. (a, b, d) are not the first step in the nursing process.
5. **(a)** is correct. (b, c, d) do not define critical thinking and are examples of times when critical thinking may be used.
6. **(d)** Evaluation determines whether goals are achieved and interventions effective. (a, b, c) are initial steps in developing the nursing care plan.
7. **(a)** The licensed practical nurse/licensed vocational nurse (LPN/LVN) can collect data. (b, c, d) are all steps in the nursing process for which the registered nurse (RN) is responsible; the LPN/LVN may assist the RN with these.

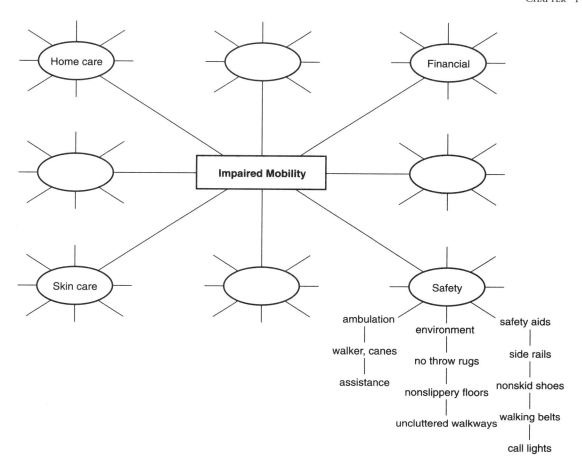

8. (**c**) is data the nurse can collect through use of the five senses. (a, b, d) are subjective data that the patient must report.

9. (**b**) indicates that the patient is concerned about freedom from injury and harm. (a) relates to basic needs such as air, oxygen, and water. (c) relates to feeling loved. (d) is related to having a positive self-esteem.

10. (**d**) is objective, realistic, and measurable with a time frame. (a, c) relate to the nursing diagnosis of impaired airway clearance. (b) relates to the nursing diagnosis of altered nutrition.

ANSWERS

▶ VOCABULARY

1. **(B)**   4. **(C)**
2. **(A)**   5. **(D)**
3. **(E)**   6. **(F)**

▶ ETHICAL AND LEGAL PRINCIPLES

1. state, protect, quality
2. caring
3. dignity, maintaining, family, right

▶ REVIEW QUESTIONS

The correct answers are in **boldface.**

1. **(b)** Laws are made to regulate citizen behaviors for the good of society. (a, c, d) are incorrect.
2. **(b)** The nurse-patient relationship is based on trust that the nurse will maintain all patient's rights. (a) is a constitutional right, not an ethical issue. (c) is a legal issue. (d) is not an ethical principle.
3. **(c)** is correct. (a, b, d) are incorrect.
4. **(a)** is correct. (b, c, d) are incorrect.
5. **(d)** is correct. (a, b, c) are incorrect.
6. **(b)** is the first step. (a,c,d) are incorrect.
7. **(a)** is correct. (b, c, d) are incorrect.
8. **(c)** is correct. (a, b, d) are incorrect.
9. **(b)** is correct. (a, c, d) are incorrect.
10. **(a)** is correct. (b, c, d) are incorrect.
11. **(d)** Criminal punishment can result in loss of freedom; (a, b, c) are related to civil liability.
12. **(a)** is correct. (b, c, d) are intentional torts.
13. **(c)** is correct; health care and legal systems can enforce treatment for contagious disease. (a) Generally patients can refuse any or all treatments, except in cases such as contagious disease. (b) The Patient's Self-Determination Act generally guarantees the right to refuse all treatments, except in certain cases. (d) Health care systems along with legal systems can force patients to take medications for contagious diseases.

3

ANSWERS

▶ VOCABULARY

1. **(B)**
2. **(C)**
3. **(I)**
4. **(G)**
5. **(D)**
6. **(E)**
7. **(F)**
8. **(J)**
9. **(H)**
10. **(A)**
11. **(K)**
12. **(L)**

▶ CULTURAL CHARACTERISTICS

1. Primary characteristics of culture include nationality, race, skin color, gender, age, and religious affiliation.
2. Secondary characteristics of culture include socioeconomic status, education, occupation, military status, political beliefs, length of time away from the country of origin, urban versus rural residence, marital status, parental status, physical attributes, sexual orientation, and gender issues.
3. Traditional practitioners are health care practitioners who are not native to the United States. They are native to some other country, although they may practice in the United States. Examples include curanderos, espirituistas, sobadors, diviners, and crystal gazers.
4. Present-oriented people accept the day as it comes with little regard for the past—the future is unpredictable. Future-oriented people anticipate a bigger and better future and place a high value on change. Some individuals balance all three views; they respect the past, enjoy living in the present, and plan for the future.

▶ CRITICAL THINKING: BATHING

1. In this patient's culture, it is improper for someone of the opposite sex to help with bathing.
2. Find a male nurse's aide, ask a family member to help, or skip the bath again.
3. Having a male aide do the bath is the best solution. If no male aide is available, the family may be approached for help, although this is not the best solution. Because this is the fourth day without a bath, skipping the bath is not a good option.

▶ REVIEW QUESTIONS

*The correct answers are in **boldface**.*

1. **(a)** is correct. Many Native-Americans are not time conscious. She may not keep her appointment if you reschedule, so give the immunizations now. (b) is incorrect; she may not keep her appointment. (c) is incorrect; she may not return to have her stitches removed. (d) is incorrect; to ensure that the children get the immunizations, give them now.
2. **(c)** is correct. Many Hispanics are openly expressive of their grief. Her bereavement behaviors are culturally congruent. Remaining with her is supportive. (a) is incorrect; there is no need to call the cardiac arrest team. (b) is incorrect; lying on the floor is more disconcerting to the nurse than it is to the bereaved woman. (d) is incorrect. This is not the best intervention. Expressive bereavement is normal. However, a later strategy may include a sedative.
3. **(b)** is correct. Cupping is a traditional Chinese practice that is harmless in most cases. (a) is incorrect. Cupping is not considered child abuse. (c) is incorrect. The situation should be reported to the mother by the school nurse. (d) is incorrect. The nurse has acted in good faith and has done nothing wrong.
4. **(a)** is correct. In Arabic countries, organs can be purchased for transplantation. This is illegal in the United States. (b) is incorrect. The patient does not have an ethical dilemma; however, the nurse may have one. (c) is incorrect. There is no need to call the administrator. (d) is incorrect. Although there is no harm in giving him the telephone number, this does not take care of the immediate response. The organ center will tell him the same thing.
5. **(c)** is correct. Initially you must assess how traditional the family's food practices are before a dietary regimen can be set up. (a) is incorrect. Giving a traditional ethnic individual an exchange list of foods does not ensure that he or she will change dietary practices to an American food exchange list. Additionally, exchange lists are not recommended. (b) is incorrect. Being able to calculate calories does not ensure that the family knows how

to balance a diabetic diet. (d) is incorrect. Although this is certainly an option for the future, the initial step is to take a dietary assessment.

6. **(d)** is correct. Patients are allowed to have a Santero visit as long as he or she does not do anything to interfere with treatment or cause a safety problem. (a) is incorrect. It is not necessary to get the supervisor's permission. However, it is a good idea to let the supervisor know that a Santero is going to visit. (b) is incorrect. All religious counselors are allowed to visit. (c) is incorrect. The patient has the right to see her own religious counselor.

7. **(d)** is correct because family is usually very important to Hispanic patients' spirituality. (a) is incorrect. Large numbers of family members in the cafeteria may cause further disruption in the cafeteria. (b) is incorrect. Large groups in the lobby may cause overcrowding for other families. (c) is incorrect. All family members should be allowed to visit. It may help to have them choose a spokesperson to control visiting for this patient.

8. **(b)** is correct. Reducing portion size decreases the overall calorie and fat consumption. (a) is incorrect; telling a patient to not purchase lard does not mean she will comply. (c) is incorrect; rarely does a person bake two separate pies. The goal is to reduce overall fat and calorie consumption. (d) is incorrect; the goal is for the patient to reduce fat and calories.

9. **(b)** is correct. Because many Appalachians believe in self-reliance and helping themselves first, this is the best answer. (a) is incorrect. Scare tactics are not appropriate; she may live whether or not she receives radiation therapy. (c) is incorrect; this statement does not encourage patient advocacy. (d) is incorrect; radiation therapy may be the best choice for this type of cancer.

10. **(b)** is correct. Changing the schedule slightly is preferable to omitting the medication. (a) is incorrect. Blood levels can be maintained on a different schedule, as long as the doses are reasonably spread out. (c) is incorrect. Omitting the medication will alter blood levels. (d) is incorrect. It does not respect the patient's religious beliefs.

ANSWERS

► VOCABULARY

1. **(E)**
2. **(D)**
3. **(F)**
4. **(B)**
5. **(A)**
6. **(C)**

► COMPLEMENTARY THERAPY: PROGRESSIVE MUSCLE RELAXATION

Purpose:

To help the patient identify subtle levels of mental and physical tension that accompany stress and learn to respond to stress with relaxation rather than tension.

Teaching Plan:

See Table 4-4 in your textbook.

► CRITICAL THINKING

1. Feverfew is used for migraine headaches, inflammation, and menstrual problems, among other things.
2. Capsaicin is used for pain associated with a variety of disorders.
3. Several sources should be consulted before taking herbs. The Internet has a lot of good information, but the source should be carefully evaluated. A pharmacist knowledgeable in herbs and herb-drug interactions, as well as the primary physician or care provider, should be consulted.
4. "Mrs. Lawless, I am concerned that your herbs could interact with your heart failure medications. I will check with your doctor and the hospital pharmacist to be sure they are safe before you take them."

► REVIEW QUESTIONS

The correct answers are in **boldface.**

1. **(d)** is correct. Progressive muscle relaxation is being added to a traditional therapy, making it complementary. (a) is incorrect. Inhalers and oral medications are both traditional therapies for asthma. (b) is incorrect. Cardiac rehabilitation is a traditional therapy. (c) would be considered an alternative therapy because the Echinacea is being used in place of a traditional therapy.
2. **(a)** is correct. Hydrotherapy would be considered alternative because it is being used in place of nonsteroidal anti-inflammatory drugs. (b) is incorrect. Because chemotherapy is still being used, the addition of the spiritual healer would be considered complementary. (c) is incorrect; antibiotics and bronchodilators are both traditional medical therapy. (d) is incorrect. Aspirin is traditional therapy for a headache.
3. **(d)** is correct. The patient should keep his or her eyes closed during imagery, so this statement indicates more teaching is needed. (a, b, c) are all parts of guided imagery.
4. **(c)** is correct. Allopathy is the proper term for traditional western medicine. (a, b, d) are all nontraditional medical practices.
5. **(b)** is correct. Chiropractors do not perform surgery. (a, c, d) are potentially true, but the nurse needs to safeguard her patient by informing her that a chiropractor is not trained or qualified to do surgery.
6. **(a)** is correct; Echinacea has been shown in some studies to be potentially effective against colds and viruses. (b) is incorrect. Feverfew is used for headaches and inflammation, among other things. (c) is incorrect. Chamomile is used for anxiety. (d) is incorrect. Ginger is used for nausea.
7. **(b)** is correct. The primary care practitioner can help determine which alternative therapies are safe. (a) is incorrect. Any therapy can be potentially unsafe. (c) is incorrect. Many alternative therapies are safe when used correctly. (d) is incorrect. Alternative and complementary therapies can be effective for chronic pain.
8. **(c)** is correct. It is least appropriate to tell the patient he will be able to reduce his pain medications; this is a possibility, but not a guarantee. (a, b, d) are all appropriate measures to take before beginning to practice any new alternative therapy.

5

ANSWERS

▶ VOCABULARY

1. diffusion
2. isotonic
3. hypertonic
4. hypovolemia
5. cation
6. hypernatremia
7. hypokalemia
8. hypocalcemia
9. Acidosis
10. alkalosis

▶ DEHYDRATION

Corrections are in **boldface.**

Mrs. White is a 78-year-old woman admitted to 7 South with a diagnosis of severe dehydration. The licensed practical nurse/licensed vocational nurse (LPN/LVN) assigned to Mrs. White is asked to collect data related to fluid status. The LPN expects Mrs. White's blood pressure to be **elevated because of the shift of fluid from tissues to her bloodstream.** The nurse also finds Mrs. White's skin to be **taut and firm,** and she notes that the **urine is copious** and dark amber. She asks Mrs. White if she knows where she is and what day it is because she knows that severe dehydration may cause confusion. In addition, she initiates **intake and output measurements** because this is the most accurate way to monitor fluid balance.

- Blood pressure will be low, not elevated, due to loss of intravascular volume.
- The skin will have poor turgor and will tent when pinched. Remember, the best place to check for tenting in the elderly patient is over the sternum or forehead.
- Urine volume will be diminished as the body attempts to conserve fluid.
- Daily weights are the most reliable indicator of fluid loss or gain.

▶ ELECTROLYTE IMBALANCES

1. (D)
2. (E)
3. (B)
4. (C)
5. (A)

▶ CRITICAL THINKING

1. Check Mr. James' vital signs. Elevated blood pressure, bounding pulse, and shallow, rapid respirations are common signs of fluid overload. If he is able to stand, weigh him to see if his weight has increased since yesterday.
2. Kidney function declines in the elderly, and the intravenous (IV) fluids may have been too much for him. Regular assessment can prevent overload from occurring.
3. The registered nurse (RN) may decide to reduce the IV rate until orders are obtained. The LPN can elevate the patient's head to ease breathing. Make sure oxygen therapy is being administered as ordered. Stay with him to help him feel less anxious. Anticipate a possible diuretic order. Continue to monitor fluid balance.
4. It is probably unrealistic to expect Mr. James' lungs to clear because he was admitted with bronchitis. However, return of lung sounds to admission baseline would signal resolution of the acute overload. Other signs would include return to admission vital signs and weight and ability to walk to the bathroom again without excessive shortness of breath.

▶ REVIEW QUESTIONS

The correct answers are in **boldface.**

1. **(b)** is the correct answer; 0.9 percent is isotonic, making 0.45 percent hypotonic. (a) is isotonic; (c, d) are hypertonic.
2. **(c)** is the correct answer. Aldosterone retains sodium and therefore water in the body. (b) Thyroid hormone and (d) insulin does not affect sodium; (a) antidiuretic hormone (ADH) retains water.
3. **(b)** is the correct answer. Failing kidneys cannot effectively excrete water, making the patient at risk for overload. (a) Meningitis, (c) psoriasis, and (d) influenza do

not cause fluid retention. Influenza can cause fluid loss if vomiting or diarrhea is present.

4. (**a**) is the correct answer. The patient with an ileostomy loses large amounts of water with continuous liquid stools. (b) Asthma, (c) diabetes, and (d) fractures do not cause fluid loss.

5. (**b**) is the correct answer. Cottage cheese is high in sodium. (a) Apples, (c) chicken, and (d) broccoli are not high in sodium.

6. (**c**) is the correct answer. Potatoes are high in potassium. (a) Bread, (b) eggs, and (d) cereal are not high in potassium.

7. (**b**) is the correct answer. Fluid gains and losses are evidenced in weight gains and losses. (a) Intake and output (I&O), (c) vital signs, and (d) skin turgor are all ways to monitor fluid balance, but they are not as reliable. I&O may be inaccurate, vital signs may be affected by other factors, and measurement of skin turgor is subjective.

8. (**a**) is the correct answer. Hyponatremia accompanied by fluid loss results in dehydration and mental status changes. (b) Hyperkalemia, (c) hypercalcemia, and (d) hypomag-nesemia are not as likely to affect fluid balance and mental status.

9. (**c**) is the correct answer. Ambulation can help prevent bone loss. Because the patient is weak and is at risk for falls and fractures, assistance should be provided. (a) Bed rest promotes bone loss, (b) fluids will not help calcium levels, and (d) the patient needs calcium, not protein.

10. (**d**) is the correct answer. The heart is most at risk for dysrhythmias. (a) Lungs, (b) kidneys, and (c) liver are not as affected.

11. (**b**) is the correct answer. He is probably hyperventilating because of the anxiety. Rebreathing carbon dioxide exhaled into a paper bag can decrease the Po_2 level and relieve symptoms of alkalosis. (a) Oxygen, (c) positioning, and (d) coughing and deep breathing all help increase oxygenation, which is not needed at this time.

12. (**b**) is the correct answer. Hypoventilation related to lung disease causes retention of carbon dioxide, which causes acidosis. (a) Hyperventilation causes alkalosis, (c) loss of acid causes alkalosis, and (d) loss of base causes acidosis, but it is not the cause in this case.

6

ANSWERS

► VOCABULARY

1. **(H)**   5. **(E)**
2. **(F)**   6. **(C)**
3. **(A)**   7. **(D)**
4. **(G)**   8. **(B)**

► PERIPHERAL VEINS

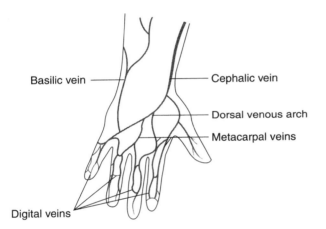

Basilic vein ——————— Cephalic vein

——— Dorsal venous arch

——— Metacarpal veins

Digital veins

► COMPLICATIONS OF IV THERAPY

1. Phlebitis
2. Infection
3. Extravasation
4. Circulatory overload
5. Infiltration
6. Septicemia
7. Pulmonary embolism
8. Air embolism

► CRITICAL THINKING

Begin with mechanical problems such as positioning of catheter by moving the extremity around to see if the intravenous (IV) is simply "positional." Check the tubing for kinks, and the clamp to be sure it is open. Next, assess the infusion site: Look for redness and signs of infiltration (such as coolness and swelling), compare extremities, and check catheter/administration hub connection to make sure it is secure. If the infusion is still not running, the catheter may be occluded with a fibrin or blood clot. The registered nurse (RN) should be consulted to confirm this assessment and decide whether the catheter should be discontinued. Attempts should not be made to flush the catheter because this will dislodge a possible clot into the circulation. The RN may attempt to milk the tubing or withdraw a clot by aspiration.

► CALCULATION PRACTICE

1. 21 gtt/min
2. 25 gtt/min
3. 83 mL/h
4. 8 mL/h
5. 42 gtt/min

► REVIEW QUESTIONS

The correct answers are in **boldface.**

1. **(a)** is the correct answer. The Intravenous Nurses Association writes the Standards of Nursing Practice for Intravenous Therapy, which guides the practice of IV therapy. (b, c, d) do not address the practice of IV therapy.
2. **(b)** is the correct answer. IV medications act rapidly because they are instantly in the bloodstream. (a) Furosemide (Lasix) can be given orally. (c) IV dosing is not necessarily more accurate. (d) Oral furosemide does not have more side effects.
3. **(b)** is the correct answer. The basilic vein is the most distal vein. The nurse should always start distally and then use more proximal veins for future IV sites. (a, c, d) are all proximal and are reserved for central insertions.
4. **(c)** is the correct answer. The site must be cleaned for at least 30 seconds if alcohol is used to effectively rid the skin of bacteria. (a, b, d) are incorrect.
5. **(a)** is the correct answer. A clot could be flushed from the cannula into the circulation and lodge in a pulmonary artery, causing a pulmonary embolism. (b) Air, not a clot, causes an air embolism. (c) Arterial spasm is caused by

injecting medication. (d) Extravasation is caused by infiltration of vesicant drugs.

6. (**c**) is the correct answer. Leakage of IV fluid into tissues causes puffiness. (a, b, d) indicate infection or inflammation.

7. (**c**) is the correct answer. 1000/8 = 125. (a, b, d) are incorrect.

8. (**c**) is the correct answer. (a, b, d) are incorrect.

9. (**b**) is correct. (a) is isotonic. (c, d) are hypotonic.

10. (**b**) is the correct answer. The date, time, IV site, type of cannula, and signature of person inserting should all be documented. (a, c, d) should all be completed before documentation.

ANSWERS

▶ VOCABULARY

Antigen is a protein marker on a cell's surface that identifies the cell as self or nonself.

Asepsis is a condition free from germs, infection, and any form of life.

Bacteria are one-celled organisms that can reproduce but need a host for food and supportive environment. Bacteria can be harmless normal flora or disease-producing pathogens.

Nosocomial infection is an infection acquired in a health care agency.

Pathogens are microorganisms or substances capable of producing a disease.

Phagocytosis is ingestion and digestion of bacteria and particles by phagocytes that ingest and destroy particulate substances such as bacteria, protozoa, and cell debris.

Virulence is the ability of the organisms to produce disease.

Viruses are small intracellular parasites that can live only inside cells and may produce disease when they enter a cell.

▶ PATHOGEN TRANSMISSION

1. (C)
2. (D)
3. (C)
4. (D)
5. (B)
6. (A)
7. (C)
8. (B)

▶ PATHOGENS AND INFECTIOUS DISEASES

1. Staphylococcus
2. Streptococcus
3. Candidiasis
4. Dermatomycosis
5. Histoplasmosis
6. Toxoplasmosis
7. Protozoa
8. Virus
9. Rickettsia
10. Fungi

▶ CRITICAL THINKING

1. Equipment-mask, gown, gloves, a sign reading "Contact Isolation," soap and paper towels, special bags for linen and trash, wash area in the room.

2. Disposable thermometer, disposable or autoclavable blood pressure (BP) cuff, stethoscope that remains in the room and can be disinfected, grooming items, bedpan, bath basin, separate container for sharps. Intravenous (IV) equipment and any other equipment needed for the care of the patient must be able to be disinfected.

3. Limit visitors; those who come must be instructed on how to implement isolation precautions. Encourage contact via telephone with family and friends who cannot visit. Maintain a cheery environment; open curtains; maintain sensory stimuli by remaining with the patient as long as possible. Encourage diversional activities, things the patient likes to do, such as TV, books, etc. Always answer call light immediately.

▶ REVIEW QUESTIONS

The correct answers are in **boldface.**

1. (**d**) This is the purpose of culture and sensitivity; contamination would make diagnosis invalid; uncontaminated cultures must be grown in the laboratory and then treated with antibiotics. (a) and (c) are true but not the primary reasons. (b) is incorrect.

2. (**c**) Washing hands before and after patient contact is considered the most important method of infection prevention. (a) Hands cannot be sterilized. (b) is a good action but it alone is not sufficient for infection control. (d) Gloves are worn only during certain procedures, when the caregiver is likely to come in contact with a moist body surface. Even when gloves are worn, hand washing before and after wearing the gloves is still essential for infection control.

3. (**a**) Surgical asepsis is aimed at the destruction of microbes before they enter the body. (b) and (d) describe medical asepsis. (c) is not related to surgical asepsis.

4. (**a**) All pathogens require moisture, food, warmth, and darkness. Some need oxygen, but others do not.

5. (**c**) The only way to obtain a sterile specimen is to catheterize the patient. (a, b, d) are incorrect because any voided specimen is contaminated.

6. (**c**) In the morning the patient is likely to have more sputum, and additionally, the specimen is likely to have more cells and bacteria. (a, b, d) are not the optimal times.

7. (**d**) A high fever indicates that the patient has developed a secondary bacterial infection. (a, b, c) are incorrect. Viral infections such as the common cold are usually associated with a low-grade fever. Symptoms of the common cold include stuffy nose with watery discharge, scratchy throat, dry cough, sneezing, and watery eyes.

8. (**a**) A culture identifies pathogen presence. (b) A drug level or peak and trough measures antibiotic levels. (c) A sensitivity report indicates what pathogens are sensitive to certain antibiotics. (d) is incorrect.

9. (**a**) is a sign of local infection. (b, d) are seen in shock. (c) is typical of a systemic infection.

10. (**b**) is a method of sterile technique. (a, c, d) are all medical asepsis practices.

11. (**c**) is correct. Nosocomial infections are acquired as a result of hospitalization. (a) is a secondary infection, (b) is a sexually transmitted disease, and (d) is incorrect.

12. (**d**) is correct. Vancomycin is the treatment of choice for Methicillin resistant staphylococcus aureus (MRSA). (a, b, c) are incorrect.

ANSWERS

► VOCABULARY

1. Acidosis
2. Anaerobic
3. Anaphylaxis
4. Antiarrhythmics
5. Cardiogenic
6. Cyanosis
7. Dysrhythmia
8. Oliguria
9. Tachycardia
10. Tachypnea

► MATCHING

1. (C)
2. (A)
3. (B)
4. (B)
5. (B)
6. (C)

► SIGNS AND SYMPTOMS OF SHOCK PHASES

Signs/Symptoms	Phases		
	Mild/Compensating	**Moderate/Progressive**	**Severe/Irreversible**
Heart rate	Elevated	Tachycardia	Slowing
Pulses	Bounding	Weaker, thready	Absent
Blood pressure	Normal	<90 mm Hg	<60 mm Hg
Systolic		*In Hypertensive, 25 percent below baseline	
Diastolic	Normal	Decreased	Decreasing to 0
Respirations	Elevated	Tachypnea	Slowing
Depth	Deep	Shallow	Irregular, shallow
Temperature	Varies	Decreased	Decreasing
		*May elevate in septic shock	
Level of consciousness	Anxious, restless, irritable, alert, oriented	Confused, lethargic	Unconscious, comatose
Skin/mucous membranes	Cool, pale	Cold, moist, clammy, pale	Cyanosis, mottled, cold, clammy
Urine output	Normal	Decreasing to <20 mL/h	15 mL/h decreasing to anuria
Bowel sounds	Normal	Decreasing	Absent

► CRITICAL THINKING

1. Stage: Severe/irreversible
   Category of Shock: Hypovolemic
   Initial Action: Notify physician, aid volume restoration by monitoring intravenous infusion
2. Stage: Mild/compensating
   Category of Shock: Septic
   Initial Action: Notify physician, maintain oxygen
3. Stage: Moderate/progressive
   Category of Shock: Cardiogenic
   Initial Action: Stop intravenous infusion, notify physician

► REVIEW QUESTIONS

*The correct answers are in **boldface**.*

1. (**c**) Notify the physician immediately because the patient is hypovolemic and needs intravenous fluids. (a) This is not the type of intravenous fluid the patient needs; an isotonic intravenous solution such as 0.9 percent normal saline would be appropriate. (b, d) are incorrect.
2. (**b**) Elevated creatinine clearance indicates possible renal damage. (a, c, d) are near normal and not indicative of a problem.
3. (**b**) The pulse elevates to compensate for decreasing cardiac output in mild shock. (a, c, d) are found in moderate shock.
4. (**a**) is correct. (b, c, d) are found in mild shock.
5. (**b**) Inform the registered nurse so the intravenous rate can be increased while the physician is being notified because the patient is hypovolemic. (a, c, d) are incorrect because the patient needs immediate intervention. (a) provides no intervention, although vital signs will be monitored continuously, and (c, d) will worsen the condition.
6. (**b**) increases blood pressure. (a, c, d) are incorrect.
7. (**b**) Decreased peripheral tissue perfusion may be seen first as slow capillary refill. (a, c, d) are incorrect.
8. (**c**) Tachypnea is compensatory to maintain normal oxygen levels when cardiac output decreases. (a) If anxiety occurs, it is not the primary cause of tachypnea. (b) Decreasing retention of carbon dioxide is not the primary reason for tachypnea, although it is a benefit. (d) is incorrect.
9. (**c**) Blood pressure is dropping and peripheral vasoconstriction occurs, resulting in less blood flow to the extremities; sympathetic nervous system compensation causes sweating to cool the body for "fight or flight." (a, b, d) are incorrect.
10. (**c**) is a 25-percent decrease from baseline. (a, b, d) are incorrect.
11. (**b**) The goal is to increase understanding when knowledge is deficient. (a, c, d) are incorrect.

9

ANSWERS

▶ VOCABULARY

1. **(D)**
2. **(C)**
3. **(F)**
4. **(A)**
5. **(I)**
6. **(H)**
7. **(J)**
8. **(E)**
9. **(B)**
10. **(G)**

▶ CULTURAL COMPETENCE

Remember that each patient is an individual and may or may not act like others from his or her cultural group.

- Native-Americans might not ask for pain medication. They may believe pain is something that must be endured.
- European-Americans may be stoic and avoid taking medication even when it is necessary. They may fear addiction or dependence.
- African-Americans may express pain more freely and may feel pain and suffering are inevitable.
- Hispanic-Americans from Puerto Rico may moan or cry. Those from Mexico may be more stoic, especially the men, who do not want to appear weak.
- Asian-Americans tend to be stoic and not express pain as freely.

▶ CRITICAL THINKING

1. Using the WHAT'S UP? format, you would assess where her pain is, how it feels, what makes it better or worse, when it began, how severe it is on a scale of 0 to 10, related symptoms, and her perception of the pain and what will relieve it.

2. Morphine is an opioid that works by binding to opioid receptors in the central nervous system.

3. Because you can expect Miss Murphy to be in pain on her operative day, it is most beneficial to administer her analgesic every 4 hours, before pain begins to recur. This will help her walk and cough and prevent postoperative complications. Often postoperative analgesics are administered via patient-controlled anesthesia (PCA).

4. Common side effects of opioids included drowsiness, nausea, and constipation. Respiratory depression and constricted pupils are signs of overdose.

5. If the morphine has been effective, Miss Murphy will be able to ambulate and cough with minimal difficulty and will rate her pain at a level that is acceptable to her.

6. According to the equianalgesic chart, the 30 mg of oral codeine in Tylenol No. 3 would be equal to about 2 mg of intramuscular (IM) morphine, a much smaller dose than she has been receiving. The physician should be contacted for a more appropriate order.

7. Relaxation, distraction, back rubs, and imagery might all be effective in addition to the morphine. She has already been using distraction as she visits with her family.

▶ REVIEW QUESTIONS

*The correct answers are in **boldface**.*

1. **(d)** is correct. Pain is whatever the experiencing person says it is, occurring whenever the experiencing person says it does. (a, b, c) may all be true in some situations but are not general definitions of pain.

2. **(c)** is correct. *Suffering* is the term used to describe the sense of threat that can accompany pain. (a, b, d) may all be present with pain, but they are not the same as suffering.

3. **(a)** is correct. Constipation is a common side effect. (b) is not common, (c) is not a side effect of opioids, and (d) is not common and is different than a side effect.

4. **(c)** is correct. The patient's self-assessment is the best measure of pain available. (a) Some patients may moan or cry, but others may not—this may be a cultural variation; (b) vital signs are most reliable when assessing acute pain; and (d) the patient's request for pain medication may be unrelated to the degree of pain.

5. **(b)** is correct. Distraction can be effective when used with analgesics. (a) Some patients may deny their pain, but not most; (c) laughing and talking do not mean pain is not present; and (d) there is no evidence that laughing changes the duration of action of medications.

6. **(a)** is correct. Acute pain may be accompanied by elevated vital signs. (b, c) are incorrect because vital signs adapt to chronic pain.

7. **(d)** is correct. Meperidine has a toxic metabolite called normeperidine, which can build up and cause cerebral irritation. (a, b, c) may all be true, but the nurse must first consider the patient's safety before trying other approaches.

8. **(c)** is correct. Pain level should be assessed before giving any analgesic, and respiratory rate should be assessed before giving any medication that can depress respirations. (a) Liver and kidney function are not routinely assessed, (b) blood glucose is not routinely assessed, and (d) physical cause of pain may not always be known.

9. **(a)** is correct. Naloxone is a narcotic antagonist. (b, c, d) are not narcotic antagonists.

10. **(c)** is correct. There is no research to justify the use of placebos to treat pain. (a, b, d) all imply that the placebo will be given. Placebos should be given only in research settings with patient consent.

11. **(c)** is correct. Most patients who are too drowsy to push the button are not in pain. Further assessment is needed to determine if he is in pain and how to proceed. (a, b) No one but the patient should ever push the button. (d) The medication should be increased only as ordered after a complete assessment and assurance that Mr. Brown is safe.

12. **(b)** is correct. The patient should always be believed. (a, c, d) may all be true, but if the nurse makes a wrong assumption, a patient in pain may go without treatment. Injuries sustained in a motorcycle accident are likely to be painful.

10

ANSWERS

VOCABULARY

1. Alopecia
2. Anorexia
3. Leukopenia
4. Xerostomia
5. Palliative
6. Chemotherapy
7. Cytotoxic
8. Neoplasm
9. Metastasizes
10. Benign

CELLS

1. True
2. False—for one protein
3. False—to the ribosomes
4. True
5. False—on the messenger RNA
6. True
7. False—only those needed for its specific functions are active
8. False—46
9. False—each cell has a full 46 chromosomes
10. False—it is also necessary for repair of tissues

BENIGN VERSUS MALIGNANT TUMORS

Benign tumors typically grow slowly, cause minor tissue damage, remain localized, and seldom recur after treatment. Cells resemble tissue of origin. Malignant tumors often grow quickly, cause damage to surrounding tissue, spread to other parts of the body (metastasize), and recur after treatment. Cells are altered to be less like their tissue of origin.

CRITICAL THINKING

1. Leukopenia: Use careful handwashing; teach Delmae and her family the importance of doing the same. Teach her to avoid crowds, people with infections, and bird, cat, or dog excreta. Avoid giving her fresh fruits or vegetables that cannot be peeled. Teach her signs and symptoms of infection to report.
2. Thrombocytopenia: Teach Delmae the importance of avoiding injury to prevent bleeding. Avoid injections. Teach her to watch for and report symptoms of bleeding, such as bruising, petechiae, or blood in urine, stool, or emesis.
3. Anemia: Provide a balanced diet, with supplements as prescribed. Administer oxygen as ordered for dyspnea. Provide opportunities to rest.
4. Stomatitis: Offer soft, mild foods. Offer frequent sips of water. Use a mouthwash such as diphenhydramine diluted in water or saline. Avoid hot, cold, spicy, and acidic foods.
5. Nausea and vomiting: Give antiemetics as ordered. Use prophylactically, not just when nausea is present. Provide mouth care before meals. Provide small, frequent meals and room-temperature or cool foods. Serve meals in a clean, pleasant environment that is free from odors and unpleasant sights. Offer hard candy. Use music or relaxation as distractions.
6. Alopecia: Offer an accepting attitude. Help the patient locate a wig or other head covering if she wishes. Tell her that her hair will grow back.

REVIEW QUESTIONS

*The correct answers are in **boldface**.*

1. (**b**) is correct.
2. (**b**) is correct.
3. (**c**) is correct.
4. (**d**) is correct. Cancer cells are confused and disorganized. (a) They are not well organized. (b) Cancer cells do not function effectively like their tissue of origin. (c) Cancer cells grow out of control.
5. (**b**) is correct. High-fat foods may increase the risk of some cancers. (a) Broccoli and cauliflower help reduce cancer risk. (c) Chicken and fish are low-fat meats that are healthy choices. (d) Cakes and breads are not problems unless they are high in fat or other high-risk ingredients.
6. (**c**) is correct. A biopsy enables the pathologist to examine and positively identify the cancer. (a) Cultures diag-

nose infection. (b) X-ray can help locate a tumor but cannot determine whether it is benign or malignant. (d) A bronchoscopy may be done, but a biopsy is necessary to positively identify the cancer.

7. **(a)** is correct. Frequent mouth care will help prevent the discomfort and dryness that accompany mucositis. (b) Cold liquids may worsen mucositis. (c) High-carbohydrate foods will not help. (d) Juices are acidic and may irritate the mucous membranes.

8. **(b)** is correct. Remember the importance of time, distance, and shielding. (a) Leaving the patient alone for 24 hours is inappropriate. (c) Body fluids should not be touched, but it is not feasible to care for the patient and avoid touching altogether. (d) A "contaminated" sign will make the patient feel isolated and afraid.

9. **(b)** is correct. Petechiae are small hemorrhages into the skin. (a) Fever is a sign of infection. (c) Pain is not a sign of bleeding. (d) Vomiting is not a sign of bleeding unless it is bloody.

10. **(a)** is correct. Washing hands frequently is an excellent way to help prevent infection in the patient at risk. (b) Avoiding injections will help prevent bleeding but will do little to prevent infection. (c) Visitors with infections should be discouraged, but the patient needs the support of family at this time. (d) Fresh fruits and vegetables can transmit infection.

11. **(d)** is correct. Alternative methods for pain control can be helpful but should never be expected to substitute for analgesics in the patient with cancer. (a) Distraction should be used with, not instead of, medication. (b) The nurse must believe the patient's report of pain. (c) Distraction can be effective when used with medication and in no way indicates that Mrs. Fitzpatrick's pain is not real.

12. **(c)** is correct. The goal of hospice is to help patients achieve a comfortable death. (a, b, d) are all aimed at curing Jack's cancer. If cure is his goal, a referral to hospice is inappropriate.

11

ANSWERS

► VOCABULARY
1. surgeons
2. perioperative
3. postoperative
4. induction
5. preoperative
6. intraoperative
7. adjunct
8. dehiscence
9. anesthesiologists
10. anesthesia
11. atelectasis
12. debridement
13. hypothermia
14. evisceration

► SURGERY URGENCY LEVELS
1. (D)   6. (A)
2. (C)   7. (B)
3. (C)   8. (A)
4. (D)   9. (C)
5. (B)   10. (A)

► NOURISHING THE SURGICAL PATIENT
*Corrections are in **boldface**.*

Healing requires increased vitamin **A and D** for collagen formation, vitamin **K** for blood clotting, and **zinc** for tissue growth, skin integrity, and cell-mediated immunity. **Protein** is essential for controlling fluid balance and manufacturing antibodies and white blood cells. Hypoalbuminemia, a low **serum** albumin, impedes the return of interstitial fluid to the venous return system, **increasing** the risk of shock. A serum **albumin** level is a useful measure of protein status.

► MEDICATIONS
1. True
2. False—the surgeon determines if the anticoagulant therapy is stopped several days before surgery, which it often is

3. False—the patient may be told by the physician to either take no insulin, the normal dose of insulin, or half of the normal dose
4. True
5. True
6. False—surgery is a great stressor for the body
7. True
8. False—circulatory collapse can develop if steroids are stopped abruptly

► INTRAOPERATIVE NURSING DIAGNOSES AND OUTCOMES
1. Free from injury
2. Maintains skin integrity
3. Maintains blood pressure, pulse, and urine output within normal limits
4. Is free of symptoms of infection
5. Reports pain is relieved to satisfactory level

See next page for answers to Wound Healing Phases.

► CRITICAL THINKING
1. For nursing interview, diagnostic testing, anesthesia interview, and preoperative teaching to ensure patient is in the best possible condition for surgery.
2. Laboratory tests: blood glucose, creatinine, blood urea nitrogen (BUN), electrolytes, complete blood count (CBC), prothrombin time (PT), partial thromboplastin time (PTT), bleeding time, type and screen, urinalysis, and pregnancy test are some common tests; oxygen saturation, electrocardiogram (ECG), chest x-ray.
3. Explain what is to be done in preadmission testing; explain preadmission prep: bathing, scrubs, preps, medications, nil per os (NPO) time, no nail polish or makeup; admission procedures the day of surgery: registration, nursing unit, emotional support, consent signed, preoperative checklist completion; intravenous (IV) line insertion, medications, surgery, postanesthesia care unit and family waiting locations, surgery time frames; postoperative care:

▶ WOUND HEALING PHASES

Phase	Time Frame	Wound Healing	Patient Effect
Phase I	Incision to second postoperative day	Inflammatory response	Fever, malaise
Phase II	Third to fourteenth postop day	Granulation tissue forms	Feeling better
Phase III	Third to sixth postop week	Collagen deposited	Raised scar formed
Phase IV	Months to 1 year	Wound contracts and shrinks	Flat, thin scar

pain control, deep breathing and coughing, leg exercises, activity, leg abduction, drains.

4. Explain admission procedures; get consent signed, preoperative checklist completion; IV insertion; give medications.

5. Greeting the patient; verifying patient's name, age, and allergies; surgeon performing the surgery; consent; surgical procedure, especially right or left when applicable, and medical history; answering questions; and alleviating anxiety. Explain what to expect in surgery: "The room may feel cool, but you can request extra blankets." "There is a lot of equipment, including a table and large bright overhead lights." "Several health care team members will introduce themselves to you." "The physician will greet you."

6. Licensed practical nurses/licensed vocational nurses (LPN/LVNs) may scrub in surgery to hand instruments to the surgeon. The LPN/LVN must know sterile technique, surgical instruments, and medications placed in the sterile field for use during surgery.

7. Maintaining the patient's airway and safety.

8. Pain control is essential to prevent physiological harm to the patient and to ensure that the patient can participate in recovery activities such as deep breathing and coughing and activity. Deep breathing and coughing prevents atelectasis and pneumonia. Leg exercises and activity prevent thrombophlebitis. Drains are inserted to prevent fluid accumulation and infection.

▶ REVIEW QUESTIONS
The correct answers are in **boldface**.

1. **(c)** The LPN/LVN can offer emotional support as needed to patients. (a) is the role of the registered nurse (RN). (b, d) are roles of the physician.

2. **(b)** The registered nurse must be informed so the surgeon can be notified. (a, c, d) are not appropriate interventions, and if the patient is extremely scared, the surgeon must be told because surgery may need to be canceled.

3. **(a)** Higher steroid levels are needed during stress to the body, which surgery produces. (b, c, d) are not complications of steroid withdrawal; circulatory collapse is.

4. **(d)** Eliminate background noise because elderly cannot filter out noise. (a) This increases glare, which will interfere with vision. (b) Large black-on-white print should be used. (c) A low tone should be used.

5. **(d)** The nurse's signature verifies that it was the patient who signed the consent after informed consent was provided by the surgeon. (a, b, c) are not the role of the nurse and are not indicated by the witnessing of the consent.

6. **(b)** Skin integrity is maintained during surgery with proper positioning and avoidance of pressure points. (a, c, d) are preoperative goals.

7. **(a)** Oxygen saturation must be above 90 percent. (b) is incorrect. (c) Patients do not have to void before postanesthesia care unit (PACU) discharge. (d) IV narcotics cannot have been given less than 30 minutes ago.

8. **(c)** Patients and a responsible adult must understand discharge instructions before discharge. (a) Patients cannot drive home. (b) Patient does not have to have home telephone but must be able to be contacted in some way for follow-up. (d) IV narcotics cannot have been given less than 30 minutes ago.

9. **(c)** Pneumonia can be prevented with lung expansion promoted by ambulation. (a, b, d) are not prevented with ambulation.

10. **(b)** Use two people to assist patient for first time in case patient is light-headed. (a) One person may not be enough to support patient if fainting occurs. (c) Patient should not self-dangle for safety. (d) Narcotics should be given about 1 hour before ambulation so patient is comfortable but hypotension is less likely.

11. **(c)** Presence of flatus occurs with normal bowel function. (a, d) indicate the bowel is not functioning. (b) is not related to bowel function.

12. **(c)** Have patient lie down to reduce pressure on the incisional area to help prevent evisceration. (a) Having patient sit upright promotes evisceration. (b) Intravenous fluids should be maintained at ordered rate and increased fluid needs anticipated because of large fluid loss occurring with dehiscence and evisceration. (d) This would not be the nurse's first action, and the patient would likely be prepared for surgery.

13. **(d)** Exhaling deeply to reach target is incorrect and would indicate need for teaching. (a, b, c) are incorrect because they are the appropriate way to use the spirometer.

14. **(a)** Sympathetic nervous system saves fluid in response to stress of surgery, which reduces urine output initially. (b, c, d) are incorrect.

15. **(b)** A fever occurring shortly after surgery is often due to atelectasis because infection takes longer to develop, so encouraging coughing and deep breathing can help prevent pneumonia. (a) An infection is not usually the cause of a fever in this time frame. (c) Tylenol is not necessary for a low-grade fever and will not help the cause. (d) Fluid intake should be maintained to help thin lung secretions.

ANSWERS

VOCABULARY

1. **(C)**	5. **(D)**
2. **(B)**	6. **(G)**
3. **(A)**	7. **(F)**
4. **(E)**	8. **(H)**

PRINCIPLES FOR TREATING SHOCK

1. True
2. False—direct
3. False—lower
4. True
5. True
6. False—do not
7. True

SIGNS AND SYMPTOMS OF INCREASED INTRACRANIAL PRESSURE

1. **(B)**	7. **(B)**
2. **(A)**	8. **(A)**
3. **(A)**	9. **(A)**
4. **(B)**	10. **(A)**
5. **(A)**	11. **(B)**
6. **(B)**	12. **(B)**

ASSESSMENT OF MOTOR FUNCTION

If the patient is unable to	The lesion is above the level of
Extend and flex arms	C-5 to C-7
Extend and flex legs	L-2 to L-4
Flex foot, extend toes	L-4 to L-5
Tighten anus	S-3 to S-5

HYPERTHERMIA

1. **(A)**	6. **(B)**
2. **(A)**	7. **(A)**
3. **(B)**	8. **(B)**
4. **(B)**	9. **(B)**
5. **(A)**	10. **(A)**

CRITICAL THINKING

1. Unresolved grieving of his wife's death.
2. Withdrawn, rarely leaves home, has not bathed, wearing soiled clothing, refrigerator is empty, curtains drawn, paces, says "I want to die." He is exhibiting cognitive, emotional, and behavioral disorganization.
3. He no longer possesses coping skills necessary to maintain usual level of functioning. His moods, thoughts, and actions are so disordered that they have the potential to lead to suicide if the situation is not quickly controlled.
4. Dysfunctional grieving related to spouse's unexpected death; risk for injury related to impaired judgment; ineffective health maintenance related to disturbed thought processes.
5. Establish an atmosphere of trust. Use active listening. Make environment safe. Reduce external sources of stimulation. Speak directly and truthfully to patient. Include supportive members of patient's family. Patient is prepared for each new development as circumstances evolve. Threatening, challenging, or arguing with disturbed patient is not done.

REVIEW QUESTIONS

*The correct answers are in **boldface**.*

1. **(c)** Respiratory distress may be experienced in anaphylactic shock because of fluid in the air passages and constricted bronchi. (a, b, c) are not common with anaphylactic shock.
2. **(a)** Arterial blood flow is assessed with capillary refill. (b, c, d) are not assessed with capillary refill.
3. **(b)** Activated charcoal would be given to help absorb the medication. (a, b, d) would not be appropriate for a semiconscious patient.

4. **(b)** Patient is alert and oriented. (a, c, d) are incorrect. Core body temperature should be within normal range. Skin should be warm and dry.

5. **(c)** (3 mg/5 mg) $\times$ 1 mL = 3/5 = 0.6 mL. (a, b, d) are incorrect.

6. **(c)** A rapid, thready pulse indicates compensation (rapid) and loss of blood volume (thready). (a, b, d) are incorrect.

7. **(c)** Airway is the first priority, then breathing, circulation, disability.

8. **(b)** The brachial artery is the proximal artery to the radial artery. (a, c, d) are not the most proximal arteries to the radial artery.

13

ANSWERS

▶ VOCABULARY

1. Respite care
2. Powerlessness
3. Chronic illness
4. Spirituality
5. Hopelessness
6. Terminal illness
7. Developmental stage

▶ CHRONIC ILLNESS AND THE ELDERLY

Corrections are in **boldface**.

The elderly constitute one of the **largest** age groups living with chronic illness. Elderly spouses or older family members are **increasingly being called on** to care for a chronically ill family member. Children of elders who themselves are reaching their **sixties** are being expected to care for their parents. These elderly caregivers **may also be** experiencing chronic illness. For elderly spouses, it is usually the less ill spouse who provides care to the other spouse. The elderly family unit is at great risk for ineffective coping or further development of health problems. Nurses should assess **all** members of the elderly family to ensure that their health needs are being met.

Elderly adults are **very** concerned about becoming dependent and a burden to others. They may become depressed and give up hope if they feel that they are a burden to others. Establishing **short-term** goals or self-care activities that allow them to participate or have small successes are important nursing actions that can **increase** their self-esteem.

▶ DYING AND GRIEVING

1. False—allows
2. True
3. False—God
4. True
5. False—is at peace and simply seeks a comfortable and dignified death

▶ CRITICAL THINKING

1. The nurse should explore Mrs. Martin's spiritual needs: Is she hopeful? What makes her feel at peace? How does she usually meet her spiritual needs? Does she have certain religious customs?
2. Spiritual distress; potential for enhanced spiritual well-being; hopelessness; powerlessness.
3. Interventions may include using the meditation room for quiet reflection or prayer, chaplain visits, or worship services; assisting Mrs. Martin with transportation to the meditation room or worship services; and providing desired reading material such as a Bible or prayer book.
4. If Mrs. Martin expresses a feeling of peace or hopefulness.

▶ REVIEW QUESTIONS

The correct answers are in **boldface**.

1. (**d**) Integrity versus despair. (a, b, c) are earlier developmental stages.
2. (**a**) stress management directly influences how a patient ages. (b, c, d) do not directly influence a patient's aging.
3. (**d**) This empowers the patient to control her own health care. (a, b, c) take control away from the patient.
4. (**b**) Home care nurses can strengthen a patient's self-care capacity by saying, "Let me assist you" instead of "Let me do this for you." (a) Being a caretaker instead of a partner is not helpful in improving self-esteem. (c) Empowering the patient instead of doing it all for the patient would be helpful. (d) Doing everything for the patient instead of assisting makes the patient feel dependent and useless.
5. (**a**) Offering praise for small patient efforts shows interest in the patient and motivates the patient to try other tasks. (b) If praise is offered only for major patient efforts, opportunities to praise small tasks are lost; if the patient never accomplishes major tasks, no praise is ever given. (c) If ADLs are done for the patient, no opportunity for independence and success is allowed for the patient. (d) Assisting patient at first sign of difficulty with ADLs allows the patient no opportunity to succeed at a difficult task.

6. (**b**) Using humor can be helpful, and this is one method of using humor. (a) Avoiding the use of humor is not beneficial because humor has been shown to enhance health. (c) A serious manner may not be as helpful in improving a patient's mood. (d) Limiting conversation to a minimum further isolates the patient.

7. (**d**) Stress decreases when the caregiver is given personal time away from the patient, which everyone needs. (a) Personal time increases. (b) Rest time increases. (c) There is no cost for most volunteer respite services.

8. (**d**) Allowing the patient to make informed decisions should foster health promotion. (a, b, c) Making the choices for the patient and family may not result in implementation of those choices because input was not obtained from them.

9. (**a**) Providing educational information empowers the patient to make informed choices. (b) Limiting visiting hours for family members isolates the patient and does not allow patient free choice. (c) Asking family members to provide care makes the patient dependent if some independence is possible. (d) Setting the goals for the patient and family takes the decision-making process away from the patient.

10. (**a**) Disorientation occurs from metabolism alterations. (b) Body temperature decreases. (c) Increased sleeping occurs from metabolism changes. (d) Oliguria occurs from decreased intake.

11. (**c**) Natural analgesia may result from reduced nerve sensitivity caused by dehydration. (a) The body stores energy rather than using it. (b) Metabolism decreases with impending death. (d) Peristalsis decreases with impending death.

12. (**d**) Hearing is the last sense to leave, so the nurse should be aware of all communication within hearing of the patient and also ensure that explanations are still given to the patient. (a, b, c) are incorrect.

13. (**a**) Peripheral vascular disease is a chronic illness. (b, c, d) are acute illnesses.

14. (**a**) Being willing and able to carry out the medical regimen is important in dealing positively with the illness. (b, c, d) would be unhelpful behaviors in adapting to a chronic illness.

15. (**b**) Malabsorption syndrome is a congenital disorder. (a, c, d) are acquired illnesses.

16. (**a**) is correct. (b, c, d) are incorrect.

14

ANSWERS

► VOCABULARY
1. Activities of daily living
2. Arrhythmia
3. Cataract
4. Attitude
5. Aspiration
6. Edema
7. Glaucoma
8. Expectoration
9. Constipation
10. Homeostasis
11. Contracture
12. Pressure ulcer
13. Nocturia
14. Extrinsic factors
15. Macular degeneration
16. Osteoporosis
17. Sensory deprivation
18. Optimal functioning
19. Reality orientation
20. Sensory overload

► AGING CHANGES
1. (A)	14. (L)
2. (C)	15. (O)
3. (E)	16. (P)
4. (F)	17. (Q)
5. (B)	18. (R)
6. (H)	19. (T)
7. (D)	20. (U)
8. (G)	21. (S)
9. (K)	22. (V)
10. (N)	23. (W)
11. (M)	24. (Z)
12. (J)	25. (X)
13. (I)	26. (Y)

► COMMUNICATING WITH THE HEARING IMPAIRED
1. True
2. False—face patient so the speaker's face is visible to patient
3. False—speak toward patient's best side of hearing
4. True
5. True
6. False—recognize that high-frequency tones and consonant sounds are lost first, z, sh, ch, d, g
7. True

► MEDICATIONS
*Corrections are in **boldface**.*

Older patients are **more** susceptible to drug-induced illness and adverse medication side effects for various reasons. They take **many** medicines for the **more than** one chronic illness that they have. Different medications interact and produce side effects that can be dangerous. Over-the-counter medicines older patients take, as well as the self-prescribed extracts, elixirs, herbal teas, cultural healing substances, and other home remedies commonly used by individuals of their age cohort, **do** influence other medications.

If an older patient crushes a large enteric-coated pill so that it can be taken in food and is easily swallowed, it **destroys** the enteric protection and can inadvertently cause damage to the stomach and intestinal system. Some patients **intentionally** skip prescribed doses in an effort to save money. When prescribed doses are not being taken as expected, problems do not clear up as quickly and new problems may result. The nurse should educate the older patient and the patient's family. Patients need to know what each prescribed pill is for, when it is prescribed to be taken, and how it should be taken.

► CRITICAL THINKING

This is a values clarification exercise, so answers are your own individualized answers that should be based on guiding principles.

1. An individual response
2. Your values and beliefs (what are they)
3. Be tactful and provide privacy during situation resolution
4. Consider professionalism issues, agency policy, patient safety
5. Consider professionalism, respect for others' values

► REVIEW QUESTIONS

*The correct answers are in **boldface**.*

1. **(c)** is the only symptom for glaucoma. (a, b, d) are incorrect.
2. **(d)** There is a decreased taste sensitivity for salt and sweet flavors. (a, b, c) are not aging changes.
3. **(b)** Peripheral vascular resistance increases with age, contributing to hypertension development. (a, c, d) decrease with aging.
4. **(b)** Circulatory status is the reason for slow, deliberate movements because gravity shifts body fluids with position change. (a, c, d) are incorrect.
5. **(a)** The older circulatory system is very sensitive to fluid-overload situations, and intravenous therapy increases the risk potential. (b, c, d) are incorrect.
6. **(c)** Whispering decreases the pitch of the sounds, making your words easier to hear for someone who has lost only high-pitched frequencies. (a, b, d) are incorrect for high-pitched hearing loss.
7. **(b)** Wax can obstruct the conduction pathway, causing a bone-conduction problem. (a, c) are not related to a bone-conduction problem, but a nerve problem.
8. **(b)** Psychological factors are the primary source of sexual dysfunction, as documented in the literature. (a, c, d) are not the primary source.
9. **(a)** This puts the patient's needs ahead of the nurse's needs. (b, c, d) do not show respect for the patient's needs.
10. **(b)** Weight-bearing exercise helps fight the degeneration of bone in osteoporosis. (a) Calcium intake should be increased. (c, d) do not have any influence on osteoporosis.

15

ANSWERS

▶ STRUCTURES OF THE CARDIOVASCULAR SYSTEM

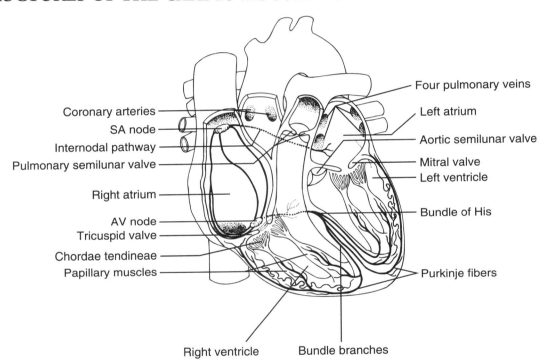

Coronary arteries
SA node
Internodal pathway
Pulmonary semilunar valve

Right atrium

AV node
Tricuspid valve

Chordae tendineae
Papillary muscles

Four pulmonary veins
Left atrium
Aortic semilunar valve

Mitral valve
Left ventricle

Bundle of His

Purkinje fibers

Right ventricle   Bundle branches

▶ CARDIAC BLOOD FLOW

A.	14	H.	7
B.	10	I.	12
C.	1	J.	8
D.	3	K.	9
E.	13	L.	11
F.	6	M.	2
G.	5	N.	4

▶ VOCABULARY

Across

2. Claudication
4. Arteriosclerosis
5. Pulse deficit
6. Ischemia
8. Homans' sign
11. Bruit
12. Dysrhythmia
13. Paresthesia
14. Bradycardia

Down

1. Thrill
2. Poikilothermy
3. Paralysis
7. Clubbing
9. Murmur
10. Preload
13. Palpation

AGING AND THE CARDIOVASCULAR SYSTEM

*Corrections are in **boldface**.*

It is believed that the "aging" of blood vessels, especially arteries, begins in **childhood.** Average resting blood pressure tends to **increase** with age and may contribute to stroke or **left-**sided heart failure. The **thinner-**walled veins, especially those of the legs, may also weaken and stretch, making their valves incompetent. With age, the heart **muscle** becomes less efficient, and there is a **decrease** in both maximum cardiac output and heart rate. The health of the myocardium depends on **its** blood supply. Hypertension causes the **left** ventricle to work harder, so it may **hypertrophy.** The heart valves may become **thickened by** fibrosis, leading to heart murmurs. Dysrhythmias become more common in the elderly as the cells of the conduction pathway become **less** efficient.

CARDIOVASCULAR SYSTEM

1. cardiovascular system
2. heart's
3. vascular system, capillaries
4. stiffen
5. lubb, diastole
6. absent, normal
7. cardiac, catheterization
8. peripheral, pain, poikilothermia
9. vascular, venography

ACUTE CARDIOVASCULAR NURSING ASSESSMENT

1. Allergies
2. Smoking
3. Pain
4. Weight gain
5. Crackles
6. Dizziness
7. Fatigue
8. Pink-tinged sputum

CRITICAL THINKING

▶ REVIEW QUESTIONS

*The correct answers are in **boldface**.*

1. **(a)**
2. **(b)**
3. **(c)**
4. **(d)**
5. **(a)**
6. **(d)**
7. **(a)** The leg reading is 10 mm Hg higher. (b, c, d) are incorrect.
8. **(b)** is the arm with the higher reading, which is what should be used. (a) The reading is lower. (c) It is not as practical to use the leg because the higher-reading arm is available, although the leg could be used. (d) The arm with the lower reading should not be used.
9. **(a)** is correct. (b, c, d) are incorrect.
10. **(c)** It normally increases to compensate for the position change. (a, b) It does not drop. (d) This indicates orthostatic hypotension.
11. **(b)** Reduced blood supply results in a lack of oxygen and nutrients that contribute to the signs seen. (a, c, d) are incorrect.
12. **(b)** Medication is used in lieu of exercise when the patient cannot tolerate exercise to simulate the increased blood flow that would occur with exercise. (a, c, d) are incorrect.
13. **(d)** Third degree heart block that interferes with normal heart rate can be treated with a pacemaker. (a, b, c) are not usually treated with a permanent pacemaker.

16

ANSWERS

VOCABULARY

1. (A)
2. (G)
3. (F)
4. (E)
5. (D)
6. (C)
7. (B)
8. (K)
9. (J)
10. (I)
11. (H)

DIURETICS

1. (C)
2. (B)
3. (A)
4. (C)
5. (B)
6. (C)
7. (A)
8. (A)

HYPERTENSION RISK FACTORS

1. False
2. True
3. False
4. True
5. False

STAGES OF HYPERTENSION AND RECOMMENDATIONS FOR FOLLOW-UP

1. False—1 year
2. True
3. True
4. False—1 month
5. True
6. False—2 months
7. True
8. False—1 month
9. True
10. True

CRITICAL THINKING

1. Weight, smoking history, diet and salt intake, alcohol use, exercise patterns, stress management, life roles, finances, knowledge base. Feedback: 5 feet 4 inches, 156 lb; does not smoke or use alcohol; salts food liberally, eats three meals and snacks, moderate fat intake; walks when time permits; deals with issues as they come, which is often in her roles as wife and mother to three children; has no prescription insurance coverage; knows very little about hypertension.

2. Individualized teaching plan for Mrs. Martin's needs should include addressing knowledge deficits through teaching according to protocols for weight management, diet and salt intake, exercise importance, stress-management techniques, and medications.

3. Informing her of the importance of controlling her hypertension; financial assessment to ensure that she has a funding source to buy medication because she may need lifelong medication.

4. Blood pressure readings on follow-up visits are within normal limits with medication.

REVIEW QUESTIONS

*The correct answers are in **boldface**.*

1. **(a)** Race is a nonmodifiable risk factor. (b, c, d) are modifiable risk factors for hypertension.

2. **(c)** Isolated systolic hypertension has been found in the elderly population when the systolic blood pressure is 160 mm Hg or more but the diastolic blood pressure is less than 95 mm Hg. (a) Primary hypertension is the result of unknown causes. (b) Secondary hypertension has an identifiable cause. (d) Malignant hypertension is severe high blood pressure.

3. **(b)** *Hypertension* is defined as a blood pressure of more than 140/90 on two separate occasions. (a) Blood pressure measurement is the heart contracting, or systolic, as well as relaxing, or diastolic. (c) Stress, activity, and emotions may temporarily raise blood pressure. (d) Peripheral vascular resistance may help determine blood pressure, but it does not define hypertension.

4. **(a)** Smoking is associated with a high incidence of stage III hypertension. (b, c) Patients who smoke may show an increase in blood pressure because nicotine vasoconstricts the blood vessels. (d) Smoking is a major risk

factor for cardiovascular disease but has not been shown to cause hypertension.

5. **(d)** is correct. (a, b, c) do not have headache as a common side effect.

6. **(b)** Stage II hypertension is classified as a systolic blood pressure of 160 to 179 and a diastolic blood pressure of 100 to 109. (a) Stage I is 140 to 159/90 to 99. (c) Stage III is 180/110.

7. **(c)** Medications for hypertension should be taken daily as directed. (a) Sunbathing may increase dehydration, a side effect of the drug. (b) Lifestyle modifications are to be continued with antihypertensive therapy. (d) The medication is keeping the blood pressure lowered and will have to be taken daily.

8. **(b)** Thiazide diuretics reduce the reabsorption of potassium, so patients should be monitored for signs of hypokalemia or muscle weakness. (a, c, d) Numb hands, gastrointestinal distress, and nightmares are not common side effects of metolazone.

9. **(a)** Enalapril maleate (Vasotec) inhibits the conversion of angiotensin I to angiotensin 11, thereby decreasing the levels of angiotensin II, which decreases vasopressor activity and aldosterone secretion. (b, c, d) The actions of enalapril maleate (Vasotec) achieve antihypertensive effects by suppression of the renin-angiotensin-aldosterone system, but not by adjusting the fluid volume, dilating vessels, or decreasing cardiac output.

10. **(c)** Cough is the common side effect of enalapril maleate. (a, b, d) Acne, heartburn, and diarrhea are not common side effects of enalapril maleate.

11. **(b)** Propanolol (Inderal) blocks the effects of beta-adrenergic stimulation, decreasing blood pressure, cardiac output, and cardiac contractility. (a, c, d) Propanolol (Inderal) does not increase heart rate, affect fluid volume, or increase cardiac contractility.

12. **(c)** Stopping propanolol (Inderal) abruptly may cause withdrawal syndrome. (a) Propanolol (Inderal) does not affect fluid volume or electrolytes unless combined with a diuretic. (b) Gastrointestinal side effects are not common. (d) Patients are instructed to avoid prolonged standing and to make position changes slowly because they may experience hypotension.

13. **(d)** Knowledge is needed to control this chronic condition. (a) Defining characteristics of activity intolerance include abnormal electrocardiographic readings and vital signs and reports of dyspnea or fatigue. (b) Ineffective airway clearance is the state in which an individual is unable to clear secretions. (c) Impaired physical mobility is a temporary limitation of the ability to move freely, which is not the focus of care for hypertension.

14. **(c)** Although a patient may feel better after taking medication, the hypertension is well controlled but not cured. (a, b, d) Hypertension can damage the target organs if it is not controlled. Accurate statements by patients regarding complications of hypertension and lifestyle modifications may indicate that patients are well informed.

15. **(a)** The Joint National Committee (JNC) recommends regular aerobic exercise to prevent and control hypertension. (b) Smoking, even low-tar cigarettes, is a risk factor for heart disease. (c) Alcohol intake is limited to 1 oz/d by the JNC. (d) A daily multivitamin supplement has not been shown to prevent or control hypertension.

17

ANSWERS

VOCABULARY

1. Chorea
2. Pericarditis
3. Myocarditis
4. Petechiae
5. Pericardiocentesis
6. Cardiac tamponade
7. Cardiomyopathy
8. Cardiomegaly
9. Myectomy
10. Thrombophlebitis

INFLAMMATORY AND INFECTIOUS CARDIOVASCULAR DISORDERS

1. (B)   4. (C)
2. (E)   5. (D)
3. (A)

RHEUMATIC FEVER AND RHEUMATIC HEART DISEASE

*Corrections are in **boldface**.*

  Rheumatic fever **is a complication of** a streptococcal infection such as a sore throat. Rheumatic fever signs and symptoms include polyarthritis, subcutaneous nodules, chorea with rapid, **uncontrolled** movements, carditis, fever, arthralgia, and **pneumonitis.** The joints become inflamed **one at a time,** resulting in polyarthritis. The **major** joints are most commonly affected, but this inflammation **does not** cause permanent damage. Subcutaneous nodules that are small, firm, and **painless** develop over bony prominences. A throat culture diagnoses **a streptococcal infection at the time of the infection.** Chronic rheumatic carditis can be a complication of rheumatic fever. The heart valves and their structures can be scarred and damaged. These changes **may occur years** after an episode of rheumatic fever and can lead to heart failure. Rheumatic fever can be prevented by detecting and treating streptococcal infections promptly with **penicillin.** The signs and symptoms of a pharynx streptococcal infection include sudden sore throat, fever **of 101°F to 104°F,** chills, throat redness with exudate, sinus or ear infection, and lymph node enlargement. Nursing care focuses on relieving the patient's pain and anxiety, maintaining normal cardiac function, and educating the patient about rheumatic heart disease.

► THROMBOPHLEBITIS

ACUTE PAIN

Interventions	Rationale	Evaluation
Assess pain using rating scale such as 0 to 10.	Self-report is the most reliable indicator of pain.	Does patient report pain using scale?
Provide analgesics and nonsteroidal anti-inflammatory drugs (NSAIDs) as ordered.	Pain is reduced when inflammation is decreased.	Is patient's rating of pain lower after medication?
Apply warm, moist soaks.	Heat relieves pain and vasodilates, which increases circulation to reduce swelling. Moist heat penetrates more deeply.	Does patient report increased comfort with warm, moist soaks? Is swelling reduced?
Maintain bed rest with leg elevation above heart level.	Elevation decreases swelling, which reduces pain.	

DEFICIENT KNOWLEDGE

Interventions	Rationale	Evaluation
Explain condition, symptoms, and complications.	Patient must have basic knowledge to comply with therapy.	Is patient able to verbalize knowledge taught?
Explain medications, therapies ordered, monthly lab test monitoring, and need for Medic Alert identification.	Compliance and safe use of medications are promoted with an adequate knowledge base.	Can patient explain medications, therapies, lab tests, purpose of Medic Alert identification?
Teach patient not to massage extremity.	Massage can dislodge an embolus.	Does patient avoid massaging extremity?

► DIAGNOSTIC TESTS FOR INFECTIVE ENDOCARDITIS

1. (G)
2. (E)
3. (C)
4. (F)
5. (B)
6. (D)
7. (H)
8. (A)

► CRITICAL THINKING

A. Enlargement of heart muscle, especially along the septum without dilation of the ventricle, which does not relax or fill easily.
B. Smaller, reduced because of decreased relaxation and size.
C. Chest x-ray.
D. It would increase contractility in a heart that does not relax easily, so filling would be decreased with even less relaxation.
E. A myectomy would remove some of the enlarged ventricle to help increase ventricular size and make relaxation easier.
F. (a) Because cardiac output is reduced, dehydration must be avoided to prevent a further decrease in cardiac output. (b) Exertion is avoided so that an increase in cardiac output, which the compromised heart is unable to provide, is not required.
G. The family will feel useful and included in the patient's care if they are taught cardiopulmonary resuscitation (CPR). They will feel a sense of control and purpose in the event that CPR is required.

► REVIEW QUESTIONS

*The correct answers are in **boldface.***

1. (**b**) A throat culture must be done to rule out a streptococcal infection, which can lead to complications. (a, c, d) are not as essential to prevent complications.
2. (**d**) is a bacterial infection that can precede rheumatic fever. (a, b, c) are incorrect.
3. (**a**) To prevent endocarditis from recurring because of increased risk from previous heart damage. (b) is not the reason they are given. (c, d) are not prevented by antibiotics.
4. (**c**) They can cause the clot to dislodge and become an embolus. (a) They do not prevent calf swelling. (b) Preventing a life-threatening complication is the priority. (d) They do not cause a clot to form.
5. (**c**) is monitored for heparin. (a, b, d) are not monitored for heparin; b and d are monitored for warfarin (Coumadin) therapy.
6. (**a**) vitamin K is the antidote. (b, c, d) are incorrect; d is the antidote for heparin.
7. (**b**) The desired outcome for pain is that it is satisfactorily relieved according to patient. (a) is the outcome for anxiety. (c, d) would not be appropriate for a patient with acute thrombophlebitis because bed rest is ordered.
8. (**b**) The next dose of warfarin (Coumadin) should be held until the physician is informed because prothrombin time (PT) monitors Coumadin effects. (a) is incorrect because the PT is elevated and could cause bleeding. (c, d) are incorrect because PT does not monitor heparin.

9. (**a**) Bed rest is essential to prevent emboli development. (b, c, d) would encourage emboli development if the affected leg is involved.

10. (**b**) is above therapeutic range. (a, c) are measured for heparin. (d) is normal.

11. (**d**) The patient is experiencing paroxysmal nocturnal dyspnea, which occurs from increased fluid returning to the heart from reclining; the fluid then builds up in the lungs. (a, b, c) are incorrect.

12. (**b**) Anorexia is a side effect of digoxin (Lanoxin). (a, c, d) are incorrect.

13. (**b**) $\dfrac{45 \text{ mg}}{60 \text{ mg}} \times 2 \text{ mL} = \dfrac{90}{60} = 1.5 \text{ mL}$. (a, c, d) are incorrect.

14. (**d**) Friction of inflamed pericardial and epicardial layers rubbing together. (a, b, c) are incorrect.

15. (**c**) Chest pain is the most common symptom, especially with deep inspiration. (a, b, d) are incorrect.

18

ANSWERS

VOCABULARY

1. (D)	11. (C)
2. (I)	12. (A)
3. (M)	13. (H)
4. (J)	14. (K)
5. (R)	15. (N)
6. (P)	16. (S)
7. (L)	17. (O)
8. (B)	18. (Q)
9. (E)	19. (T)
10. (G)	20. (F)

ATHEROSCLEROSIS

1. A fatty streak appears on the lining of an artery. This buildup of fatty deposits is known as *plaque*. Plaque has irregular, jagged edges that allow blood cells and other material to adhere to the wall of the artery. With time, this buildup can cause stenosis of the vessel, which leads to partial or total occlusion of the artery. When this occurs, the area distal to it can become ischemic due to lack of blood flow. This buildup will become calcified and harden, leading to damage of the vessel with loss of elasticity and compliance.

2. Cigarette smoking, hypertension, elevated serum cholesterol, diabetes mellitus, obesity, stress, and sedentary lifestyle.

3. Assess readiness to learn. Example for smoking: Explain what occurs when one smokes, including changes to vessels and effect on blood flow. Determine when patient craves cigarettes most, and teach patient to try a different activity to distract from smoking. Teach patient to avoid caffeine products—chocolate, cocoa, and caffeinated soft drinks. Avoid stimulants. Increasing fluid intake, especially during the first 3 days of quitting smoking, will help wash nicotine out of the system. Have patients read books instead of magazines; magazines have many cigarette ads.

MYOCARDIAL INFARCTION

Corrections are in boldface.

Myocardial infarction (MI) is the death of a portion of the **heart muscle** caused by a blockage or spasm of a coronary artery. When the patient has an MI, the affected part of the muscle becomes damaged and can no longer function properly. Ischemic injury takes **several hours** before complete necrosis and infarction take place. The ischemic process affects the subendocardial layer, which is **most** sensitive to hypoxia. Myocardial contractility is depressed, so the body attempts to compensate by triggering the **autonomic** nervous system. This causes an **increase** in myocardial oxygen demand, which further depresses the myocardium. After necrosis, the contractility function of the muscle is **permanently** lost. If treatment is initiated at the **first sign** of an MI, the area of damage can be minimized. If prolonged ischemia is allowed to take place, the size of the infarction can be quite **large.**

The area that is affected by an MI depends on which coronary artery is involved. The left anterior descending (LAD) branch of the left main coronary artery is the area that feeds the **anterior** wall. The right coronary artery (RCA) feeds the **inferior** wall and parts of the atrioventricular node and the sinoatrial node. An occlusion of the RCA leads to abnormalities of impulse conduction and formation. The left circumflex coronary artery feeds the **lateral** wall and part of the posterior wall of the heart.

Pain is the **most** common complaint. The pain **may radiate** to one or both arms and shoulders, the neck, and the jaw. The patient usually **denies** that an MI is occurring. Other symptoms may include restlessness; a feeling of impending doom; nausea; diaphoresis; and cold, clammy, ashen skin. The only symptom that might be present in the elderly patient may be a **sudden onset of shortness of breath.**

The three strong indicators of an MI are patient history, abnormal electrocardiographic (ECG) readings, and **troponin I** levels.

Initially, patients are kept on bed rest to **decrease** myocardial oxygen demand. Patients are medicated promptly when complaining of chest pain. **Morphine sulfate** is the most widely used narcotic. It helps decrease anxiety, **slows** respirations, and has a **vasodilation** effect on coronary arteries. Oxygen is given usually at **2 L/min** via nasal cannula. Nitroglycerin sublingual, topical, or by intravenous drip can also be administered. Thrombolytic therapy is a frequent option of **lysing** a clot that is occluding a coronary artery.

A nursing care plan should include factors that may contribute to **increased** cardiac workload. Changes in diet, stress reduction, regular exercise program, cessation of smoking, and following a medication schedule require extensive patient and family teaching.

➤ PHARMACOLOGICAL TREATMENT

1. (**D**)   6. (**F**)
2. (**C**)   7. (**I**)
3. (**A**)   8. (**E**)
4. (**G**)   9. (**H**)
5. (**B**)

➤ CRITICAL THINKING

1. (**a**) is correct.
2. Associated with arterial occlusive disease. This is pain in the calves of the lower extremities associated with activity or exercise. With poor blood supply to the muscles, they are unable to receive increased oxygen to meet the demand of increased activity. As ischemia increases, a cramping-type pain develops.
3. When activity stops, the muscle does not have the increased oxygen demand, so the pain begins to subside with rest.
4. Smoking contributes to loss of high-density lipoproteins, which are the best type to have present to decrease the risk of cardiovascular disorders. The rate of progressive damage to vessels is increased with smoking. Smoking also contributes to vasoconstriction, which leads to angina and cardiac dysrhythmias.

➤ REVIEW QUESTIONS

The correct answers are in **boldface.**

1. (**d**) A stress ECG demonstrates the extent to which the heart tolerates and responds to the additional demands placed on it during exercise. The heart's ability to continue adapting is related to the adequacy of blood supplied to the myocardium through the coronary arteries. If the patient develops chest pain, dangerous cardiac rhythm changes, or significantly elevated blood pressure, the diagnostic testing is stopped. (a, b, c) are incorrect.
2. (**d**) When a patient is apprehensive and afraid, the nurse should listen and encourage the patient to express his or her feelings. This can ease the mental burden and help the patient feel less overwhelmed, alone, and helpless. Listening is an active process even if the patient does most of the talking. (a) Learning is impaired during times of anxiety. (b) Avoiding the subject may indicate to the patient that the nurse does not care. (c) How others have done ignores the fact that for this person, the experience is unique.
3. (**c**) People who are allergic to shellfish also may be sensitive to iodine, which is the base for the radiopaque dye used for the arteriogram. Notify the physician if the patient is allergic to either of these. The physician may cancel the procedure or take other precautions, such as the administration of an antihistamine or other emergency medication. (a, b, d) are not related to the test dyes used.
4. (**a**) If nitroglycerin tablets are fresh, the patient should feel a tingling or fizzing in the mouth. Tablets usually need to be replaced about every 3 months. (b, d) Nitroglycerin tablets do not disintegrate or change color when old. (c) Aspirin smells like vinegar when it becomes old.
5. (**b**) Fresh vegetables without added salt are low in sodium. (a, c, d) are high in sodium.
6. (**c**) Pulmonary edema. These symptoms are classic signs of pulmonary edema. (a, b, d) Respiratory distress may be observed, but the frothy sputum is symptomatic of pulmonary edema.
7. (**b**) Capillary refill is normally less than 3 seconds. (a, c, d) are all symptomatic of atherosclerosis.
8. (**c**) 30 percent. (a, b, d) are incorrect.
9. (**c**) Lack of sufficient oxygen to the myocardium is the cause of chest pain. (a) causes wasting of heart muscle. (b) causes dysrhythmias. (d) will not cause chest pain unless oxygen supply is insufficient to meet the workload.
10. (**a**) Hypertension can be controlled with proper diet, exercise, and medications. (b, c, d) cannot be changed.
11. (**b**) Coconut oil is saturated. (a, c, d) are examples of unsaturated fats.
12. (**c**) Edema, moderate to severe, is a manifestation of venous insufficiency. (a, b, d) are all found with venous insufficiency.
13. (**b**) Pain is the outstanding symptom. (c) Cramping is also a feature to a lesser extent. (a, d) Numbness and swelling are not characteristic.
14. (**b**) Arteriolar vasoconstriction. (a, c, d) are not descriptive of Raynaud's disease.

19

ANSWERS

▶ VOCABULARY

1. annuloplasty
2. commissurotomy
3. insufficiency
4. regurgitation
5. stenosed
6. valvuloplasty

▶ MITRAL VALVE PROLAPSE

*Corrections are in **boldface**.*

During ventricular **systole,** when pressures in the left ventricle rise, the leaflets of the mitral valve normally remain **closed.** In mitral valve prolapse (MVP), however, the leaflets bulge backward into the left **atrium** during systole. Often there are **no** functional problems seen with MVP. However, if the leaflets do not fit together, mitral **regurgitation** can occur with varying degrees of severity.

MVP tends to be hereditary, and the cause is **unknown.** Infections that damage the mitral valve may be a contributing factor. It is the most common form of valvular heart disease and typically occurs in **women** age 20 to 55. Most patients with MVP have **no** symptoms. Symptoms that may occur include chest pain, dysrhythmias, palpitations, dizziness, and syncope.

No treatment is needed unless symptoms are present. Stimulants and caffeine should be avoided to prevent symptoms. Information on endocarditis prevention is essential.

▶ VALVULAR DISORDERS

1. False—narrowing
2. True
3. True
4. False—allows
5. True
6. False—mitral, aortic
7. True
8. False—late
9. True
10. True
11. True
12. True
13. False—enlarges
14. True
15. False—new protocols consider antibiotics for some invasive procedures per protocols

▶ CRITICAL THINKING

1. Aging.
2. Ask if there is a history of rheumatic fever.
3. The left ventricle increases atrial kick; the left ventricle hypertrophies to increase contractility.
4. Left ventricular failure.
5. Decreased coronary artery blood flow results from the reduced cardiac output at the same time that the left ventricular workload is increased. This imbalance in oxygen supply and demand results in angina.
6. Prophylactic antibiotics.
7. Hypertrophy is a compensatory mechanism.
8. Sudden death may occur from aortic stenosis, so the valve is replaced.

▶ REVIEW QUESTIONS

*The correct answers are in **boldface**.*

1. **(b)** Impaired emptying of blood from the left ventricle occurs because the blood cannot easily leave the left ventricle through the narrowed aortic valve. (a) The aortic valve is narrowed. (c) Backflow of blood into the left atrium occurs with mitral regurgitation. (d) Impaired emptying of the left atrium occurs with mitral stenosis.
2. **(a)** Backflow of blood into the left atrium occurs through the mitral valve, which does not close tightly. (b, c, d) are incorrect.
3. **(c)** Ventricular hypertrophy occurs to help maintain cardiac output. (a, b, d) are incorrect.
4. **(b)** Left ventricular failure results in decreased cardiac output, which reduces oxygen to the tissues and causes fatigue. (a, c, d) are incorrect.
5. **(a)** Furosemide helps prevent pulmonary edema, a complication of decreased cardiac output and heart failure. (b, c, d) help prevent complications not related to decreased cardiac output.

6. (**d**) Cardiac catheterization measures chamber pressures. (a, b, c) do not.
7. (**c**) The patient's goal would be to be able to verbalize knowledge of disorder. (a, b, d) are incorrect.
8. (**a**) Assessing the patient's learning priorities helps ensure that he is motivated to learn because his needs and not the nurses' needs are being met. (b, d) do not promote learning and may hinder it. (c) is not correct.
9. (**a**) Wearing Medic Alert identification is essential in case of a bleeding problem or loss of consciousness. (b) An increased intake of green leafy vegetables can counteract the warfarin (Coumadin's) effects because they contain vitamin K, the antidote for Coumadin. (c) Blood test appointments are monthly. (d) An electric razor is to be used when shaving.
10. (**a**) If the patient understands to breathe normally when moving, Valsalva's maneuver will not occur. (b, c) are incorrect. (d) results in Valsalva's maneuver.
11. (**d**) Dyspnea and coughing are indicators of heart failure because of fluid congestion in the lungs, so you would listen to lung sounds to see if crackles are present. (a, b, c) are incorrect.

20

ANSWERS

► VOCABULARY

1. (S)	12. (J)
2. (I)	13. (P)
3. (E)	14. (A)
4. (O)	15. (G)
5. (H)	16. (N)
6. (D)	17. (C)
7. (L)	18. (Q)
8. (K)	19. (T)
9. (U)	20. (R)
10. (B)	21. (F)
11. (M)	

► COMPONENTS OF A CARDIAC CYCLE

► HEART RATE

1. 100
2. 110
3. 80

► CARDIAC CONDUCTION

1. (E)	13. (V)
2. (I)	14. (T)
3. (L)	15. (N)
4. (R)	16. (C)
5. (X)	17. (S)
6. (U)	18. (P)
7. (Q)	19. (D)
8. (A)	20. (G)
9. (W)	21. (J)
10. (M)	22. (K)
11. (H)	23. (F)
12. (O)	24. (B)

► ELECTROCARDIOGRAM INTERPRETATION

A.

1. Rhythm: Regular
2. Heart rate: 100 beats per minute
3. P waves: Smoothly rounded and upright in lead II, precede each QRS complex, alike
4. PR interval: 0.14 seconds
5. QRS interval: 0.06 seconds
6. Electrocardiogram (ECG) interpretation: Normal sinus rhythm

B.

1. Rhythm: Regular
2. Heart rate: 56 beats per minute
3. P waves: Smoothly rounded and upright in lead II, precede each QRS complex, alike
4. PR interval: 0.20 seconds
5. QRS interval: 0.08 seconds
6. ECG interpretation: Sinus bradycardia

CRITICAL THINKING

1. Assess patient: vital signs, heart sounds; note symptoms; place on heart monitor per agency protocol.
2. Report the patient findings to the registered nurse or physician. Elevate head of bed (HOB) for comfort, monitor vital signs, maintain oxygen per nasal cannula at 2 L/min per agency protocol, remain with patient to help alleviate anxiety.
3. Hypokalemia or ischemia causing irritability of the heart.
4. Light-headedness, feel heart skipping, chest pain, or fatigue.
5. ECG, oxygen, administration of potassium, electrolyte levels, may consider antidysrhythmic agent if symptomatic.

REVIEW QUESTIONS

*The correct answers are in **boldface**.*

1. (**c**) The complete heartbeat consisting of contraction or systole and relaxation or diastole of the atria and ventricles. (a, b) The circulation of the blood is a result of the action of the cardiac cycle. (d) is the contraction portion of the cardiac cycle.
2. (**b**) Assess patient. Monitored rhythms can be deceptive. Always "treat the patient, not the monitor." (a, c, d) may be appropriate actions *after* the patient is assessed, if indicated.
3. (**c**) The superior and inferior vena cavae. (a) delivers the blood back to the left side of the heart after oxygenation in the lungs. (b) receives the blood pumped from the left ventricle into the systemic circulation. (d) is a part of the heart's own circulation.
4. (**d**) is correct. (a) controls the flow of blood from one heart chamber to another and into the pulmonary and systemic circulations. (b) is the sac covering the heart. (c) collects blood to then be pumped out of the heart into the circulation.
5. (**a**) The left ventricle is the largest chamber. (b) The right ventricle is smaller. (c, d) Both the right and the left atria are smaller than either ventricle.
6. (**d**) The T wave represents ventricular *repolarization*, or the resting state of the heart. The U wave is frequently seen in patients with hypokalemia. (b) represents ventricular depolarization. (c) represents atrial *depolarization*.
7. (**b**) 40 to 60 beats per minute is the inherent rate for the atrioventricular node. (a) is the inherent rate for the ventricles. (c) is the normal rate for the sinoatrial node. (d) is not a normal heart rate.

8. (**c**) Sinus rhythms identify the impulse as having originated in the sinoatrial node. (a) Escape beats are late beats occurring when a more rapid focus fails to initiate a beat. (b) A block occurs when the normal conduction pathway of the heart is disturbed. (d) Ectopic rhythms are abnormal beats.
9. (**b**) Digoxin (Lanoxin) slows the heart rate and increases the force of contraction. (a) To decrease ectopic beats, you would give an antiarrhythmic such as procainamide or lidocaine intravenously, or quinidine orally. (c) To relieve chest pain, you would give nitroglycerin sublingually or intravenously. (d) To raise blood pressure, you would give a vasopressor such as dopamine or dobutamine.
10. (**a**) Atrial fibrillation can cause interruptions in the movement of blood through the heart and the formation of a thrombus, with serious consequences. (b) Swelling of hands and feet, often an early sign of heart failure, could be a less serious result of atrial fibrillation. (c, d) are not the result of atrial fibrillation.
11. (**d**) Both are appropriate treatments for atrial fibrillation. (a) Lidocaine is not an appropriate treatment, and oxygen only for the symptoms of extremely fast or slow atrial fib while correcting the dysrhythmia. (b) Nitroglycerin is not an appropriate treatment, and bed rest only to conserve energy while correcting the dysrhythmia. (c) Isuprel is not a treatment for atrial fibrillation.
12. (**a**) Three or more premature ventricular contractions (PVCs) in a row constitute ventricular tachycardia. (b) Bigeminy is a PVC every second beat. (c) Trigeminy is a PVC every three beats. (d) Multifocal PVCs are PVCs arising from different foci in the ventricle and therefore vary in appearance.
13. (**d**) In a hemodynamically stable patient, treatment with medication is the first choice. (a) Cardioversion would be tried only if other measures did not work. (b) Pacing is seldom an option for this. (c) Defibrillation is not appropriate treatment.
14. (**c**) is the correct answer. (a) is the name of the rhythm of a dying heart with wide QRS complex and slowing irregular rate. (b) is a pattern with no ventricular activity. (d) is the absence of a firing mechanism in the sinus node.
15. (**c**) Elevate the head of the bed and start oxygen by nasal cannula, both to improve oxygenation because oxygen hunger is a common cause of heart irritability. (a) An ECG is next after the previously stated actions. (b) Call the physician next. (d) is not an appropriate action; in fact, it would likely cause harm by compromising breathing by pressure of the diaphragm on the heart and lungs.

21

ANSWERS

▶ VOCABULARY

1. Pulmonary edema (Acute Heart Failure)
2. Cor pulmonale
3. splenomegaly, hepatomegaly
4. peripheral vascular resistance
5. Paroxysmal nocturnal dyspnea
6. preload
7. afterload
8. Orthopnea

▶ FLUID ACCUMULATION PATTERNS

Left-sided Heart Failure

Left ventricle → left atrium → pulmonary veins → lungs

Right-sided Heart Failure

Right ventricle → right atrium → vena cavae → jugular vein distention → hepatomegaly → splenomegaly → peripheral edema

▶ SIGNS AND SYMPTOMS OF HEART FAILURE

1. (L)   5. (R)
2. (R)   6. (L)
3. (L)   7. (R)
4. (R)   8. (L)

▶ CRITICAL THINKING

1. Left-sided heart failure leading to backward fluid accumulation in lung tissues and decreased cardiac output.

2. Left: dyspnea, cough, crackles, orthopnea. Right: jugular vein distention, peripheral edema.

3. (a) Potent diuretic to reduce fluid congestion and fluid returning to the heart (preload) to improve cardiac output. (b) Positive inotropic agent to strengthen heart's contraction. It also slows the heart rate, allowing better emptying of the ventricle. Cardiac output is increased. (c) Restricting sodium may reduce fluid volume and aid in reducing edema. (d) Provides greater availability of oxygen to the tissues by increasing the percentage of oxygen in inhaled air.

4. Mr. Donner is experiencing acute heart failure—pulmonary edema. Fluid accumulation in his lungs is severe and requires immediate treatment.

5. (a) Decreases fluid returning to the heart (preload) to ease the heart's workload and improve cardiac output. (b) Provides greater availability of oxygen in inhaled air. (c) Potent diuretic when given intravenously (IV) has a quicker onset of action to reduce the amount of fluid congestion and fluid returning to the heart to improve cardiac output. (d) Positive inotropic agent given IV has a quicker onset of action to strengthen the heart's contraction. (e) Sedative action reduces anxiety, and given IV it has a quicker onset of action.

6. Excess fluid volume related to (r/t) pump failure; clear breath sounds and free of edema. Activity intolerance r/t fatigue; tolerates activity with appropriate increases in heart rate, blood pressure, and respirations. Sleep pattern disturbance r/t nocturnal dyspnea; awakens refreshed and is less fatigued during day. Impaired gas exchange r/t pump failure; maintains clear lung fields. Anxiety r/t dyspnea; verbalizes decrease in anxiety. Self-care deficits (total) r/t fatigue and dyspnea; activities of daily living (ADLs) completed with assistance. Ineffective management of therapeutic regimen r/t lack of knowledge; states understanding of treatment plan and willingness to follow it.

7. Signs and symptoms of heart failure; medications; purpose, monitoring (heart rate, potassium), side effects; diet; energy conservation; daily weights.

▶ REVIEW QUESTIONS

*The correct answers are in **boldface**.*

1. (**b**) Decreased cardiac output occurs with heart failure, leading to reduced oxygenation of the tissues and therefore fatigue. (a, c, d) all result from heart failure, as does fatigue. They do not cause the fatigue.

2. (**d**) The heart is failing as a pump to move blood forward. (a) occurs in cardiac arrest, (b) occurs in a myocardial infarction, (c) is the opposite of what occurs with heart failure.

3. (**c**) Fluid in the lungs is heard as crackles. (a, b, d) are related to right-sided heart failure.

4. (**a**) If fluid accumulates from heart failure, weight will increase and is detectable by daily weights. (b) would be monitored for problems with an adequate caloric intake, not a fluid problem. (c) would be monitored for the effects of digitalis toxicity. (d) would be monitored for ascites development.

5. (**c**) 0.25 mg by mouth (PO) is the usual adult daily dose of digoxin (Lanoxin). (a, b) are less than the usual daily dose of Lanoxin. (d) is greater than the usual daily dose of Lanoxin.

6. (**b**) Lanoxin increases the strength of the heart's contraction. This allows better emptying of the ventricle, which improves cardiac output and increases blood flow to the kidneys, so increased urine output occurs. (a) If urine output decreases, the Lanoxin has not improved cardiac output to increase blood flow to the kidneys. (c) Lanoxin slows the heart rate. A rapid heart rate occurs to compensate for reduced cardiac output. (d) A slow heart rate is expected with Lanoxin, but below 50 is slower than desired for effectiveness.

7. (**a**) Hypokalemia may predispose to Lanoxin toxicity. (b, c, d) do not predispose to Lanoxin toxicity.

8. (**a**) Poor appetite is a common sign of Lanoxin toxicity. (b) Diarrhea is a side effect of Lanoxin. (c) Yellow lights, not halos, are a sign of toxicity. (d) Bradycardia occurs with toxicity.

9. (**d**) Furosemide is a loop diuretic that may deplete electrolytes, especially potassium, so ongoing monitoring of potassium is necessary. (a, b, c) are not affected directly by furosemide and are not monitored for this therapy.

10. (**a**) Morphine sulfate is given to relieve the patient's anxiety caused by the dyspnea of pulmonary edema. (b) Chest pain is usually associated with a myocardial infarction, not pulmonary edema. (c) It does not strengthen the heart's contraction. (d) It may decrease blood pressure.

11. (**d**) the right ventricle enlarges from the extra workload that occurs from the increased pulmonary pressures while ejecting blood into the pulmonary artery. (a, b, c) are not directly affected by pulmonary pressures.

12. (**c**) is a common sign of pulmonary edema. (a, b) are associated with right-sided heart failure. (d) Tachycardia occurs in pulmonary edema as a compensatory mechanism.

13. (**d**) Inotropic agents strengthen the heart's contractions. (a) An agent that slows the heart rate is a chronotropic agent. (b) An inotropic agent does not increase heart rate. (c) Conduction time is not affected by the inotropic property of a medication.

14. (**a**) Furosemide is a potent diuretic that works quickly when given IV to increase urine output. (b, c, d) are not the reasons a diuretic is given.

15. (**b**) An anxious patient is comforted by the presence of the nurse and does not want to be left alone. (a) would increase oxygen needs and increase dyspnea and anxiety. (c, d) could make the dyspneic patient feel more confined, increasing dyspnea and anxiety.

22

ANSWERS

▶ VOCABULARY

1. (I)
2. (J)
3. (B)
4. (C)
5. (F)
6. (D)
7. (A)
8. (E)
9. (H)
10. (G)

▶ CARDIAC SURGERY

Across

1. Endocarditis
2. Atelectasis
3. Aneurysm
4. Communication
5. Bowel infarction
6. Pain
7. Three
8. Ninety
9. Contusion
10. Glucose

Down

1. Deficient knowledge
2. Encephalopathy
3. Bleeding
4. Commissurotomy
5. Tissue
6. Postcardiotomy
7. Gastric distention
8. Myxoma
9. Saphenous
10. Total parenteral nutrition

▶ PREOPERATIVE CARDIAC SURGERY ADMISSION TESTING

1. Routine
2. Not routine
3. Routine
4. Routine
5. Routine
6. Not routine
7. Not routine
8. Routine
9. Not routine
10. Not routine

▶ CARDIOPULMONARY BYPASS

Corrections are in **boldface.**

Using the cardiopulmonary bypass (CPB) pump can present its own unique set of complications. Before going on the pump, the patient is **anticoagulated** with heparin until the prothrombin time (PTT) is **five** to **six** times greater than normal. The effects of the heparin are reversed with **protamine sulfate,** the antidote for heparin, immediately **before** coming off the pump. However, heparin is absorbed and stored in organs and tissue and can be sporadically released hours after surgery, thus predisposing the patient to excessive **bleeding.** Air embolism is a risk that is **minimized** by the pump being primed with lactated Ringer's solution. The priming solution increases circulating volume, which then results in a shifting of fluid into the interstitial tissue and edema formation. These fluid shifts can continue up to 6 hours after surgery and can cause **hypotension.**

▶ CRITICAL THINKING

1. Arterial blood gases, pulmonary function tests.
2. Immediately, and repeat or reinforce information when family members arrive.
3. Yes, if he is asking for the information.
4. Insulin requirements will increase due to the stress of surgery, increasing the endogenous production of glucose while decreasing the production of insulin.
5. He may require more frequent suctioning, a longer period of intubation, and mechanical ventilation because of his history of chronic obstructive pulmonary disease.

▶ REVIEW QUESTIONS

*The correct answers are in **boldface**.*

1. **(b)** is correct. (a, c, d) are not functions of the CPB machine.
2. **(b)** is correct. (a, c, d) are incorrect.
3. **(c)** is correct. (a, b, d) are not caused by lactated Ringer's solution, and they are not usual problems that occur immediately after cardiac surgery.
4. **(d)** is correct. (a) is not a surgical treatment. (b) is a mitral annuloplasty. (c) is not a surgical treatment.
5. **(d)** is correct. (a) Hypotension tends to occur more frequently than hypertension, and both are usually transient unless there is pre-existing hypertension. (b, c) are complications but do not occur as frequently as bleeding.
6. **(a)** The highest time for rejection is immediately after surgery occurs. The risk decreases over time, although it is still possible.
7. **(d)** is correct. (a, b, c) He is complaining of pain in his midsternal chest area, not in his head, lower abdomen, or lateral chest.
8. **(c)** is correct. (a, d) He is not at risk of a sternal fracture or pneumothorax occurring after the trauma. (b) He is not at risk of a myocardial infarction after the trauma unless he had a pre-existing heart condition.
9. **(a)** is correct. (b) Chest tubes are not inserted into the pericardium, where the blood is building, although this would help a pneumothorax. (c) might be the treatment of a sternal fracture. (d) would probably be included in the treatment of a myocardial infarction.
10. **(d)** is correct. (a, b, c) are progressive, more of a chronic disease process.
11. **(c)** is correct. (a, b, d) There usually is not enough blood loss to produce anemia or hypovolemia leading to shock.
12. **(b)** is correct. (a) is when a piece of grafting material is used to join an artery and a vein. (c) is a malformation of the blood supply in the brain. (d) is the graft or material that is used to join the artery and vein in an arteriovenous shunt.
13. **(c)** is correct. (a, b, d) are all qualities of pulses.
14. **(a)** is correct. (b, c, d) are complications of cardiac surgery but are not the most common.
15. **(b)** is correct. (a, c, d) will not reinflate the alveoli, which are collapsed from atelectasis.

23

ANSWERS

▶ VOCABULARY
1. Ecchymosis
2. Lymphedema
3. petechiae
4. Purpura
5. thrombocytopenia

▶ LYMPHATIC SYSTEM
1. (B)   4. (A)
2. (D)   5. (C)
3. (E)

▶ STRUCTURES OF THE LYMPHATIC SYSTEM

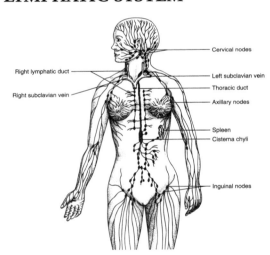

Right lymphatic duct
Right subclavian vein
Cervical nodes
Left subclavian vein
Thoracic duct
Axillary nodes
Spleen
Cisterna chyli
Inguinal nodes

▶ HEMATOPOIETIC SYSTEM
1. (J)   6. (C)
2. (F)   7. (D)
3. (B)   8. (A)
4. (G)   9. (H)
5. (I)   10. (E)

▶ CRITICAL THINKING
1. Fever may indicate a febrile or hemolytic reaction. Back pain is an early symptom of hemolytic reaction. Respiratory distress may signal circulatory overload or anaphylaxis. Crackles are a symptom of circulatory overload. Hives indicate an urticarial reaction.
2. Even though 20 breaths per minute may be normal, it is an increase for Mr. Foster. A thorough assessment should be done and the registered nurse notified, in case this is an early sign of a reaction.
3. The maximum time blood can hang is 4 hours from the time it is picked up from the blood bank.

▶ REVIEW QUESTIONS
The correct answers are in boldface.
1. (**a**)
2. (**d**)
3. (**d**)
4. (**b**)
5. (**c**) is correct. The partial thromboplastin time (PTT) is monitored for heparin therapy. (a, b) are used to monitor warfarin therapy. (d) indicates platelet function.
6. (**d**) is correct. Cryoprecipitate contains clotting factors. (a, b, c) do not contain clotting factors.
7. (**b**) is correct. The international normalized ratio (INR) should be between 2 and 3. 1.6 is low. (a) The patient is unlikely to bleed with a low INR. (c) The dose should be altered only by the physician. (d) Vitamin K might be given if the INR is prolonged.
8. (**a**) is correct. Blood flows more easily through a larger-gauge needle. (b, c, d) are too small and may damage red blood cells (RBCs).
9. (**c**) is correct. The transfusion must be stopped immediately because these are symptoms of a possible deadly hemolytic reaction. (a) A physical assessment would be nice, but this is an emergency and there is not time. (b) There is no time for a good pain assessment. (d) An analgesic can be administered after emergency care has stabilized the patient.
10. (**b**) is correct. A bone marrow biopsy is painful. (a) Explaining the procedure to the family should be done, but it is not as important as pain control for the patient. (c) The patient is observed for bleeding after, not before, the procedure. (d) The physician can drape the site.

24

ANSWERS

► VOCABULARY

1. False	6. False
2. True	7. True
3. True	8. True
4. True	9. False
5. False	10. True

► CRITICAL THINKING

1. Mr. Frantzis is in the final stage of his disease, and he has opted for no treatment. Rehabilitation is no longer a goal. On days when he is feeling especially tired, it would be appropriate to bring him his breakfast in bed. A liquid supplement that is easy to drink might also be helpful.

2. Do a complete pain assessment using the WHAT'S UP? format. The pain might be sternal or rib tenderness from crowding of bone marrow. Administer analgesics as ordered.

3. Not all runny noses are infectious. Find out if the nursing assistant has a cold. If so, reassign Mr. Frantzis' care to another assistant, because he is at risk of infection.

4. Mr. Frantzis may be developing confusion if the leukemia has invaded the central nervous system. Clarify with him who Jennifer is, and assess him for confusion (keep in mind that you may look like someone named Jennifer, and he may not be confused at all). If he is becoming confused, institute measures to keep him safe.

5. Provide good mouth care after each meal and as required. Use a soft toothbrush or a swab if irritation is severe. Avoid giving him foods that are irritating, acidic, or extremely hot or cold. Remove his dentures for cleaning and at bedtime. Inspect his mouth carefully while dentures are out.

► SICKLE CELL ANEMIA

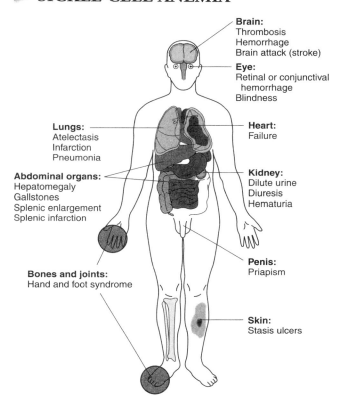

Brain:
Thrombosis
Hemorrhage
Brain attack (stroke)

Eye:
Retinal or conjunctival
  hemorrhage
Blindness

Lungs:
Atelectasis
Infarction
Pneumonia

Heart:
Failure

Abdominal organs:
Hepatomegaly
Gallstones
Splenic enlargement
Splenic infarction

Kidney:
Dilute urine
Diuresis
Hematuria

Penis:
Priapism

Bones and joints:
Hand and foot syndrome

Skin:
Stasis ulcers

► REVIEW QUESTIONS

The correct answers are in **boldface.**

1. **(b)** is correct. Red meat is high in iron. (a, c, d) are not as high in iron.

2. **(b)** is correct. Hemoglobin carries oxygen to tissues; hemoglobin level is reduced in anemia. (a) Oxygen transport to tissues is the problem. (c) Oxygen, not nutrients, is the problem. (d) Anemia does not cause lung damage.

3. **(d)** is correct. The conjunctivae are pale in a patient with anemia. (a, b, c) are not necessarily pale in anemia, especially in a dark-skinned patient.

4. **(a)** is correct. The patient with anemia may experience palpitations as an early compensatory mechanism. (b, c, d) are later signs.

5. **(b)** is correct. Chilling and exercise may both contribute to hypoxemia and a crisis. (a, c, d) do not cause hypoxemia.

6. **(a)** is correct. Infarction of small bones in the fingers and toes causes unequal growth. (b, c, d) are not symptoms of hand-foot syndrome.

7. **(c)** is correct. The best measure of effective teaching is actual change in behavior, as evidenced by the patient using an electric razor. (a, b, d) are all good measures of learning, but they are not as convincing as the actual change in behavior.

8. **(b)** is correct. Often the patient knows best when bleeding is occurring, and treatment should be initiated as soon as possible. (a) Deep palpation may injure tissue and worsen bleeding. (c) An x-ray will waste valuable time when the patient could be receiving treatment. (d) Heat is a vasodilator and could increase bleeding. Also, waiting before beginning treatment is not recommended.

9. **(d)** is correct. Multiple myeloma attacks bone, making it prone to fractures. (a, b, c) are not directly related to multiple myeloma.

10. **(a)** is correct. Fluids help minimize complications of hypercalcemia. (b) Respiratory problems are not related to hypercalcemia. (c) Activity should be encouraged to keep calcium in the bones. (d) Heat will not affect calcium.

25

ANSWERS

VOCABULARY

1. lymphoma
2. Lymph nodes
3. B, T
4. splenomegaly
5. splenectomy

HODGKIN'S DISEASE

*Corrections are in **boldface**.*

Joe is a 28-year-old construction worker diagnosed with stage I Hodgkin's disease. He initially went to his physician because of a **painless** lump in his neck. He is also experiencing **low-grade fevers** and weight loss. The diagnosis was confirmed by the presence of Reed-**Sternberg** cells by the lab. He expresses his fears to his nurse, who tells him that **although Hodgkin's disease is a cancer,** it is often curable. Joe takes a leave from work and begins **curative** radiation therapy.

REVIEW QUESTIONS

*The correct answers are in **boldface**.*

1. (**d**) is correct. Fatigue is subjective and is best by the patient. (a, b, c) may be indirectly related to fatigue, but they rely on the nurse's interpretation.

2. (**a**) is correct. Going to church will place the patient in a crowd of people, which will increase risk of exposure to infection. (b, c, d) do not expose the patient to infection.

3. (**c**) is correct. This can assist her to identify support systems that can help her cope. (a, b) offer false reassurance. (d) is inappropriate because there is no evidence that she is terminal at this time. It may be addressed at a time when she is coping better.

4. (**a**) is correct. Vitamin K can help correct clotting problems and prevent bleeding during surgery. (b, c, d) are not affected by vitamin K.

5. (**b**) is correct. A high incision often discourages deep breathing and coughing because of the resulting pain. This can result in infection. (a) platelet count does not increase risk of infection; (c, d) early ambulation and discharge may help prevent infection.

6. (**d**) is correct. Fever is a sign of infection. (a, b, c) are not signs of infection.

7. (**c**) is correct. Vaccines will help guard against infection. (a, b) do not help prevent infection; (d) is unnecessary.

26

ANSWERS

▶ VOCABULARY

1. Dyspnea
2. Crepitus
3. Thoracentesis
4. Barrel chest
5. Respiratory excursion
6. Adventitious
7. Tracheotomy
8. Tidaling
9. Apnea
10. Tracheostomy

▶ ANATOMY

1, 6, 8, 5, 2, 4, 10, 3, 7, 9, 11

▶ VENTILATION

1, 4, 3, 6, 2, 5, 7

▶ ADVENTITIOUS LUNG SOUNDS

1. (E)   4. (D)
2. (A)   5. (C)
3. (F)   6. (B)

▶ CHEST DRAINAGE

Suction chamber

Water seal chamber

Drainage collection chamber

THE RESPIRATORY SYSTEM

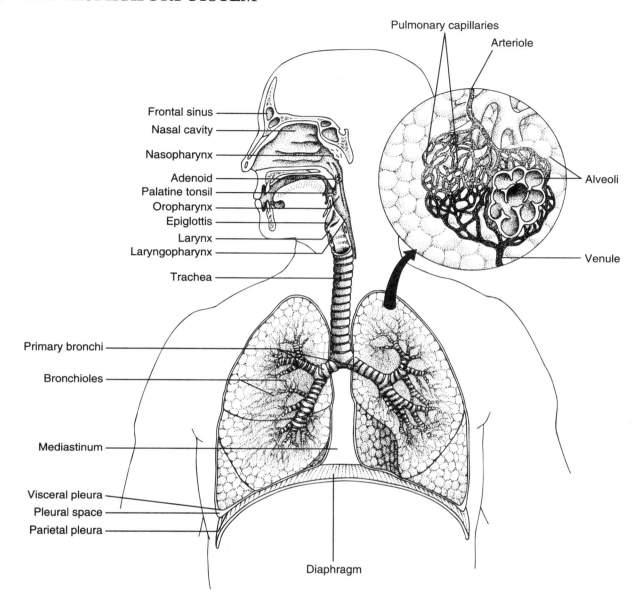

Pulmonary capillaries

Arteriole

Frontal sinus

Nasal cavity

Nasopharynx

Adenoid

Palatine tonsil

Oropharynx

Epiglottis

Larynx

Laryngopharynx

Trachea

Alveoli

Venule

Primary bronchi

Bronchioles

Mediastinum

Visceral pleura

Pleural space

Parietal pleura

Diaphragm

CRITICAL THINKING

1. Mr. Howe's cough should be assessed using the WHAT'S UP? technique. He should be asked how it feels, how bad it is, what makes it better or worse, and when it started. In addition, he should be asked about amount, color, odor, and consistency of sputum.
2. Night sweats, cough, and weight loss are typical symptoms of tuberculosis (TB). Bloody sputum is also common. These symptoms should alert the nurse to ask the physician about the likelihood of TB and the need for isolation to protect staff and other patients.
3. A chest x-ray and sputum culture and sensitivity will be ordered. Additional tests for TB are discussed in Chapter 28.
4. Mr. Howe should be kept nil per os (NPO) according to institution policy before the bronchoscopy. An injection of atropine may be ordered to dry secretions. After the test, Mr. Howe's vital signs and respiratory status will be monitored. Mr. Howe will remain NPO until his gag reflex returns. The nurse should consult the physician's orders for additional postprocedure instructions.

REVIEW QUESTIONS

*The correct answers are in **boldface**.*

1. (**d**) is correct.
2. (**b**) is correct.
3. (**d**) is correct.
4. (**b**) is correct.
5. (**c**) is correct.
6. (**c**) is correct. Cilia help remove potential pathogens. (a, b, d) are not affected by changes in cilia.
7. (**b**) is correct. Wheezes sound like a violin. (a) crackles sound like Velcro. (c) A friction rub sounds like leather rubbing together. (d) Crepitus is not a lung sound.

8. **(b)** is correct. The first concern is increasing oxygenation, and replacing the oxygen will help. (a, c) may be appropriate, but oxygen should be tried first. (d) 72-percent is not normal.

9. **(a)** is correct. Pursed lip breathing helps excrete carbon dioxide. (b, c, d) are not promoted by pursed lip breathing.

10. **(d)** is correct. "Good lung down" has been shown to increase oxygenation. (a, b, c) do not increase oxygenation.

11. **(a)** is correct. Assistance with cleaning the catheter two to three times a day should be provided. (b) Transtracheal oxygen usually prevents the need for another oxygen source. (c) Removal of the catheter for this length of time may cause the tract into the trachea to close. (d) A transtracheal catheter is not hooked to humidification.

12. **(d)** is correct. Chest physiotherapy (CPT) helps mobilize secretions. (a) CPT does not affect chest muscles. (b) CPT does not use humidification. (c) CPT does not promote expansion.

13. **(c)** is correct. Reducing the level of wall suction will reduce the bubbling. (a) Bubbling in the water-seal chamber, not the suction chamber, indicates a system leak. (b) There is no need to replace the system. (d) Increasing the water level will increase the level of suction.

27

ANSWERS

► VOCABULARY

1. laryngectomee
2. epistaxis
3. exudate
4. rhinoplasty
5. dysphagia
6. rhinitis

► NASAL SURGERY

1. Wake Mr. Jones and examine his throat. He may be swallowing blood. Vital signs should also be checked for signs of blood loss. Make sure that he is in semi-Fowler's position.
2. "You may need to ask your physician for an antihistamine or cough suppressant. If you must sneeze, be sure to do so with your mouth open. A stool softener and plenty of liquids and fiber can help keep your stools soft."
3. "Aspirin and related drugs such as ibuprofen can increase your risk for bleeding and should be avoided." Acetaminophen is preferred if it is not contraindicated.

► CRITICAL THINKING

1. Influenza is caused by a virus. Antibiotics will not be effective. Antibiotics must be used with discretion to prevent the development of resistant strains of bacteria.
2. Fever and illness can lead to dehydration. Fluids will also help thin respiratory secretions so that they are more easily expectorated.
3. Fever may be beneficial if it is not too high. Ask the physician at what temperature she recommends acetaminophen. Some sources say to give it only if fever reaches above 103° F or if discomfort is severe.
4. Influenza is contagious, so if symptoms are the same, it would be reasonable to provide the same care as was recommended for your son. It is probably not necessary to take her to the doctor unless additional symptoms develop or symptoms persist.
5. The elderly are more at risk for complications of influenza, especially pneumonia. She should see her physician.

► REVIEW QUESTIONS

*The correct answers are in **boldface**.*

1. (**a**) is correct. Facial tenderness is a symptom of a sinus infection. (b, c, d) are not symptoms of sinus infection.
2. (**c**) is correct. Rest will help the immune system fight the infection. Humidity will help loosen secretions. (a, d) are effective for pulmonary, not sinus, secretions; (b) is not a nursing intervention.
3. (**d**) is correct. Interventions were aimed at comfort. (a, b, c) do not evaluate effectiveness of comfort measures.
4. (**d**) is correct. Dysphagia and hoarseness are common symptoms of cancer of the larynx. (a, b, c) may possibly develop later or as complications, but they are not early symptoms.
5. (**c**) is correct. A patent airway is always a priority. Remember your ABCs (airway, breathing, circulation). (a, b, d) are important but will not be of any use if the airway is not patent.
6. (**a**) is correct. If a patient places a finger over his laryngectomy, he will cut off his air supply. (b, c, d) are all options for communication for a patient with a laryngectomy.
7. (**a**) is correct. Narcotics depress the respiratory rate and cough reflex, which would increase risk for postoperative complications. (b) Narcotics do not increase secretions; (c) they do not cause stomal edema; and (d) narcotics can be addicting, but not when they are taken for legitimate pain.
8. (**c**) is correct. Pollutants in the tracheostomy can cause infection and irritation. (a) He will be taught to suction his tracheostomy as needed; (b) this is not a therapeutic statement; and (d) he will need to do routine tracheostomy care.
9. (**d**) is correct. A sitting position will help reduce bleeding. Leaning forward will allow the blood to drain out of the nose so that bleeding can be monitored. (a, c) Lying down increases pressure in the nose and may increase bleeding, and (b) extending the neck will allow blood to drain down the back of the throat and be swallowed, making it impossible to monitor the severity of the bleeding.
10. (**d**) is correct. Epinephrine is a vasoconstrictor. (a) Raising the blood pressure (BP) can increase bleeding; (b) it may dilate bronchioles, but this will not help bleeding; and (c) epinephrine does not enhance clotting.

28

ANSWERS

▶ VOCABULARY

Across

3. ARDS (acute respiratory distress syndrome)
4. Paradoxical
7. Hemoptysis
9. MDI (metered dose inhaler)
10. Mucous
13. Thoracotomy
18. NMT (nebulized mist treatment)
20. Pleurodesis
21. Bleb
22. TB

Down

1. AP (anteroposterior)
2. Ectopic
3. Antitussive
5. Adjuvant
6. ABG (arterial blood gases)
8. Anergy
11. Status
12. Exudate
14. Hemothorax
15. Tachypnea
16. Induration
17. Risk
19. SOB

▶ RESPIRATORY MEDICATIONS

1. (**B**)   5. (**A**)
2. (**D**)   6. (**C**)
3. (**E**)   7. (**G**)
4. (**F**)

▶ CRITICAL THINKING

1. A complete respiratory assessment should be done. Edith's respiratory symptoms can be assessed using the WHAT'S UP? format. Degree of dyspnea can be rated on a scale of 0 to 10. Lung sounds are auscultated. Activity tolerance is assessed. Skin color is noted.
2. A 48 pack-year history can mean two packs a day for 24 years, or three packs a day for 16 years, and so on. Multiply packs per day by number of years for pack-years.
3. Emphysema causes destruction of alveolar membranes and adjacent capillaries, reducing the surface area available for gas exchange. Reduced gas exchange results in hypoxia, which causes dyspnea.
4. Edith's lung sounds will most likely sound diminished.
5. Edith probably has a chronically high P_{CO_2}, making a low P_{O_2} her stimulus to breathe. If a high flow rate of oxygen is administered, it will reduce her stimulus to breathe.
6. Emphysema increases the risk for occurrence of bullae and blebs. Rupture of these can cause pneumothorax.
7. Fowler's, semi-Fowler's, or orthopneic (leaning over bedside table) positions increase room for lung expansion and help reduce dyspnea. Sitting in a chair may also help if it is not too tiring.
8. Edith has probably had many lectures on the evils of smoking. Assess her knowledge of the relationship between her illness and her smoking. If she is willing, her physician can be asked for an order for nicotine patches and medication, and she can be referred to a local stop-smoking program (check yellow pages). Assist her to identify a friend who has quit smoking for support.

▶ REVIEW QUESTIONS

The correct answers are in **boldface***.*

1. (**a**) is correct; 86 percent is low, and the patient would benefit from supplemental oxygen. (b) 86 percent is not normal. (c) 86 percent does not warrant emergency treatment unless additional symptoms are present. (d) Walking in the hall will further reduce his Sa_{O_2}.
2. (**a**) is correct. A bronchoscopy is an endoscopic procedure. (b, c, d) A bronchoscopy does not involve dyes or x-rays.
3. (**d**) is correct. The patient's throat will have been numbed and irritated by the scope. A gag reflex must be

present before he can safely eat. (a) Breakfast should be held until the gag reflex returns. (b) There is no dye. (c) The patient did not receive a general anesthesia. Any sedation given should be gone before he returns to his room.

4. **(b)** is correct. Smoking and chemicals can increase the risk of cancer. (a, c, d) do not increase cancer risk.

5. **(b)** is correct. Radiation for lung cancer is palliative. (a) Surgery is the treatment for cure. (c) He will probably require oxygen eventually. (d) Treatment may slow the spread but will probably not totally prevent it.

6. **(a)** is correct. Airways are inflamed and spastic in asthma. (b) Asthma does not cause fluid collection. (c) Asthma constricts rather than stretches airways. (d) Asthma is not caused by infection, although infection may exacerbate it.

7. **(b)** is correct. Emphysema destroys alveoli, causing loss of elasticity and air trapping. (a) Inflammation and secretions are more characteristic of bronchitis. (c) Capillaries are damaged in emphysema, but the entire blood supply is not destroyed. (d) Large sacs of sputum are not present in emphysema.

8. **(d)** is correct. Corticosteroids have potent anti-inflammatory action. (a, b, c) are not affected by corticosteroids.

9. **(a)** is correct; 2 L/min is the maximum rate for patients with chronic respiratory disease. (b, c, d) are too high and may reduce respiratory drive.

10. **(c)** is correct. Intravenous morphine can reduce acute dyspnea. (a) Cortisone is slower acting. (b) Meperidine (Demerol) will not help. (d) A beta blocker may worsen dyspnea.

11. **(b)** is correct. It is the only placement that keeps the system below the patient's chest. (a, c, d) all risk having the system above the patient's chest, which can cause return of drainage to the chest.

12. **(a)** is correct. Bubbling in the water-seal chamber indicates an air leak. (b) will reduce bubbling in the suction control chamber. (c) Vigorous bubbling is not expected in the water-seal chamber. (d) Asking the patient to cough will not correct the problem.

13. **(b)** is correct. Auscultating lung sounds will help determine whether the lung is re-expanding. (a, c, d) may all be appropriate, but they do not monitor whether the chest-drainage system is helping.

14. **(a)** is correct. Smoking is a major risk factor for many kinds of lung disease. (b, c, d) are risk factors for a variety of problems, but they are not as significant as smoking in causing lung disease.

29

ANSWERS

▶ **FUNCTIONS OF THE GASTROINTESTINAL SYSTEM**

1. lower esophageal
2. ileocecal
3. pyloric
4. small
5. stomach
6. large
7. small
8. esophagus
9. external anal
10. salivary
11. teeth, tongue
12. villi
13. rectum

▶ **STRUCTURES OF THE GASTROINTESTINAL SYSTEM**

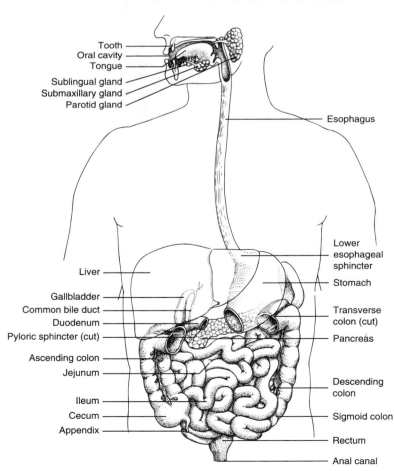

Tooth
Oral cavity
Tongue
Sublingual gland
Submaxillary gland
Parotid gland
Esophagus
Lower esophageal sphincter
Liver
Stomach
Gallbladder
Common bile duct
Duodenum
Transverse colon (cut)
Pyloric sphincter (cut)
Pancreas
Ascending colon
Jejunum
Descending colon
Ileum
Cecum
Sigmoid colon
Appendix
Rectum
Anal canal

► VOCABULARY

1. Endoscope
2. Bowel sounds
3. Colonoscopy
4. Gavage
5. Impaction
6. Guaiac
7. Fluoroscope
8. Steatorrhea
9. Gastric analysis
10. Gastroscopy

► LABORATORY TESTS

1. **(E)**
2. **(D)**
3. **(B)**
4. **(A)**
5. **(C)**

► BOWEL PREPARATION

Corrections are in **boldface.**

A **bowel** preparation is required for several procedures that visualize the lower bowel. This preparation is important for effective test results. An incomplete bowel preparation may prevent the test from being done or cause the need for it to be repeated. This can result in the patient's **delayed** discharge and **increased costs.** The patient usually receives a **clear liquid** diet 24 hours before the test, and a **warm** tap-water enema or Fleet enema is given **until returns are clear.** Elderly or debilitated patients should be carefully assessed during the administration of multiple enemas, which can fatigue the patient and **decrease** electrolytes. In patients with bleeding or **severe diarrhea,** the bowel preparation may not be ordered by the physician.

► CRITICAL THINKING

1. The total parenteral nutrition (TPN) rate should be started at a lower rate and gradually increased until the ordered rate is reached. This is necessary to allow body systems and the pancreas time to adjust to the high dextrose concentration.

2. The high dextrose percentage can cause the patient to be hyperglycemic, so it is necessary to monitor serum glucose levels to detect this and treat it with insulin. If the patient becomes hyperglycemic, it does not indicate that he or she is diabetic. When the high dextrose percentage is stopped, the patient's blood glucose returns to baseline levels. If insulin is given, it is used only temporarily to cover the hyperglycemia.

3. (a) Dextrose of 12 percent or less may be given in peripheral veins; (b) dextrose greater than 12 percent must be given in a central vein such as the subclavian or jugular vein because the high glucose concentration is irritating to veins.

4. It is important to run TPN on an infusion pump to carefully control the rate. It is important not to allow the TPN to go in too quickly, or hyperglycemia and then dehydration from the high blood sugar can result. Dehydration occurs from the body's attempt to dilute and eliminate the high levels of blood sugar.

5. TPN should never be increased to catch it up if it is behind schedule because the patient would become hyperglycemic and dehydrated.

6. When TPN is discontinued, the infusion must be slowly weaned off to prevent hypoglycemia from occurring if the dextrose was abruptly stopped. This weaning must take several hours and may take up to 48 hours.

7. When TPN is ordered to be stopped, the patient is fed if not contraindicated to prevent hypoglycemia from occurring when the dextrose is stopped.

8. *Possible nursing diagnosis:* Imbalanced nutrition: less than body requirements.
   Outcome: Patient will maintain ideal body weight or gain weight toward goal weight.
   Interventions:
   Obtain baseline patient weight and identify ideal body weight.
   Identify barriers to nutrient ingestion.
   Weigh patient weekly and report changes to physician.
   Administer and monitor TPN as ordered according to TPN protocols.
   Monitor lab values such as albumin and absolute lymphocyte levels.
   If patient is receiving TPN, monitor blood glucose levels.
   Teach patient about TPN and necessary management of it if it is used in the home setting.

► REVIEW QUESTIONS

The correct answers are in **boldface.**

1. **(b)**
2. **(b)**
3. **(a)**
4. **(c)**
5. **(c)** Hypoactive bowel sounds occur less than 5 to 30 per minute. (a) There are some bowel sounds, so they are not absent; (b) hyperactive bowel sounds occur at a rate greater than 30 per minute; (d) the rate of 4 per minute is less than normal.
6. **(c)** Bowel sounds must be auscultated for 5 minutes in each quadrant to be considered absent. (a, b) A time period less than 5 minutes is considered inadequate to conclude that bowel sounds are absent; (d) listening for 15 minutes is an excessive amount of time to auscultate bowel sounds.
7. **(c)** Stool cultures must be collected using sterile technique so as not to introduce any pathogens to the specimen that would alter the test results. (a, b, d) can be done using clean technique.
8. **(b)** A flat plate x-ray can be done with food in the stomach or feces in the bowel, which does not impair visibility of the structures and has no risk for aspiration. (a, c, d) all require clear visibility or may have a risk of aspiration.
9. **(a)** Barium can produce constipation if it is not diluted. (b) is incorrect because there is no pain during or after a barium swallow; (c) is incorrect because nutritional intake is not excessive as a result of the barium ingestion;

(d) is incorrect because the barium can produce constipation, not diarrhea, if it is not diluted.

10. **(c)** The chalky barium will cause the patient's stool to look white for 1 to 3 days after the procedure. (a) Stools usually gradually return to a brown color; (b, d) are not associated with the color of barium and are not normal stool colors.

11. **(b)** The gag reflex must return before the patient eats or drinks to prevent aspiration. (a) Keeping the patient nil per os (NPO) does not rest the vocal cords; (c) there is no reason to keep the throat after an esophagogastroduodenoscopy (EGD); (d) an absent gag reflex does not stimulate vomiting.

12. **(d)** The patient sits upright to facilitate the tube moving down into the stomach by gravity. (a, b, c) do not facilitate insertion of the nasogastric (NG) tube by gravity and would inhibit the tube insertion.

13. **(c)** Disturbed body image is expressed by how patients see themselves and the pride they take in their appearance. (a, b, d) do not address the embarrassment the patient expresses.

14. **(b)** Swallowing helps insertion by closing the epiglottis, thus preventing the NG tube from slipping into the trachea, which could obstruct the airway and be dangerous to the patient. (a, c) close the throat, preventing passage of the tube into the esophagus; (d) has no effect on the insertion of the NG tube.

30

ANSWERS

▶ VOCABULARY

1. *Helicobacter pylori*
2. Anorexia
3. Gastritis
4. Aphthous stomatitis
5. Bulimia nervosa
6. Dumping syndrome
7. Gastrectomy
8. Obesity
9. Hiatal hernia
10. Gastrojejunostomy

▶ GASTRITIS

1. (A)   5. (B)
2. (B)   6. (A)
3. (A)   7. (C)
4. (C)   8. (A)

▶ PEPTIC ULCER DISEASE

*Corrections are in **boldface**.*

Most peptic ulcers are caused by the **bacteria *Helicobacter pylori*.** Peptic ulcers are commonly found in the **duodenum.** Symptoms of peptic ulcers include burning and a gnawing pain in the **epigastric region.** There is pain and discomfort on an **empty** stomach, which may be relieved by **ingesting** food. Peptic ulcers **can** be cured. Medication treatment for most peptic ulcers should include **antibiotics** as indicated.

▶ GASTRECTOMY

Vagus nerve
Distal portion resected

Stomach joined to jejunum

Stomach joined to duodenum

Total resection of cancerous stomach

Esophagus
Diaphragm
Jejunum
Duodenum

► CRITICAL THINKING

1. Your first action is to prevent Mrs. Sheffield from aspirating. You maintain her side-lying position and remind her to remain in this position, propping her with pillows so she does not aspirate.

2. Your next action is to take her vital signs.

3. You determine that Mrs. Sheffield is in the early stages of hypovolemic shock (increased pulse and respirations, decreased temperature and blood pressure, and diaphoresis), and her gastric bleeding needs to be stopped immediately. You maintain her intermittent low-wall suction to aspirate the gastric output, thus preventing further gastric distention. You also maintain her intravenous (IV) setting to compensate for her fluid loss.

4. You notify the physician of Mrs. Sheffield's condition.

5. Current vital signs; signs and symptoms—diaphoresis, nausea, slightly distended abdomen; intake and output—vomitus (amount and color), nasogastric output (amount and color), IV (solution and rate), urine output since return to your unit; other data: the time Mrs. Sheffield returned from the postanesthesia care unit, her vital signs, and your general assessment of her on return to your unit.

6. Apply oxygen at 2 L via nasal cannula and reassure the patient that her condition is being closely monitored and that her physician is taking her back to surgery to repair her abdomen. Then order the laboratory work. Gather the equipment necessary to transport Mrs. Sheffield with oxygen, an emesis basin, and some extra blankets.

► REVIEW QUESTIONS

The correct answers are in **boldface.**

1. **(a)** Confusion is a common side effect of cimetidine, especially in the elderly. (b, c, d) are not side effects of cimetidine.

2. **(a)** Anorexia is a symptom of chronic gastritis type B. (b) Dysphagia is seen in gastroesophageal reflux disease. (c) Diarrhea is not a sign of chronic gastritis type B. (d) A feeling of fullness can occur in patients with dumping syndrome.

3. **(d)** Gastrectomy is the only effective treatment for gastric cancer. (a) Gastroplasty reduces the size of the stomach to treat morbid obesity. (b) Gastrorrhaphy is suturing of the stomach wall. (c) Gastric stapling is a surgical treatment for obese patients.

4. **(b)** Diaphoresis is a common sign of hypovolemic shock. (a) Hypotension, not hypertension, is a sign of hypovolemic shock. (c) The pulse would be weak and thready, not bounding. (d) There would not be edema associated with hypovolemic shock.

5. **(c)** A low-fat diet is advised to decrease the fat content in the stool. (a) A bland diet may decrease irritation of the bowel, but the patient's problem stems from inadequate mixing of food with pancreatic and biliary secretions to digest fats, and a low-fat diet would be more

helpful for this. (b) A high-carbohydrate diet does not prevent fat from being introduced in the diet. (d) A pureed diet would not be helpful because it could contain fat.

6. **(d)** Diet management and exercise are the first interventions used to promote weight loss in the obese patient because they are noninvasive. Also, monitoring the patient in a diet and exercise program gives the health care provider information about the patient's metabolism, food preferences, food habits, rate of weight loss, and activity tolerances. (a) is a surgical procedure that would be considered if noninvasive interventions were not successful. (b, c) are not surgical procedures used for treating obesity; they are used for diseases such as cancer.

7. **(a)** Eating small, frequent meals that can pass easily through the esophagus prevents the rapid filling of the stomach and thus heartburn and regurgitation. (b) The patient should avoid reclining for 1 hour after eating because reclining would promote reflux, not prevent it. (c) The patient should sleep in an elevated position to prevent reflux by raising the head of the bed on 6-inch blocks and using pillows. (d) Eating before bedtime should be avoided so the stomach is empty, to prevent reflux.

8. **(d)** Start the oxygen first. Use Maslow's hierarchy to help prioritize interventions. Oxygen administration will increase the amount of oxygen in the vascular system, thus increasing the oxygen to the tissues. (a) The IV should be hung next to help restore and maintain volume. (b) The laboratory can be called to draw blood for a complete blood cell count while other interventions are occurring, which will give you a hemoglobin level that will indicate oxygen-carrying capacity. (c) While his blood is being drawn and processed, insert the nasogastric tube, which will decompress his stomach, and keep the head of his bed up 30 to 45 degrees to prevent aspiration of any emesis.

9. **(a)** A painless ulcer is common early in oral cancer. (b) White painful ulcers describe aphthous stomatitis (canker sore). (c) Feeling of fullness occurs with hiatal hernia or esophageal cancer. (d) Heartburn occurs with hiatal hernia.

10. **(b)** Esophageal dilation is performed to enlarge the esophagus and allow food to pass the obstruction caused by the tumor. (a) Gastrectomy is done for stomach cancer. (c, d) Radical or modified neck dissection is performed for oral cancer that has metastasized to cervical lymph nodes.

11. **(d)** Foods that cause discomfort need to be identified so they can be avoided. (a) Large meals promote reflux, so small meals should be eaten. (b) Sleeping flat without pillows promotes reflux, so the patient should be elevated. (c) Lying down after each meal would promote reflux, so the patient should sit up for 2 hours after a meal.

31
ANSWERS

▶ VOCABULARY

1. (L)
2. (J)
3. (B)
4. (K)
5. (A)
6. (D)

7. (H)
8. (I)
9. (C)
10. (E)
11. (G)
12. (F)

▶ OSTOMIES

*Corrections are in **boldface**.*

1. Michelle Braun is a 16-year-old with ulcerative colitis. She is taking cortisone and **sulfasalazine (Azulfidine).** She is on a **low-**residue diet. She is now admitted to the hospital for a colectomy and **permanent end ileostomy.** You monitor her intake and output (I&O), daily weights, and electrolytes. You also assess for signs of inflammation in her joints, skin, and other parts of her body. You teach her to **increase** fluids following surgery, **but it is not feasible** to limit the number of stools she has daily.

2. James Key is a 46-year-old with a new sigmoid colostomy. Following surgery you assess his stoma every shift for 3 days to ensure that it remains **pink** and moist. You explain that the stool will be **formed** and that **irrigation is optional.** You contact the dietitian to provide a list of the high-fiber foods that he should eat.

▶ CRITICAL THINKING

1. Assess Mrs. Hendricks' abdomen for normal bowel sounds, distention, tenderness, and other signs of problems. Assess her diet, exercise, fluid intake, and other possible factors that may have caused constipation.

2. Because Mrs. Hendricks has arthritis, she may not be getting much exercise. Lack of teeth probably prevents her from eating many fresh fruits or vegetables. Poor fluid intake and certain medications may also be factors. Chronic laxative abuse can be a factor, but Mrs. Hendricks only takes Milk of Magnesia occasionally.

3. Mrs. Hendricks is only 1 day behind her normal bowel movement schedule. This is not a major concern. However, you should intervene to prevent the problem from becoming worse. Unrelieved constipation can lead to fe-

cal impaction, megacolon, and complications related to use of the Valsalva's maneuver.

4. Before giving Mrs. Hendricks more Milk of Magnesia, you can try giving her some prune juice, walk her in the halls if she is able, and have her sit on the toilet or bedside commode (avoid use of bedpan) to attempt to have a bowel movement. Placing her feet on a footstool while sitting on the toilet may also help.

5. Prevention is the best treatment for constipation. Place Mrs. Hendricks on a regimen of 2 g bran with her cereal each morning. Include pureed fresh fruits and vegetables as much as possible in her diet. Encourage fluids and assist her to walk in the halls several times each day. Establish a regular time each day (or two) for Mrs. Hendricks to have the bathroom to herself for a bowel movement. Offer a warm drink such as a cup of coffee or tea or warm water before this time. If these measures do not work, add Metamucil to her daily regimen. Avoid the Milk of Magnesia, Senna (Sennakot), and enema as much as possible.

▶ REVIEW QUESTIONS

*The correct answers are in **boldface**.*

1. **(b)** is correct. Ulcerative colitis affects the colon and rectum. (a) is a better description of diverticulitis; (c) describes Crohn's disease; and (d) is not true of ulcerative colitis.

2. **(d)** is correct. Complete blood count (CBC) should be monitored because ulcerative colitis can cause bleeding; electrolytes are monitored because of loss with diarrhea. (a) monitors liver problems, (b) monitors muscle damage, and (c) monitors pancreas function.

3. **(d)** is correct. Fresh fruits and vegetables can exacerbate diarrhea. (a, b, c) can all exacerbate diarrhea symptoms.

4. **(c)** is correct. Total parenteral nutrition (TPN) is the only way to adequately feed a person for an extended period without using the gut. (a, b) both require a functional bowel; (d) provides inadequate nutrition for an extended period.

5. **(a)** is correct. A low-fiber diet increases risk of diverticulosis. (b, c, d) do not increase risk for diverticulosis.

6. (**a**) is correct. Foods with seeds may need to be avoided. (b, c, d) do not exacerbate diverticulosis.

7. (**c**) is correct. A bowel obstruction can cause nausea and vomiting. (a, b) are not related to diverticulitis. There is no evidence that (d) is correct.

8. (**d**) is correct. The loop can be replaced after the resected area of bowel has healed. (a) transverse ostomies do not usually drain constant liquid stool, (b) there is no such thing as a looped bag, and (c) the ostomy will drain stool.

9. (**a**) is correct. Fluids are needed to replace those lost in liquid stools. (b, c, d) can all increase liquid stools and fluid loss.

10. (**b**) is correct. Pouches are made of odor-proof plastic. (a) nothing will absorb all odor, (c) effluent does have an odor, and (d) daily pouch changes are hard on skin and not recommended.

32

ANSWERS

▶ VOCABULARY

1. **(F)**	6. **(B)**
2. **(H)**	7. **(C)**
3. **(I)**	8. **(E)**
4. **(J)**	9. **(G)**
5. **(D)**	10. **(A)**

▶ PANCREAS

1. Trypsin
2. Lipase
3. Amylase

▶ LIVER

1. **(C)**
2. **(H)**
3. **(D)**
4. **(I)**
5. **(E)**
6. **(B)**
7. **(J)**
8. **(G)**
9. **(F)**
10. **(A)**

▶ ANATOMY

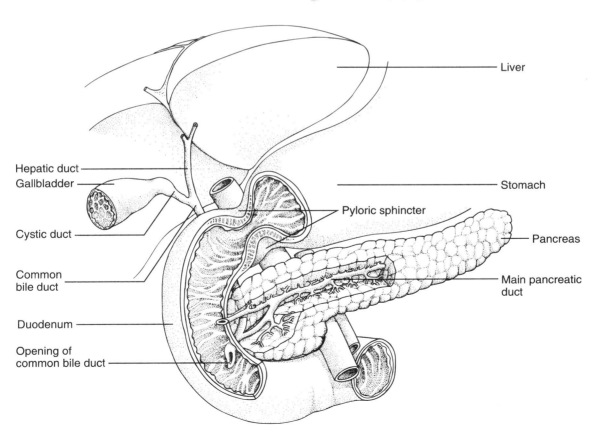

Hepatic duct

Gallbladder

Cystic duct

Common bile duct

Duodenum

Opening of common bile duct

Pyloric sphincter

Liver

Stomach

Pancreas

Main pancreatic duct

► CRITICAL THINKING

1. She may scratch frequently, have thin reddish-purple vein lines on her face and arms, have a distended abdomen, appear extremely thin, belch frequently, or sit leaning forward holding her abdomen.

2. She might complain of itching, abdominal pain (particularly upper midepigastric or right-upper-quadrant pain), nausea, vomiting, diarrhea, abnormal weight loss or gain, fatigue, feeling "bloated," stools that are foul smelling and clay colored, or urine that is dark amber or tea colored.

3. Mrs. White should be asked if anyone in her family has a history of diabetes, cancer, or bleeding tendencies as a result of liver, gallbladder, or pancreas disease because some families have a high incidence of these disorders. A social history should determine alcohol or recreational drug use, over-the-counter drug use, and exposure to substances such as industrial chemicals, farm pesticides, or other materials that are known to damage the liver.

4. The common laboratory tests to detect liver, gallbladder, and pancreas disease should include serum alanine and aspartate aminotransferase, amylase, ammonia, bilirubin, and prothrombin time. Additional laboratory tests may include urine amylase, urine bilirubin, and fecal fat.

5. The nurse should explain that Mrs. White will be asked to take nothing by mouth after midnight of the day the sonogram is scheduled. She will be asked to lie on a table and a clear gel will be applied to her abdomen. A "wand," or transducer, of the sonograph machine is then rubbed over her abdomen while high-frequency sound waves are beamed through the wand. The procedure is painless and should take about one-half hour. She will require no further care for the test after the test is completed.

► REVIEW QUESTIONS

*The correct answers are in **boldface**.*

1. (**c**) is correct.
2. (**d**) is correct.
3. (**a**) is correct.
4. (**c**) is correct.
5. (**c**) is correct. Jaundice causes itching, which can result in scratching and impaired skin integrity. (a, b, d) are not true.
6. (**b**) is correct. Increased serum bilirubin level is associated with decreased liver function. (a, c, d) are not true.
7. (**a**) is correct. Serum amylase increases in pancreatic diseases. (b, c, d) do not increase in pancreatic disease.
8. (**a**) is correct. Normal frequency is every 5 to 15 seconds. (b, c, d) would all be hypoactive.
9. (**b**) is correct. These are spider angiomas because they are at various locations. (a) Striae are silvery. (c) Caput medusae extend out from the umbilicus. (d) Ascites is collection of fluid in the abdomen.
10. (**d**) is correct. Both shellfish and radiopaque dye contain iodine. (a, b, c) radiopaque dye does not have ingredients in common with bee stings, adhesive tape, or citrus fruits.

33

ANSWERS

▶ VOCABULARY

1. (D)
2. (C)
3. (J)
4. (E)
5. (G)
6. (K)
7. (L)
8. (A)
9. (I)
10. (B)
11. (H)
12. (F)

▶ LIVER

Across

2. HBV
6. Caput medusae
9. TIPS
10. Asterixes
11. HAV

Down

1. Encephalopathy
2. Hepatorenal
3. Portal
4. Hepatitis
5. RUQ
6. Cirrhosis
7. Ascites
8. Varices

▶ GALLBLADDER

1. (D)
2. (F)
3. (G)
4. (E)
5. (A)
6. (H)
7. (I)
8. (J)
9. (B)
10. (C)

▶ PANCREAS

1. (A) Serum glucose may elevate because damage to the islets of Langerhans causes decreased insulin production.
2. (A) The digestive enzyme amylase is released in large quantities by the inflamed pancreas.
3. (N)
4. (A) Pleural effusion is caused by a local inflammatory reaction to the irritation from pancreatic enzymes.
5. (N)
6. (A) Serum albumin is decreased, usually from decreased protein metabolism.
7. (A) A positive Cullen's sign indicates hemorrhage from pancreatic destruction.
8. (A) Urinary output of less than 30 mL/hr usually indicates shock from circulatory collapse.
9. (A) Indicates neuromuscular irritability from decreased serum calcium levels.
10. (A) Indicates malabsorption of dietary fats from decreased lipase.

▶ CRITICAL THINKING

1. The data collected about Ms. Smith that support the diagnosis of chronic liver failure are a grossly distended abdomen, jaundiced sclera and skin, multiple bruises, and 2+ pitting edema of the lower extremities. Ms. Smith also scratches her arms and legs frequently, indicating itching. Her laboratory data indicate that her serum bilirubin, ammonia, and prothrombin time are elevated and that her serum albumin, total protein, and potassium are below normal.
2. The nurse notes that Ms. Smith is irritable, has difficulty answering questions, and appears to doze off often during the interview. Other observations that the nurse might make include asterixis, increasing difficulty in arousing the patient, muscle twitching, and fetor hepaticus.
3. The 2+ pitting edema and abdominal distention are of concern because the decreased amount of serum albumin produced by the failing liver permits fluid to seep into the abdominal cavity and other body tissues.
4. The nurse expects the physician to order a severely restricted protein diet for the hepatic encephalopathy. In addition, the patient may be ordered saline or magnesium sulfate enemas, neomycin, or lactulose to rid the body of excess ammonia.
5. The nurse can anticipate that the physician will order a vasoconstrictor drug such as vasopressin for Ms. Smith. If the vasoconstrictor does not stop the bleeding from the esophageal varices, a Senstaken-Blakemore tube may be ordered. Further, the physician may decide to do injection sclerotherapy in an attempt to prevent further episodes of bleeding.
6. The nurse must observe for aspiration or suffocation, such as increased respiratory rate and effort, increased confusion and irritability, noisy breathing, pallor, or cyanosis.

The nurse also carefully monitors the inflation pressure of the esophageal balloon to ensure that the pressure remains under 25 mm Hg to prevent erosion of the esophagus.

7. The nurse observes the patient's emesis, stool, and urine at least every 8 hours for blood. Ms. Smith is observed for any increase in bruising or bleeding from the gums. The nurse also monitors any blood clotting laboratory studies such as the prothrombin time.

8. The nurse measures Ms. Smith's abdomen daily and records the circumference. Ms. Smith is weighed daily and the weight recorded. The nurse reports any weight gain or increase in circumference promptly. Because Ms. Smith will usually be ordered a low-sodium diet and will have fluids restricted, the nurse carefully monitors and records intake and output. Ms. Smith's vital signs and mental status are assessed every 4 hours and any changes reported promptly. If diuretics are ordered, the nurse administers them as scheduled.

9. Ms. Smith is told that acetaminophen (Tylenol) is to be avoided because it is toxic to the liver and may cause further damage.

▶ REVIEW QUESTIONS

*The correct answers are in **boldface**.*

1. (**c**) is correct. This is a low-sodium meal. (a, b, d) are all high in sodium.

2. (**d**) is correct. The gastric balloon helps keep the tube in place. (a, b, c) are all appropriate interventions.

3. (**b**) is correct. Straining will further increase pressure and may cause bleeding. (a, c, d) are not appropriate.

4. (**b**) is correct. Standard precautions protect the nurse from exposure to disease. (a) reverse isolation protects the patient, not the nurse; (c, d) do not protect from blood exposure.

5. (**d**) is correct. Hepatitis B virus (HBV) is the most common cause. (a, b, c) are not the most common causes.

6. (**a**) is correct. These are symptoms of hepatic encephalopathy. They are not symptoms of (b, c, d).

7. (**b**) is correct; 20 to 60 percent of patients rebleed.

8. (**a**) is correct. Females are more at risk for gallbladder disease. (b, c, d) are also risk factors.

9. (**d**) is correct. Meperidine (Demerol) is most helpful. (a, b, c) morphine may cause painful spasms.

10. (**d**) is correct. Pro-Banthine is an antispasmotic agent that may help relieve biliary colic. (a) will worsen gallbladder spasms, (b) will not help, and (c) is used to dissolve stones.

11. (**c**) is correct. Excessive alcohol intake is associated with pancreatitis. (a, b, d) are not associated with pancreatitis.

12. (**a**) is correct. Patients describe their pain as dull, boring, and beginning in the mid-epigastrium and radiating to the back. (b, c, d) are not characteristic of pancreatitis.

34

ANSWERS

▶ **VOCABULARY**

1. (C)
2. (A)
3. (D)
4. (B)

5. (H)
6. (F)
7. (E)
8. (G)

▶ **ANATOMY**

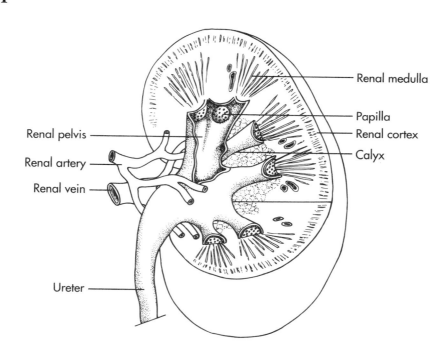

Renal pelvis

Renal artery

Renal vein

Ureter

Renal medulla

Papilla

Renal cortex

Calyx

▶ SAMPLE URINALYSIS RESULTS

Patient A: urinary tract infection
Patient B: dehydration, deficient fluid volume
Patient C: liver disease

▶ RENAL DIAGNOSTIC TESTS

1. False—intravenous pyelogram
2. False—renal ultrasound
3. False—urine culture and sensitivity
4. True
5. False—allergic reactions are possible; can be nephrotoxic

▶ CRITICAL THINKING

1. These are classic symptoms of stress incontinence.
2. She should be taught how to perform Kegel exercise. She also should be referred to a urologist or gynecologist who specializes in incontinence. She may benefit from medications or surgery.
3. Functional incontinence. She would have been continent if she had been able to call the nurse in time.
4. She should receive a call light that she can feel and that is pinned to the front of her gown. It would also be helpful if she had a roommate who could turn on the call light for her.
5. Fluids should not be restricted. Fluid restriction can result in concentrated urine, which is more irritating to the urinary tract, and cause incontinence. Some people become continent only by increasing their fluid intake and setting up a regular pattern of voiding. Fluid restriction before bedtime may be helpful.

▶ REVIEW QUESTIONS

The correct answers are in **boldface.**

1. (**a**)
2. (**b**)
3. (**c**)
4. (**b**)
5. (**d**)
6. (**a**) is correct. The perineum should be washed before collecting a urine sample from a female to decrease con-tamination of the specimen. (b, c, d) are not necessary for a routine urine specimen.
7. (**a**) is correct. The elevated specific gravity is seen with dehydration, because the urine is more concentrated. When a patient is dehydrated, the amount of urine that the patient makes is decreased, which makes the urine more concentrated. A small amount of bacteria is normally found in the urinalysis. (b, c) A small amount of bacteria does not indicate infection. (d) No blood was noted on the results.
8. (**d**) is correct. The elevated blood urea nitrogen level reflects reduced kidney function. (a, b, c) are incorrect.
9. (**b**) is correct. The patient should be nil per os (NPO) before undergoing an intravenous pyelogram (IVP) so the dye is more concentrated for better visualization of renal structures. After the IVP, the nurse should force fluids to clear the dye from the kidneys. (a, c, d) are not restricted.
10. (**a**) is correct. It is important that the nurse determine whether the patient is able to urinate. There may be edema of the urethra after a cystoscopy, which can result in urinary retention. (b, c, d) are not necessary.
11. (**a**) is correct. Urge incontinence is associated with difficulty retaining urine once the urge to urinate is sensed. (b) is stress incontinence. (c) is not a specific type of incontinence. (d) is total incontinence.
12. (**c**) is correct. It is important to keep the catheter taped to prevent movement of the catheter, which increases the chance of introducing bacteria into the urine and trauma to the urethra. (a) increases risk of infection. (b) is not necessary. (d) A full bag increases risk of backflow and contamination.
13. (**d**) is correct. With total incontinence, the patient is unable to control urination and an adult incontinence brief is appropriate. (a) Cranberry juice would be helpful to decrease onset of a urinary tract infection, but the patient would still be incontinent of urine. (b) A urinal will not help if the patient cannot tell when he or she has to go. (c) Kegel exercises will not help total incontinence.

35

ANSWERS

▶ VOCABULARY
1. Urethritis
2. Cystitis
3. Pyelonephritis
4. urethroplasty
5. calculi
6. Nephrolithotomy
7. hydronephrosis
8. nephrostomy
9. nephrectomy
10. nephrosclerosis

▶ URINARY TRACT INFECTIONS
1. The usual cause of urinary tract infections (UTIs) in women is contamination in the area from the close proximity of the rectum to the urinary meatus. Women who void infrequently are predisposed to UTIs.
2. The usual cause of UTIs in men is the presence of prostatic hypertrophy leading to obstruction of urinary flow predisposing to infection.
3. The patient should be advised to drink large amounts of water and a glass of cranberry juice daily. If the patient cannot void frequently, he or she should drink less water.
4. The single most important thing a patient with a history of UTIs should do is void frequently to prevent stasis and then infection of urine.
5.

	Cystitis	Pyelonephritis
Symptoms	Dysuria; frequency; urgency; cloudy, foul-smelling urine; sometimes hematuria	Dysuria; frequency; urgency; cloudy, foul-smelling urine; sometimes hematuria; also chills and fever, flank pain, and general malaise
Urinalysis results	Increased bacteria, white blood cells (WBCs); positive nitrites; positive leukocyte esterase	Increased bacteria, WBCs; positive nitrites, positive leukocyte esterase; may also have casts in the urine
Prognosis	Good with treatment; can become chronic condition with repeat infections	Acute pyelonephritis has a good prognosis; with repeat infections the patient can develop chronic pyelonephritis with scarring and eventual destruction of the kidneys

▶ URINARY TRACT OBSTRUCTIONS

1. The most common symptom of cancer of the bladder is hematuria because cancerous tissue readily bleeds.
2. The most common risk factor for cancer of the bladder is smoking because of continual exposure of the bladder mucosa to the carcinogenic by-products of smoking.
3. The most common symptom of cancer of the kidney is bleeding, again because cancerous tissue bleeds readily, just as in cancer of the bladder.
4. The urine of a patient with an ileal conduit is cloudy because of the presence of mucus, because a portion of the small intestine is used and it continues to secrete mucus.
5. To care for a patient with an ileal conduit, an appliance is kept on at all times that either holds urine or drains into a Foley bag. When the appliance needs changing, it is necessary to use a wick to catch urine until the appliance can be applied. See text for how to apply an appliance to a patient with an ileal conduit.
6. The most important care of a patient with a kidney stone is to strain all urine to catch the stone. Pain relief measures are also very important.
7. The patient with a calcium oxalate kidney stone should avoid foods high in calcium, such as large quantities of milk, and sources of oxalate, such as colas and beer. It can also be helpful to keep the urine acidic. The patient with a uric acid kidney stone should avoid foods that are high in purines, such as organ meats and sardines.

▶ CRITICAL THINKING

1. Mrs. Zins is having incidences of hypoglycemia because she is developing renal failure. The kidney helps degrade insulin and excrete it from the body. As the kidneys fail, smaller amounts of insulin are needed because it is not removed from the body.
2. It is important that Mrs. Zins not receive orange juice as would normally be done for a hypoglycemic patient, because her potassium level is already high. Instead, cranberry juice or another carbohydrate source should be given.
3. Diabetes causes atherosclerotic changes in the kidney vessels. In addition, diabetes causes an abnormal thickening of the glomerulus, which damages the glomerulus. The diabetic patient is predisposed to frequent pyelonephritis (kidney infections), which can damage the kidney. Also, the diabetic patient can develop a neurogenic bladder, which predisposes the patient to both infection and obstruction of the urinary system.
4. Good control of diabetes, keeping blood sugars within a defined range, can decrease the development of diabetic complications including development of renal failure.
5. Nursing diagnoses that would be relevant for Mrs. Zins include excess fluid volume (she has edema, weight gain, and jugular vein distention) and fatigue (she states she feels exhausted and also has a Hgb [hemoglobin level] of 7.2).
6. The serum creatinine of 5.4 is most diagnostic of renal failure. A 24-hour creatinine clearance is more diagnostic, but this laboratory test is not available in this case study.
7. Mrs. Zins is anemic because her kidneys have decreased or stopped production of a substance called erythropoeitin, which stimulates the bone marrow to make red blood cells. It is also possible that she has slowly been bleeding through her gastrointestinal tract, a common occurrence in renal patients.
8. The three most important assessments when caring for a patient with renal failure are: daily weight, intake and output (with fluid restriction if prescribed), and monitoring laboratory test for dangerous levels of electrolytes.
9. Mrs. Zins would probably be on a defined diabetic diet that was also low sodium, low potassium, decreased protein, and fluid restricted. If her phosphorus level was elevated, she would also be put on a low phosphorus diet. This is one of the most restrictive diets possible and is very difficult to follow.

▶ RENAL FAILURE

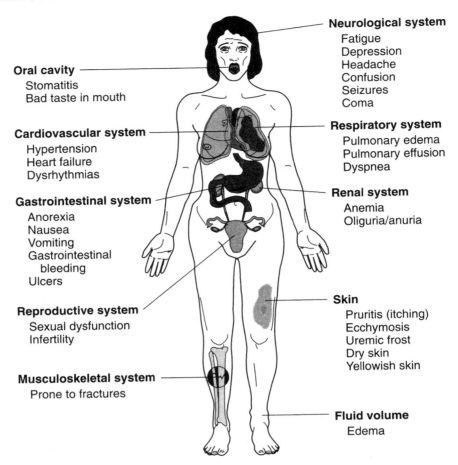

Neurological system
Fatigue
Depression
Headache
Confusion
Seizures
Coma

Oral cavity
Stomatitis
Bad taste in mouth

Respiratory system
Pulmonary edema
Pulmonary effusion
Dyspnea

Cardiovascular system
Hypertension
Heart failure
Dysrhythmias

Renal system
Anemia
Oliguria/anuria

Gastrointestinal system
Anorexia
Nausea
Vomiting
Gastrointestinal
   bleeding
Ulcers

Skin
Pruritis (itching)
Ecchymosis
Uremic frost
Dry skin
Yellowish skin

Reproductive system
Sexual dysfunction
Infertility

Musculoskeletal system
Prone to fractures

Fluid volume
Edema

▶ REVIEW QUESTIONS

*The correct answers are in **boldface**.*

1. **(d)** is correct. Hematuria is the most common symptom of cancer of the bladder. (a) nocturia or (b) dysuria may occur related to a resulting infection, or (c) retention may occur because of obstruction, but these are not the most common symptoms.

2. **(d)** is correct because the mucus is normally found in the urine of a patient with an ileal conduit. This is because a portion of the small bowel is used to make the conduit, and that portion of bowel continues to secrete mucus. (a, b, c) are not necessary.

3. **(c)** is correct because often the first and most obvious sign of acute renal failure is a decrease in urine output. (a) the blood pressure may elevate later as the patient continues into renal failure, but the urine output is most significant. (b, d) may occur in some patients, but they are not the most common.

4. **(b)** is correct because a 24-hour creatinine clearance is most diagnostic of renal failure; a result of 5 mL per hour means that the patient has approximately 5 percent of normal kidney function. (a, c, d) would be elevated in the patient with renal failure, but the creatinine clearance is most diagnostic.

5. **(d)** is correct because it is the only food listed without significant potassium in it. (a, b, c) are all high in potassium.

6. **(d)** is correct because there is a sudden decrease in urine output, and the patient has symptoms of urinary retention, which are distention and pain in the suprapubic area. (a) Decreased renal perfusion would be an appropriate answer if the patient had not had symptoms of urinary retention; (b, c) would not cause the symptoms of urinary retention.

7. **(b)** is correct. Beer is high in oxalate, which predisposes the patient to calcium oxalate kidney stones. (a, c, d) are not especially high in oxalate or calcium.

8. **(c)** is the correct answer because the patient should collect the specimen partway through urination. (a, b, d) are all relevant to other diagnostic tests of the urine but not relevant to a midstream culture.

9. **(b)** is the correct answer because the most serious complication of a high potassium level is cardiac dysrhythmias. (a, c, d) may be present in renal failure but are not associated with high potassium levels.

10. **(c)** is the correct answer because the daily weight is the single best determinant of fluid balance in the body. (a, b, d) are also important, but daily weight remains most significant.

11. **(b)** is the correct answer because orange juice is high in potassium, and the patient's potassium level is already high. (a, c) would still give the patient too much potassium; (d) it would be important to check the kind of diet later, but the first priority is to protect the patient from a dangerously high potassium level.

12. **(a)** is the correct answer because there is a larger blood flow, and dialysis is more efficient. (b) All blood access sites can clot, (c) it is harder to access a graft than a two-tailed subclavian, and (d) either site can be damaged by trauma.

13. **(b)** is the correct answer because the patient must be weighed following dialysis to determine fluid balance. (a, c, d) are not relevant.

14. **(b)** is correct because this is the mechanism by which dialysis works. (a, c, d) do not describe how dialysis works.

15. **(c)** is correct because these are symptoms that are seen with fluid retention related to untreated renal failure. (a, b, d) are not symptoms of fluid excess and renal failure.

16. **(d)** is correct because hematuria is the most common symptom of trauma to the kidney because the kidney has a very large blood supply. (a, b, c) are not symptoms of trauma.

17. **(b)** is correct because the patient has symptoms of too much fluid in the body, which is fluid volume excess. (a, c, d) are not relevant. In certain situations a nursing diagnosis of noncompliance may have caused the symptoms, but there is not enough information in the question to make this diagnosis.

36

ANSWERS

▶ VOCABULARY

1. Glycogen
2. Hyperglycemia
3. Affect
4. exophthalmos
5. Feedback

▶ ENDOCRINE GLANDS AND HORMONES

▶ HORMONES

1. (J)
2. (Q)
3. (A)
4. (H)
5. (E)
6. (M)
7. (P)
8. (K)
9. (I)
10. (C)
11. (N)
12. (F)
13. (G)
14. (D)
15. (O)
16. (B)
17. (L)

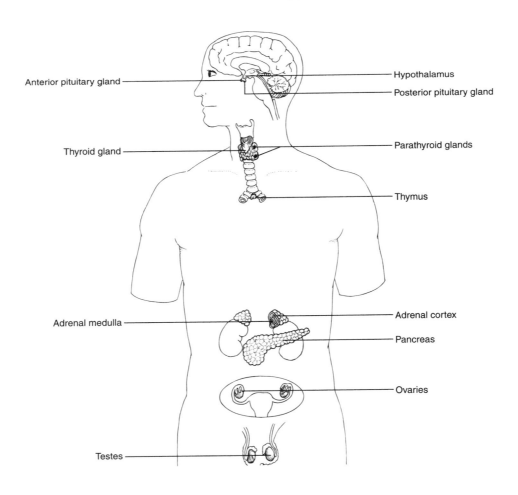

Anterior pituitary gland

Thyroid gland

Adrenal medulla

Testes

Hypothalamus

Posterior pituitary gland

Parathyroid glands

Thymus

Adrenal cortex

Pancreas

Ovaries

▶ REVIEW QUESTIONS

*The correct answers are in **boldface**.*

1. (**b**) is correct.
2. (**d**) is correct.
3. (**a**) is correct.
4. (**c**) is correct.
5. (**b**) is correct.
6. (**c**) is correct. The final urine voided at 24 hours must be added to the specimen. (a) The first, not the last, urine voided is discarded. (b) A separate container is not necessary. (d) All 24 hours of urine produced is necessary for the test.

7. (**a**) is correct. A history is appropriate. (b) could cause release of hormone and exacerbate symptoms. (c) evaluates diabetes, not thyroid function. (d) A buffalo hump is present when there is too much cortisol, not thyroid hormone.
8. (**c**) is correct. This answers her question. Further testing must be done to determine a definite diagnosis. (a) She may have cancer of the thyroid, but she needs further testing; also, the nurse does not make a medical diagnosis. (b) is not true. (d) A cold spot is not normal.

37

ANSWERS

VOCABULARY

1. euthyroid
2. goiter
3. polydipsia
4. polyuria
5. pheochromocytoma

6. dysphagia
7. myxedema
8. Nocturia
9. amenorrhea
10. ectopic

HORMONES

Disorder	Hormone Problem	Signs and Symptoms
Diabetes insipidus	Antidiuretic hormone (ADH) deficiency	Polyuria
Syndrome of inappropriate ADH (SIADH)	ADH excess	Water retention
Cushing's syndrome	Steroid excess	Moon face
Addison's disease	Deficient steroids	Hypotension
Grave's disease	High T_3 and T_4	Exophthalmos
Hypothyroidism	Low T_3 and T_4	Weight gain
Pheochromocytoma	Epinephrine excess	Labile hypertension
Hyperparathyroidism	High calcium	Muscle weakness
Dwarfism	Growth hormone (GH) deficiency	Short stature
Acromegaly	GH excess	Growing feet
Hypoparathyroidism	Low calcium	Tetany

CRITICAL THINKING

1. Because Sam has too much ADH, he will be retaining water. An appropriate nursing diagnosis would be excess fluid volume.
2. The best way to monitor fluid balance is by daily weights, at the same time each day, on the same scale, and in about the same clothes. In addition to daily weights, intake and output, vital signs, urine specific gravity, lung sounds, and skin turgor can be monitored.
3. Sam will retain water, which will reduce the osmolality of his blood. This in turn can cause cerebral edema, increased intracranial pressure, and seizures.
4. Sam's side rails should be padded. If a seizure occurs, he should be protected from harming himself (see Chapter 46).
5. Sam's urine will be very concentrated because he is not excreting much water.
6. When Sam is effectively treated, his urine will look more dilute because he will be excreting more water.
7. A head injury can directly or indirectly damage the pituitary gland, placing the patient at risk for reduced ADH secretion and DI.
8. Polyuria and polydipsia are symptoms of both DI and DM.
9. Judy's urine specific gravity will be low because she is excreting too much water.
10. Judy's serum osmolality will be high because she is losing water and becoming dehydrated.
11. Judy is at risk for deficient fluid volume.
12. Judy should watch for signs of fluid overload, such as increasing weight and concentrated urine.

► THYROID DISORDERS

1. (O)	7. (R)
2. (O)	8. (R)
3. (R)	9. (O)
4. (R)	10. (R)
5. (O)	11. (R)
6. (O)	12. (O)

► REVIEW QUESTIONS

The correct answers are in **boldface.**

1. (**c**) is correct. Negative feedback causes the pituitary to produce more thyroid stimulating hormone (TSH). (a) TSH does not take the place of T_3 and T_4, (b) TSH will not directly affect the metabolic rate, and (d) fat cells do not make TSH.

2. (**c**) is correct. Mrs. Waley is experiencing fatigue. (a) there is no evidence in the data that Mrs. Waley is overeating, (b) weight gain does not necessarily affect gas exchange, and (d) there is no evidence that Mrs. Waley is experiencing depression.

3. (**a**) is correct. Tachycardia can occur if she gets too much Synthroid. (b, c) are not side effects of Synthroid; and (d) she should lose weight, not gain weight, on Synthroid.

4. (**b**) is correct. Body fluids will be radioactive. (a, c) are not necessary; and (d) exposure to even small doses of radioactivity should be minimized.

5. (**a**) is correct. Numb fingers and muscle cramps are symptoms of tetany. (b, c, d) are not symptoms of tetany.

6. (**c**) is correct. Thyrotoxicosis causes blood pressure, pulse, temperature, and respiratory rate to rise. (a, b, d) are not affected by thyrotoxicosis (peripheral pulses may be indirectly affected).

7. (**c**) is correct. Fluids will help prevent kidney stones. (a, b, d) will not help.

8. (**d**) is correct. It is the only outcome that addresses pain. (a, b, c) may all be appropriate, but they are not related directly to the nursing diagnosis.

9. (**c**) is correct. Acromegaly is caused by an excess of GH. (a, b, d) do not cause acromegaly.

10. (**b**) is correct. Buffalo hump and easy bruising are often present in Cushing's syndrome. (a, c, d) are not symptoms of Cushing's syndrome.

11. (**a**) is correct. Vital signs are important because the patient with pheochromocytoma has labile hypertension. (b, c, d) are all part of a routine assessment, but they are not most important for the patient with unstable hypertension.

12. (**c**) is correct. Addison's disease is associated with fluid loss. (a, b, d) are not relevant.

38

ANSWERS

▶ VOCABULARY

1. Glycosuria
2. Hyperglycemia
3. Hypoglycemia
4. Kussmaul's
5. Polyphagia
6. Polydipsia
7. Nocturia
8. Peak
9. Duration
10. Tight

▶ HYPOGLYCEMIA AND HYPERGLYCEMIA

1. (O)   5. (O)
2. (R)   6. (R)
3. (R)   7. (O)
4. (R)   8. (R)

▶ LONG-TERM COMPLICATIONS OF DIABETES

1. (E)   5. (G)
2. (B)   6. (F)
3. (D)   7. (C)
4. (A)

▶ CRITICAL THINKING

1.

2. Keeping the blood glucose level too low can increase risk of hypoglycemia, especially in a patient who has had diabetes for some time. If autonomic neuropathy is present, symptoms of hypoglycemia may go unnoticed, making hypoglycemia even more risky. The physician should always be consulted for desired glucose range.

3. Jennie is exhibiting symptoms of hypoglycemia. It occurred at 4 P.M. because Jennie is on human N insulin, which peaks in the afternoon. In addition, she probably has not had supper yet, which further increases her risk of hypoglycemia. You should notify the registered nurse and follow hospital policy, which usually directs the nurse to check the blood glucose level and provide a quick source of glucose such as juice or glucose tablets.

4. It appears that the treatment has been effective; 80 mg/dL is probably okay, especially if a meal tray is to be served soon. Check to be sure her meal is on its way, and watch her for further symptoms.

5. Common causes of hypoglycemia include skipping or delaying meals, eating less than prescribed at a meal, and more exercise than usual.

6. Because she is receiving insulin on a schedule, it is important to eat regularly to prevent periods during which there is insulin but not enough glucose in her blood.

7. Obesity causes insulin resistance. Losing weight has probably decreased Jennie's insulin resistance, making her insulin dose more effective.

8. Glucotrol stimulates insulin production and increases tissue sensitivity to insulin.

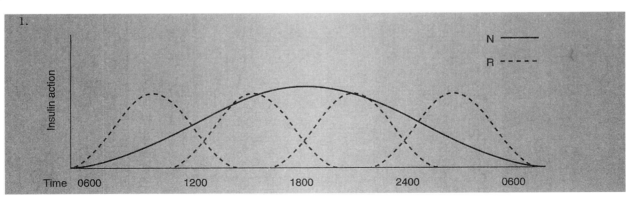

1.

9. Sulfonylureas are administered 30 minutes before breakfast and 30 minutes before supper if twice-a-day dosing is ordered. This allows absorption of medication before eating.

10. Jennie has type 2 diabetes. If she had type 1 diabetes, she would not be able to take oral hypoglycemics.

▶ REVIEW QUESTIONS

*The correct answers are in **boldface**.*

1. **(b)** is correct. Only individuals with type 2 diabetes can control diabetes with diet and exercise alone. (a) Type 1 treatment is insulin. (c) Insulin-dependent diabetes mellitus is the same as type 1. (d) Gestational diabetes occurs in pregnant women.

2. **(c)** is correct. Micronase increases tissue sensitivity to insulin. (a, b, d) can all potentially raise blood glucose levels, an undesirable result.

3. **(d)** is correct. If a patient forgets a prescribed oral hypoglycemic, blood sugar levels will go up. Fatigue, thirst, and blurred vision are the only symptoms of hyperglycemia. (a, b) are symptoms of hypoglycemia. (c) is not related to diabetes.

4. **(b)** is correct; 100 to 140 mg/dL would be considered acceptable by most practitioners. (a) is too low. (c, d) are too high.

5. **(d)** is correct. Insulin is given subcutaneously most of the time. (a) Insulin is never given orally because it would be digested. (b, c) It is rarely given intramuscularly and occasionally is given intravenously, but these are not the most common routes.

6. **(b)** is correct. Insulin should never be given without first evaluating the blood glucose level. (a, c, d) may all be significant for the person with diabetes, but they are not immediately necessary before administering insulin.

7. **(b)** is correct. The peak action time of NPH is 6 to 12 hours after administration. (a) is the onset of NPH. (c) is the duration of long-acting insulin. (d) is incorrect.

8. **(c)** is correct. The peak of regular insulin is 2 to 5 hours. (a, b, d) are incorrect.

9. **(c)** is correct. These are symptoms of hypoglycemia. (a, b, d) are not associated with hypoglycemia.

10. **(a)** is correct. Raisins contain sugar, which will raise the blood glucose level. (b, d) are protein foods and will affect the blood glucose level only very slowly. (c) is not a food.

11. **(d)** is correct. Glucagon stimulates the liver to convert glycogen to glucose, which raises the blood glucose level. (a, b, c) are all related to hyperglycemia, which would be worsened by glucagon.

12. **(a)** is correct. Obesity is a major risk factor for type 2 diabetes. (b) A viral infection may be related to type 1 diabetes. (c) Binge eating does not cause diabetes. (d) Hypertension may be a complication of diabetes, but it does not increase the risk of diabetes.

13. **(d)** is correct. Oatmeal and bread are both bread/starch exchanges. (a, b, c) are not starch exchanges.

39

ANSWERS

▶ VOCABULARY

1. hysteroscopy
2. insufflation
3. digital rectal examination
4. gynecomastia
5. hypospadias
6. hydrocele
7. varicocele
8. libido
9. menarche
10. mammography

▶ ANATOMY AND PHYSIOLOGY

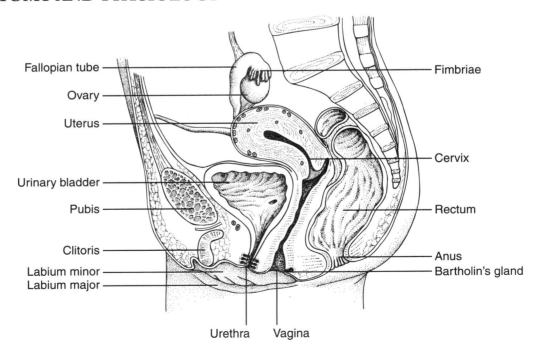

Fallopian tube — Fimbriae

Ovary

Uterus — Cervix

Urinary bladder

Pubis — Rectum

Clitoris — Anus

Labium minor — Bartholin's gland
Labium major

Urethra   Vagina

FEMALE REPRODUCTIVE STRUCTURES

1. **(E)**   5. **(B)**
2. **(G)**   6. **(A)**
3. **(F)**   7. **(D)**
4. **(C)**

MALE REPRODUCTIVE SYSTEM

4, 2, 5, 1, 3

DIAGNOSTIC TESTS

1. **(B)**   4. **(F)**
2. **(A)**   5. **(D)**
3. **(C)**   6. **(E)**

CRITICAL THINKING

1. "Even though you had prostate surgery, unless you had your entire prostate gland removed, some of the tissue will grow back, and a rectal examination is still important. We can check with your doctor to see what kind of surgery you had."

2. Examine her abdomen, and check her medical record for the report of her procedure. Most likely she had carbon dioxide (CO_2) pumped into her abdomen as part of the procedure, to enhance visualization of structures. Explain to her why her abdomen is distended, and have her lie flat to decrease migration of CO_2. If there is no record of CO_2 insufflation, something may indeed be wrong, and further assessment and reporting to the nurse or physician are indicated.

3. Prepare to assist with cultures to send to the lab. Ask if she uses protection during intercourse. Tell her she may have to refrain from sexual activity until the source and communicability of her discharge are determined.

4. Depending on how Mr. Brown shared this initial information, you probably have a good idea how comfortable he is sharing additional information. If not, you can ask if he would like to discuss the matter further. A good question to ask might be why he is no longer sexually active. If it is not by choice, he may be experiencing erectile dysfunction from complications of diabetes. If physical problems are preventing sexual activity, inform him that there are many treatments available. If Mr. Brown wishes, talk with his physician about a consultation with a urologist or other expert.

REVIEW QUESTIONS

The correct answers are in **boldface.**

1. **(a)**
2. **(b)**
3. **(a)**
4. **(d)**
5. **(c)**
6. **(b)** is correct. Breast self-examination (BSE) should be done monthly. (a) is more often than necessary; (c, d) are too infrequent.
7. **(d)** is correct. Digital rectal examination (DRE) is done by a physician at a routine visit. (a, b, c) It is unreasonable to expect such frequent physician visits; testicular self-examination (TSE) can be done at home more often.

8. **(b)** is correct. A cystourethrogram involves a catheter, dye, and x-rays. (a, c, d) are not correct.

9. **(b)** is correct. The patient should empty her bladder before the Pap smear. (a, c, d) are not necessary for Pap smears.

10. **(a)** is correct. A portion of the BSE is done while lying down. (b, c, d) are inappropriate.

11. **(c)** is correct. A charcoal swab is used for gonorrhea. (a, b, d) are used for other tests.

12. **(d)** is correct. A mammogram shows a lesion, but it cannot diagnose specifically what the lesion is. Additional tests are needed. (a, b) are not true; (c) mammogram is not the best test but is a good screening tool.

13. **(c)** is correct. Patients with metal in their bodies should avoid magnetic resonance imaging (MRI). (a) Radiation is not used with MRI, (b) MRI does not use sound waves, and (d) chemicals are not injected into body cavities.

14. **(d)** is correct. Wet mounts must be viewed immediately. (a, b, c) are not wet mounts.

ANSWERS

▶ VOCABULARY

1. (C)	6. (G)
2. (D)	7. (A)
3. (B)	8. (F)
4. (J)	9. (H)
5. (E)	10. (I)

▶ BREAST SURGERIES

1. (E)	4. (B)
2. (A)	5. (D)
3. (C)	

▶ MENSTRUAL DISORDERS

1. (E)	4. (B)
2. (C)	5. (D)
3. (A)	

▶ MASTECTOMY CARE

Errors are in **boldface.**

You are assigned to care for Mrs. Joseph, who is 1 day postoperative following a right radical mastectomy. **You know that she is not anxious,** because she had a left mastectomy a year ago and **knows everything to expect.** You listen to her breath sounds and find them clear, so it is **not necessary to have her cough and deep breathe.** You encourage her to **lie on her right side** to prevent bleeding. You use her **right arm for blood pressures,** because both arms are affected and the right one is more convenient. You also encourage her to **avoid use of her right arm** to prevent injury to the surgical site. You provide a balanced diet and plenty of fluids to aid in her recovery.

It is impossible to know if Mrs. Joseph is anxious without assessing her. Most likely she is anxious because a second mastectomy probably was done for a recurrence of cancer. She needs a lot of support. A referral to Reach to Recovery or another appropriate support group would be helpful. Also, never assume that because a patient has had a procedure before, she knows everything to expect. Assess her

knowledge level and teach accordingly. The incision on her chest may hurt when she coughs and deep breathes, increasing her risk of pulmonary complications. She should receive analgesics and encouragement to cough and deep breathe every hour. Lying on her right side may make elevation of her right arm difficult. She should assume a position in which her arm can be elevated on a pillow to decrease swelling. Neither arm should be used for blood pressures after mastectomies; consult with the physician about the advisability of using the left arm or possibly her legs. She should be taught to exercise her arm using exercises recommended by the institution.

▶ CRITICAL THINKING

1. Some factors affecting her frequent yeast overgrowths may include poor nutrition, inadequate blood glucose control, overly restrictive clothing, overheating of the genital area from long periods of sitting, immune system deficiency, a strain of yeast that is resistant to her usual treatment, and antibiotic use (many young people take antibiotics regularly for acne control).

2. Some suggestions to help her prevent this problem in the future might include wearing loose-fitting skirts and light cotton underwear for bus trips, changing positions frequently and sitting with her legs apart under her skirt, getting out and walking (if this is practical) when the bus stops, mentioning any antibiotic use to the physician, emphasizing the recurrent nature of this problem to her physician, and assessment for immune system problems if other infections are also frequent. One main area to explore with her is her blood glucose control. Find out why she is not testing often enough, and help her to plan strategies to improve testing regularity. If she is financially unable to afford the test materials, find out if there are support options available to her (the local Diabetes Association chapter or hospital diabetes clinic may be able to help you find this information). Emphasize the benefits of adequate blood glucose control for many body systems as well as this disorder.

▶ REVIEW QUESTIONS

The correct answers are in **boldface.**

1. **(d)** is correct. The male partner must agree to use the condom. (a, b, c) are not true of condoms.
2. **(b)** is correct. The vagina is acidic. (a, c) are incorrect.
3. **(c)** is correct. A douche may wash away signs of the pathogen. (a) Better visualization is nice, but it does not help identify the pathogen. (b, d) are not true.
4. **(a)** is correct. Receiving estrogen without progestins increases risk of cancer. (b, c, d) do not increase risk of cancer.
5. **(b)** is correct. Elevation of the arm reduces swelling. (a, c, d) may worsen swelling.
6. **(c)** is correct. Multiple sexual partners increases the risk of cervical cancer. (a) There is no evidence that tight underwear increases cancer risk. (b) Papanicolaou smears detect cancer early. (d) Late onset of sexual activity may reduce risk of some diseases.
7. **(a)** is correct. Her reaction shows anger over her diagnosis, a normal grieving response. (b, c, d) may be true, but there is no evidence to support them in the question.
8. **(b)** is correct. Women who have not been pregnant have higher rates of breast cancer. (a, c, d) have all been associated with breast cancer.
9. **(a)** is correct. This therapy affects hormone function. (b, c, d) do not work by affecting estrogen.
10. **(d)** is correct. Nausea will decrease intake. (a, b, c) will not increase intake. Unpeeled fresh fruits and vegetables may be contraindicated in a patient at risk for infection due to chemotherapy, but in general, the patient should be able to eat whatever sounds good.
11. **(d)** is correct. These are signs of infection. Prompt reporting is necessary so a culture can be done and antibiotics ordered. (a) Another day or two allows time for the infection to spread. (b) is not normal. (c) is unprofessional and will unnecessarily worry the patient.
12. **(c)** is correct. Coffee contains caffeine, which can worsen premenstrual syndrome (PMS) symptoms. (a, b, d) help PMS symptoms.

41

ANSWERS

▶ VOCABULARY

1. cystoscopy
2. prostatectomy
3. retrograde ejaculation
4. priapism
5. Phimosis
6. Smegma
7. circumcision
8. Cryptorchidism
9. testicle
10. scrotum
11. epididymis
12. orchitis
13. erectile dysfunction
14. varicocele
15. vasectomy

▶ DISORDERS OF THE MALE REPRODUCTIVE SYSTEM

1. (C)
2. (E)
3. (A)
4. (B)
5. (J)
6. (G)
7. (D)
8. (F)
9. (H)
10. (I)

▶ ERECTILE DYSFUNCTION

1. Medication
2. Stress
3. Hypertension
4. Transurethral resection of the prostate (TURP)
5. Heart failure
6. Multiple sclerosis

▶ CRITICAL THINKING

1. Use the WHAT'S UP? format to assess Mr. Washington's symptoms. The most important question is what he means by "can't pass water" and how long it has been since he last urinated. If he truly can pass no urine, the situation is an emergency. You can also observe for bladder distention, but palpation may be best done by the physician because of the risk for injury. Ask if he has ever been told he has prostate problems. If it has been long since he urinated last or the bladder appears distended, have the physician see the patient as soon as possible.

2. In an older man, prostate enlargement is a common cause of urinary problems. Benign prostatic hypertrophy and cancer of the prostate gland are two possibilities.

3. Be prepared to assist with Foley catheter insertion. It may be difficult to get past an enlarged prostate, so the physician may need to be involved. The catheter can maintain urine flow until Mr. Washington is transferred to the hospital for further diagnostic tests and possible surgery. Find out how Mr. Washington got to the urgent care center and arrange a ride to the hospital if ordered.

4. If urine flow continues to be blocked, hydronephrosis, infection, and rupture of the bladder can occur.

5. "A special scope will be inserted into your penis that will chip away the enlarged parts of the prostate gland. You will be anesthetized so you won't feel it. Afterward you can expect to have a catheter in your bladder for several days."

6. The catheter has several purposes. It allows urine to drain, places pressure on the resected gland to minimize bleeding, and provides a route to irrigate the bladder so clots can be removed. When totaling intake and output (I&O), irrigation solution should be included in the intake measurement because it is impossible to separate urine from solution in the output.

7. Bladder spasms are very painful, and the patient will inform you if they are occurring. Spasms may also cause leakage of urine around the catheter. Anesthetics and antispasmodic medications such as belladonna and opium (B&O) suppositories can help the discomfort. Irrigation of the catheter can flush out clots that can increase spasms. Relaxation exercises may also help.

8. Tell Mr. Washington that some episodes of incontinence may occur, but that they should subside in a few weeks. Teach him to do Kegel's exercises to increase sphincter tone. He should not restrict fluids because this can increase risk for urinary tract infection (UTI). A condom catheter or penile pad may help catch urine until incontinence improves. This problem could have been prevented by careful discharge teaching, letting Mr. Washington know what to expect and what to do about it.

▶ REVIEW QUESTIONS

*The correct answers are in **boldface**.*

1. (**a**) is correct. Incomplete bladder emptying is a symptom of benign prostatic hypertrophy (BPH). (b) erectile dysfunction is not a symptom of BPH; (c, d) are signs of kidney disease.

2. (**c**) is correct. Sexual function is occasionally affected. (a) does not answer his question; (b, d) imply that dysfunction is expected, which is not true.

3. (**b**) is correct. The B&O suppository will relieve bladder spasms. (a) Demerol relieves pain but not spasms, (c) warming the solution is not recommended, and (d) notifying the physician STAT is not necessary—bladder spasms are an expected occurrence.

4. (**c**) is correct. The catheter needs to be kept free of clots so that it drains the bladder. (a) irrigation does not stop bleeding, (b) antibiotics are not normally in the irrigating solution, and (d) irrigation does not affect urine production.

5. (**b**) is correct. Kegel's exercises will help strengthen sphincter tone. (a) restricting fluids increases risk of infection, (c) reinserting the catheter will only delay the problem, and (d) incontinence may last several weeks.

6. (**d**) is correct. Asking an open-ended question will help Mr. Blaker share his concerns at his level of comfort. (a) The information provided does not support a diagnosis of impaired communication; (b) not all patients are helped by verbalizing concerns; and (c) this does not allow Mr. Blaker to identify his own concerns.

7. (**b**) is correct. The scrotum will be painful and swollen. (a, c, d) are not symptoms of epididymitis.

8. (**d**) is correct. Ice, not hot packs, is used to reduce swelling and pain. (a, b, c) are all appropriate measures.

9. (**c**) is correct. Always replace the foreskin to prevent impairment of circulation and the possibility of not being able to replace it later. (a) Never leave the foreskin retracted; (b) the foreskin should be retracted if possible to wash the area; and (d) mild soap, not alcohol, should be used.

10. (**a**) is correct. Monthly TSE is one method to detect testicular cancer. (b) DRE is used to detect prostate enlargement; (c) an annual physical examination is advised, but it does not take the place of monthly checks; and (d) ultrasound is not done routinely to detect testicular cancer.

ANSWERS

VOCABULARY

1. (D)
2. (B)
3. (C)
4. (E)
5. (A)
6. (F)

INFLAMMATORY DISORDERS

1. (A)
2. (C)
3. (B)
4. (E)
5. (D)

TRANSMISSION OF SEXUALLY TRANSMITTED DISEASES

1. (C)
2. (B)
3. (A)
4. (D)

BARRIER METHODS FOR SAFER SEX

1. Latex condoms are less likely to break during intercourse than other types. Lubrication decreases the chances of breakage during use, but only water-soluble lubricants should be used, because substances such as petroleum jelly (Vaseline) may weaken the condom. Condoms should never be inflated to test them, because this can weaken them. Condoms should be applied only when the penis is erect. Either condoms with a reservoir tip or regular condoms that have been applied while holding approximately ½ inch of the closed end flat between the fingertips allow room for expansion by the ejaculate without creating excessive pressure, which might break the condom. The penis should be withdrawn after ejaculation before the erection begins to subside while holding the top of the condom securely around the penis to avoid spillage. Condoms should never be reused and should be discarded properly after use so others will not come in contact with the contents.

2. Female condoms should be applied before any penetration occurs (even pre-ejaculation fluid can contain microorganisms). Lubrication decreases the chances of breakage during use, but only water-soluble lubricants should be used, because substances such as petroleum jelly may weaken the condom. Female condoms should never be reused and should be discarded properly after use so others will not come in contact with the contents.

3. These may provide some protection for the cervix only. They are not effective barriers against sexually transmitted disease (STD) infection.

4. These may provide some barrier protection for manual and oral sexual activity. Although some groups suggest that male condoms may be split down one side and opened or rubber dental dam material may be taped over areas that have lesions to avoid direct contact with blood and body fluid, especially during sadomasochistic sexual activity; this *very high-risk behavior* is not recommended.

5. Anal intercourse is a *very high-risk activity* for transmission of many types of STDs, as well as many intestinal organisms, and is not recommended. Homosexual networks advise wearing double condoms and using water-soluble lubricants, preferably containing nonoxynol-9, to decrease the risk somewhat if engaging in this type of sexual activity.

CRITICAL THINKING

1. Misunderstandings may include the following:
   a. The mistaken idea that one blood test can diagnose all STDs
   b. Ignorance about the time that may be required to treat STDs (if the disease is treatable at all)
   c. Lack of understanding of the importance of interview information for diagnosing STDs
   d. Lack of understanding of the importance of physical examination for diagnosing STDs

2. The woman is an adult (and we assume is capable of making her own decisions). James is not her guardian and has no more right to information about her than anyone else in the waiting room. He may be notified by a public health authority that he has been listed as a sexual contact by someone (anonymous) who has tested positive for a particular STD. However, if they have not yet become sexually intimate, he is not actually a contact. The only ethi-

cal and legal way that he can find out the information is by her choice (without coercion) to tell him.

3. Before any testing is done, both people should see the physician separately, be interviewed, be examined, and perhaps have samples taken for investigation. The physician should then order the tests that he or she deems necessary and counsel each patient about the test procedures, possible outcomes and treatments, and the expected time frame for return of results. A return visit may be arranged for a time after the physician should have received notification of results.

4. No, James is not going to get his answer about whether he has a contagious STD today. Even if he is a virgin, he may possibly have contracted an STD prenatally, so he must wait for test results. Recent exposure to some STD agents may not show positive results for a long period.

► REVIEW QUESTIONS

*The correct answers are in **boldface**.*

1. (**c**) is correct. Syphilis has three stages. (a, b, d) are not correct.

2. (**b**) is correct. Standing with arms crossed does not convey openness or trust and may be perceived as judgmental. (a) Addressing a patient by name is professional behavior. (c) Eye contact enhances communication unless inappropriate for a patient's cultural background. (d) Every patient has a right to privacy and confidentiality.

3. (**a**) is correct. Cytotoxins are poisons. (b, c, d) would all enhance rather than treat the disorder.

4. (**b**) is correct. The nurse should remain nonjudgmental. Once a diagnosis is made, teaching can be done to prevent further problems for the mother and baby. (a, c, d) are all true.

5. (**b**) is a myth. Not all people with STDs have poor hygiene. (a, c, d) are all true statements.

6. (**b**) is correct. Lifelong monogamy for both partners is the best protection against STDs. (a) Oral contraceptives do not provide protection against STDs. (c, d) can reduce the risk of STD transmission but are not as effective as lifelong monogamy.

7. (**d**) is correct. A chlamydia collection kit is used. (a, b, c) are not used.

8. (**b**) is correct. A Venereal Disease Research Laboratory slide test (VDRL) and an rapid plasma reagin test for syphilis. They do not test for (a, c, d).

9. (**b**) is correct. Penicillin is the treatment of choice for *Trichomonas*. (a, c, d) are not effective against *Trichomonas*.

10. (**b**) is correct. Feelings of depression and shame characterize herpes syndrome. (a, c, d) are not symptoms of herpes syndrome.

11. (**c**) is correct. Human papillomavirus causes genital warts. (a, b, d) cause other viral disorders.

12. (**b**) is correct. Papanicolaou smears are done to diagnose cancer, although they can identify some other abnormal cells. (a, c, d) are incorrect.

13. (**b**) is correct. History of an STD does not necessarily provide immunity.

14. (**c**) is correct. No barrier completely eliminates STD risk. (a) A condom is not infallible. (b) This is a foolish statement because it does not discourage risky behavior. (d) Stress may reduce immune system effectiveness, but this also does not discourage risky behavior.

15. (**c**) is correct. Urethritis causes painful urination and discharge. (a, b, d) are not symptoms of urethritis.

43

Answers

▶ STRUCTURE OF NEUROMUSCULAR JUNCTION AND SARCOMERES

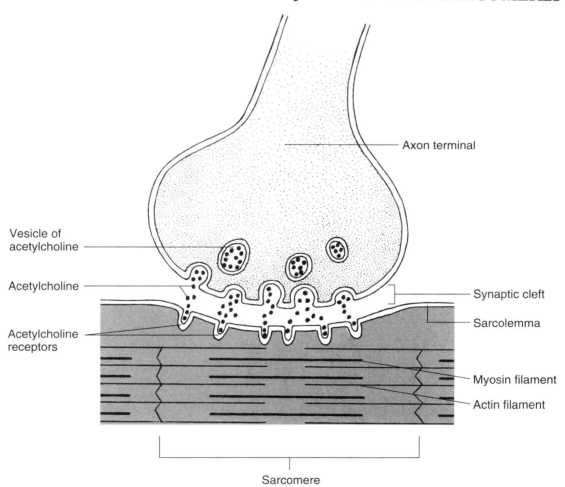

Vesicle of acetylcholine

Acetylcholine

Acetylcholine receptors

Axon terminal

Synaptic cleft

Sarcolemma

Myosin filament

Actin filament

Sarcomere

335

▶ NEUROMUSCULAR JUNCTION
1. (C, E)   3. (B, D)
2. (A, F)

▶ SYNOVIAL JOINTS
1. (E)   4. (B)
2. (C)   5. (D)
3. (A)

▶ VOCABULARY
1. (C)   6. (F)
2. (A)   7. (H)
3. (D)   8. (G)
4. (E)   9. (J)
5. (B)   10. (I)

▶ DIAGNOSTIC TESTS
1. (C)   7. (F)
2. (A)   8. (H)
3. (B)   9. (J)
4. (E)   10. (I)
5. (D)   11. (K)
6. (G)

▶ CRITICAL THINKING
1. Allergies, past health, medications, surgeries, injury, cause and mechanism of injury (how injured will indicate other injuries to look for; mechanism of injury—twisting, crushing, stretching).
2. Inspection: injury, asymmetry, mobility and range of motion, swelling, deformity and limb length, ecchymosis. Palpation: skin temperature, crepitation, tenderness, sensation.
3. X-rays of his leg and any other areas of potential injury based on the history. Complete blood count (CBC) to identify loss of blood. Additional tests may be ordered based on findings.

4. Any procedures to be done, tests to be done, need to report symptoms, pain relief issues, answer any questions.

▶ REVIEW QUESTIONS
*The correct answers are in **boldface**.*

1. (c)
2. (b)
3. (a)
4. (c)
5. (b)
6. (b) *Crepitation* is the term used for a grating sound heard in a joint. (a) A friction rub is associated with either pleural or pericardial inflammation or fluid accumulation. (c) An effusion is a collection of fluid in a space. (d) Subcutaneous emphysema is leaking air that is felt under the skin.
7. (c) Joint movement should immediately be stopped to prevent further joint injury. (a, b, d) would move the joint, causing possible injury.
8. (b) Ability to prepare food is an instrumental activity of daily living (ADL), which is part of a functional assessment. (a, c, d) are not items assessed in a functional assessment.
9. (d) A hematoma may develop following a biopsy. (a) does not occur from a biopsy. (b) Crackles are heard in the lungs. (c) An infection would not develop immediately, it would occur several days later.
10. (a) Bleeding into soft tissue is a complication of a biopsy. (b, c, d) relate to pain control.
11. (b) Stiff, sore joints are one of the early symptoms of rheumatoid arthritis. (a, d) are not early symptoms. (c) is not a related symptom.
12. (b) The patient should be nil per os (NPO) after midnight the night before surgery. (a) No food should be eaten after midnight. (c, d) are responsibilities of the physician.

44

ANSWERS

VOCABULARY
1. Arthritis
2. Arthroplasty
3. Synovitis
4. Arthrocentesis
5. Hyperuricemia
6. Scleroderma
7. Vasculitis
8. Polymyositis
9. Avascular necrosis
10. Replantation
11. Hemipelvectomy
12. Fasciotomy
13. Osteomyelitis
14. Osteosarcoma

FRACTURES
1. **(K)**   7. **(E)**
2. **(J)**   8. **(D)**
3. **(I)**   9. **(C)**
4. **(H)**   10. **(B)**
5. **(G)**   11. **(A)**
6. **(F)**

PROSTHESIS CARE EDUCATION
1. False—6 months
2. False—water
3. True
4. True
5. False—grease, prosthetist
6. True
7. False—same

HEALTH PROMOTION FOR PATIENTS WITH GOUT
1. Purine, sardines
2. Avoid
3. Fluids
4. Aspirin, aspirin
5. Avoid
6. Stress

PROGRESSIVE SYSTEMIC SCLEROSIS
Corrections are in **boldface.**

Progressive systemic sclerosis (PSS), **formerly** called systemic scleroderma, is similar to systemic lupus erythematosus in that it can affect **multiple** body organs and other connective tissues. PSS is **not** as common as lupus but has a higher mortality rate.

PSS is characterized by **inflammation** that develops into fibrosis (scarring), then sclerosis (**hardening**) of tissues. Autoimmunity is the likely cause. Like some of the other systemic connective tissue diseases, abnormal antibodies damage **healthy** tissue.

PSS affects **women** more than men, usually between 30 and 50 years of age. The disease tends to progress **very rapidly** and does not respond well to treatment. Spontaneous remissions and exacerbations occur.

► CRITICAL THINKING

IMPAIRED PHYSICAL MOBILITY RELATED TO HIP PRECAUTIONS AND SURGICAL PAIN

Intervention	Rationale	Evaluation
Reinforce transfer and ambulation techniques.	Activity is restricted due to hip precautions and weight-bearing limitations.	Does patient transfer and ambulate as instructed by physical therapy?
Place overhead frame and trapeze on bed; teach patient how to use it.	Patient mobility is increased and pain decreased with use of trapeze for movement.	Does patient use overbed frame and trapeze for movement?
Assess the patient for and take measures to prevent complications of immobility: Turn patient every 2 hours and check skin. Keep heels off of bed. Teach patient to deep breathe and cough every 2 hours; also teach use of incentive spirometer. Apply thigh-high elastic stockings. Give anticoagulants as ordered. Get patient out of bed as soon as possible. Ambulate patient as early as possible. Remind patient to practice leg exercises.	Immobility complications can occur if preventive measures are not used.	Does patient experience complications of immobility?

► REVIEW QUESTIONS

The correct answers are in **boldface.**

1. (**b**) Buck's traction is skin traction. (a, c, d) are examples of skeletal traction.
2. (**b**) Palming the cast to move it prevents indentations being made in the wet cast with fingertips. (a, c, d) are incorrect.
3. (**c**) Giving a test dose of gold is important to assess for an allergic reaction. (a, b, d) are incorrect.
4. (**d**) A test dose is given to assess for an allergic reaction. (a, b, c) are incorrect.
5. (**d**) The morphine should be prepared now so it is ready promptly when 3 hours is up; 15 mg should be given because the pain level is at the maximum and is occurring before the minimum ordered time interval. (a) Applying ice to the cast may be helpful, but because the pain is at the maximum, it will not provide enough relief. (b) There are no abnormalities to report to the physician at this time. (c) Removing the pillow may increase pain if swelling increases.
6. (**d**) This is a sign of hip dislocation. (a, b, c) are incorrect.
7. (**d**) Liver is an organ meat high in purines. (a, b, c) are not high-purine foods.
8. (**a**) can cause an attack of gout. (b, c, d) are incorrect.
9. (**c**) The erythrocyte sedimentation rate is a general screening test for systemic inflammation. (a, b, d) are incorrect.
10. (**a**) occurs commonly in patients with lupus. (b, c, d) are not common nursing diagnoses for lupus.
11. (**b**) It should be wrapped in a cool moist cloth and sealed in a plastic bag. (a) It should be cool and moist. (c) It is not placed on dry ice, which is also not readily available. (d) is not readily available or moist.

45

ANSWERS

VOCABULARY

1. dysphagia
2. Radiculopathy
3. paresthesia
4. decorticate
5. decerebrate
6. Anisocoria
7. nystagmus
8. contractures
9. dysarthria
10. aphasia

DIAGNOSTIC TESTS

1. A myelogram is an x-ray examination of the spinal canal after injection of contrast material into the subarachnoid space. Before the procedure ask the patient about allergies to contrast media. Make sure that a consent form has been signed. Check institution policy for nil per os (NPO) guidelines. Following the procedure the patient is maintained on bed rest, positioned with the head elevated or according to physician orders (based on type of dye used). Fluids are encouraged to rid the body of dye.

2. An electroencephalogram (EEG) uses electrodes attached to the scalp to monitor the electrical activity of the brain. Before the procedure, make sure the patient's hair is clean and dry. Check with the physician for any medications to hold. After the procedure, monitor for seizures, especially if seizure medications were held. Wash the adhesive from the hair as soon as possible before it becomes hard and difficult to remove.

3. A lumbar puncture involves a needle into the spinal fluid to collect cerebral spinal fluid (CSF) for analysis. Before the procedure you may ask the physician for an order for an analgesic or sedative if the patient is especially anxious. Make sure that a consent form has been signed. Assist the patient into a side-lying position with knees flexed and back arched. Some physicians prefer the patient sitting on the edge of the bed leaning over a bedside table. Stay with the patient to offer reassurance and assist the physician with specimens. Following the procedure follow orders for 6 to 8 hours of bed rest, and encourage fluids. Monitor the puncture site for leakage of CSF. Notify the physician if a headache occurs.

4. Magnetic resonance imaging (MRI) uses magnetic energy to produce images of tissues. It is not an x-ray. Ask patients if they have any metal in their bodies (pacemakers, joint replacements, foreign bodies)—if so they cannot have an MRI. Instruct the patient that he or she will be in a tunnel-like machine for a possibly prolonged time. If the patient is claustrophobic, notify the physician for a sedative or alternative orders. If the patient is in pain, request analgesic orders for before the procedure. No special aftercare is necessary.

5. Computed tomography (CT) produces images of layers ("slices") of tissue. It requires that the body or body part be within the scanner, which may be difficult for claustrophobic people. The physician may use contrast material. Find out if this is planned, and ensure the patient has no allergies to contrast material, iodine, or shellfish. The physician should be notified if kidney function is compromised, because kidneys excrete the dye. Check institution policy to know whether the patient should be kept NPO before the procedure. If dye is used, the patient should be prepared to expect a feeling of warmth during the injection. Following any procedure using dye, fluids should be encouraged. If dye is not used, no special aftercare is necessary.

▶ ANATOMY

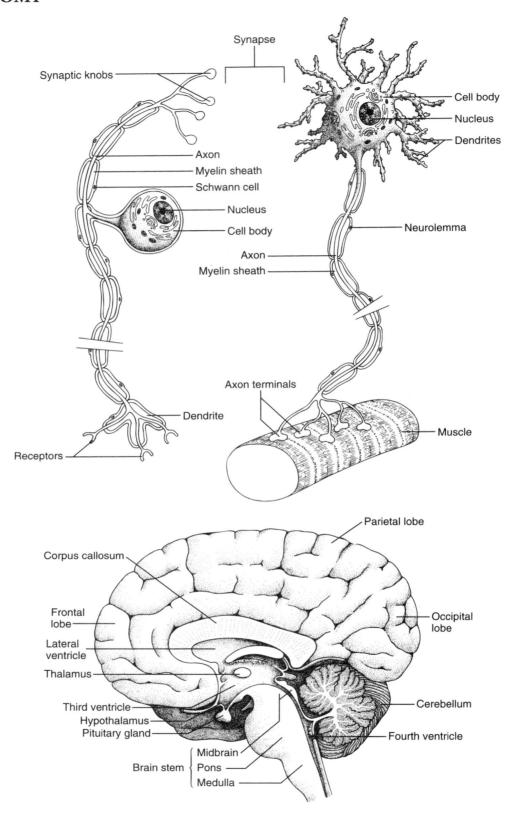

ANATOMY

1. (E)
2. (D)
3. (A)

4. (C)
5. (B)

ASSESSMENT OF CRANIAL NERVES

1. (C)
2. (D)
3. (B)

4. (A)
5. (E)

CRITICAL THINKING

1. After checking her transfer records for previous activity level, check muscle strength in her legs and feet. Ask how she got up to the bathroom at the hospital. Then have a second nurse or aide help in dangling her at the bedside and slowly standing before attempting to ambulate. If she is unable to dangle or stand, use a bedpan or bedside commode until she becomes stronger. Document how she did and how much assistance she needed in the plan of care.

2. Again, ask how she ate at the hospital, keeping in mind that her answers may not be reliable. Check for a gag reflex. Make sure she is sitting straight up to eat, preferably in a chair. Try small sips and bites first. Stay with her for the first meal to monitor her swallowing. Because she is weak on one side, check her mouth after each bite for pocketing of food.

3. Ask questions to assess orientation, such as the month and year, where she is, and who familiar visitors are.

Check recent and remote memory. (What did you have for lunch? What is your mother's name?) Clarify her question. She may have a perfectly legitimate reason to ask for the cookies.

4. Blood pressure is affected by muscle tone. A weak arm may have a lower pressure.

REVIEW QUESTIONS

The correct answers are in **boldface.**

1. **(b)**
2. **(b)**
3. **(b)**
4. **(a)**
5. **(b)**
6. **(d)**
7. **(a)**
8. **(a)**
9. **(c)** is correct. The patient is positioned on his or her side to expose the spinal column for puncture. (a, b, d) are not necessary for a lumbar puncture (LP).
10. **(a)** is correct. The patient lays flat for 6 to 8 hours to prevent headache following LP. (b) The patient should drink fluids, not be NPO; (c) pedal pulses are not significant following LP; and (d) the patient is kept flat for 6 to 8 hours, not elevated for 24 hours.
11. **(d)** correctly describes an MRI. (a) describes an electromyography, (b) describes an EEG, and (c) describes a brain scan.

46

ANSWERS

▶ VOCABULARY
1. **(I)**   6. **(D)**
2. **(F)**   7. **(E)**
3. **(A)**   8. **(C)**
4. **(G)**   9. **(H)**
5. **(B)**   10. **(J)**

▶ DRUGS USED FOR CENTRAL NERVOUS SYSTEM DISORDERS
1. **(B)**   4. **(E)**
2. **(A)**   5. **(D)**
3. **(C)**

▶ ALZHEIMER'S DISEASE
1. **(C)**   3. **(D)**
2. **(B)**   4. **(A)**

▶ CENTRAL NERVOUS SYSTEM DISORDERS
1. **(I)**   6. **(B)**
2. **(F)**   7. **(H)**
3. **(A)**   8. **(J)**
4. **(E)**   9. **(D)**
5. **(G)**   10. **(C)**

▶ SPINAL DISORDERS
Radiating pain to the ankle, footdrop, and the inability to walk on the toes are all indications of dysfunction of a lumbar nerve root. Deltoid weakness and diminished triceps reflex indicate dysfunction of a cervical nerve root.

▶ CRITICAL THINKING
Brain Attack

1. A brain attack is the infarction of brain tissue caused by the disruption of blood flow to the brain. Considering Mrs. Saunders' history, the cause of her attack was most likely ischemic, the result of atherosclerosis.

2. Hemiplegia.
3. Left, because her right side is paralyzed.
4. She was a smoker, she has a history of atherosclerosis and hypertension, and she is overweight.
5. Expressive aphasia.
6. Her score on the Glasgow Coma Scale is 11. Symptoms of rising intracranial pressure (ICP) include headache, vomiting, dilated pupil on the affected side, increasing weakness or paralysis, decorticate or decerebrate posturing, decreasing level of consciousness, increasing systolic blood pressure and respiratory rate, and increasing and then decreasing pulse rate.
7. A thrombolytic medication may have been used in the emergency department if Mrs. Saunders arrived within 3 hours of onset of her symptoms. The nurse would continue to monitor for side effects. Heparin may be ordered as an anticoagulant; antiplatelet drugs may be ordered for long-term prevention of recurrent stroke, and antihypertensives may be ordered to control blood pressure.
8. Many diagnoses fit Mrs. Saunders' situation. An example is impaired physical mobility related to flaccid right side. Measures to prevent complications related to immobility include repositioning every 1 to 2 hours, maintaining good body alignment with pillows, consulting physical therapy for exercise recommendations, range-of-motion exercises, and possibly a sling to prevent harm to her weakened shoulder muscles.
9. Reposition every 1 to 2 hours, maintain good nutrition and fluid intake, apply a pressure-reduction mattress to the bed, keep skin clean and dry, and check frequently for incontinence.
10. Because Mrs. Saunders understands spoken words, ask her if she has to go to the bathroom. Usually if a patient is attempting to get out of bed, there is a reason for it. See if she can nod yes or no in response. She might also be able to point to the bedside commode or bathroom. A picture board might also be helpful.
11. Gag and swallow reflexes can both be checked. A cotton swab at the back of the throat should elicit a gag reflex. If she gags, try a small sip of water before giving her food.

12. Ask for a consultation with the speech therapy department or other swallowing expert for recommendations specific to Mrs. Saunders. Many patients do better with pureed foods and thickened liquids. Be sure she is sitting straight up, preferably in a chair, to eat. Have her tilt her head forward while swallowing. Have her swallow each bite twice. After each bite, remind her to check the right side of her mouth for food that is not noticed.

13. Involve her family in her care. Give them small tasks to do for her. Encourage them to attend physical and other therapies with her. Explain what will happen at the rehabilitation facility. Assist the family to identify resources that can help when she is discharged to home. Consult with the social worker or discharge planner to provide them with additional information.

14. Antiplatelet drugs such as ticlopidine (Ticlid).

Spinal Cord Injury

1. These are the hallmark signs of spinal cord injury. Loss of vasomotor control results in vasodilation. This causes hypotension. Dilated blood vessels allow more exposure of blood to the skin surface, thereby cooling the blood and causing hypothermia. Bradycardia results from disruption of the autonomic nervous system.

2. Mr. Granger no longer has full use of his respiratory muscles. Therefore, he is not able to take deep breaths.

3. (a) Cervical traction will keep his cervical spine immobile and prevent further damage to the spinal cord. (b) Administration of vasopressors may be necessary to maintain blood pressure at a level that is adequate for tissue perfusion. Intravenous fluids may be inadequate to maintain blood pressure and may result in fluid overload. (c) Loss of innervation to the bladder may result in urine retention. An indwelling catheter is used to prevent bladder rupture or urinary reflux.

4. Edema of the spinal cord, fatigue of respiratory muscles, or both are reducing Mr. Granger's already compromised respiratory function. As he feels more short of breath, he becomes more anxious, fearing that his condition is worsening. Explain to him that this is a common short-term complication of spinal cord injury. Reassure him that if mechanical ventilation is required, it will not necessarily be a permanent condition.

5. Expect that Mr. Granger will be intubated or have a tracheostomy placed to allow for mechanical ventilation. Expect the ventilation to be necessary until the spinal cord edema has subsided.

6. *Ineffective breathing pattern.* The goal is that Mr. Granger will not experience hypoxia or respiratory arrest. Monitor his pulse oximetry and respiratory pattern frequently. At the first sign of restlessness, anxiety, or shortness of breath, inform the physician.

   Impaired physical mobility. The goal is for all of Mr. Granger's care needs to be met. He will be unable to care for himself independently. Whenever possible, give Mr. Granger choices as to how and when care will be performed. Include his significant others as much as he and they wish.

7. Mr. Granger needs simple explanations of what has happened to him and what his prognosis is. He also needs to begin to learn to direct his care. This will improve his ability to function outside of the hospital.

▶ REVIEW QUESTIONS
The correct answers are in **boldface.**

1. **(b)** It is most likely due to a herniated lumbar disk. (a, b, c) Bone or muscle injury and impaired circulation do not cause a radicular pain distribution.
2. **(c)** Drowsiness is a common side effect. (a, b, d) are not common side effects.
3. **(b)** Rest and cautious exercise are recommended; vigorous exercise may exacerbate the injury. (a, c, d) are all appropriate interventions.
4. **(c)** Inability to move the left leg would not be expected and should immediately be reported to the physician. (b) Decreased range of motion, (a) incisional pain, and (d) muscle spasm are common temporary results of microdiskectomy.
5. **(d)** The safest plan is to make sure another staff member is available to assist in assessing the patient's ability to ambulate. (a, b, c) Patients with right hemisphere infarcts often underestimate the extent of their deficits.
6. **(c)** Break the task into simple steps. (a) Performing the task for her and (b) telling her not to worry about it do not help increase her independence. (d) Patients in the rehabilitation unit should not be expected to teach one another.
7. **(a)** Hydrocephalus is a common consequence of subarachnoid hemorrhage. (b, c) would not typically make the patient lethargic or irritable. (d) would result in loss of consciousness and labile vital signs.
8. **(b)** Subarachnoid hemorrhage frequently affects memory function. (a, c, d) are short-term complications of subarachnoid hemorrhage.
9. **(b)** The earlier the antibiotics are started, the more likely the patient will survive the bacterial meningitis. (a, d) are not correct because antibiotics are never given to determine whether the patient will have an adverse reaction. (c) Resistant bacteria develop from inappropriate antibiotic use, not early use.
10. **(c)** Encephalitis is a disease entity by itself, not a symptom. (a, b, d) are all possible symptoms of arteriovenous malformation rupture.
11. **(b)** A structured environment provides a quiet setting with minimal distractions. (a, c, d) could potentiate the patient's agitation.
12. **(a)** is correct. Decreasing level of consciousness (LOC) is a symptom of increasing ICP. (b, c) Sympathetic and parasympathetic responses and (d) increased cerebral blood flow do not cause decreased LOC.
13. **(c)** Widening pulse pressure warns of increasing ICP. (a, b, d) do not occur in increasing ICP.
14. **(d)** is correct. Mannitol is an osmotic diuretic, so urine output should be monitored. (a, b, c) can be monitored but are not specific to mannitol.
15. **(b)** is correct. Elevation of the head of the bed reduces ICP. (a, c, d) all can potentially increase ICP.

47

ANSWERS

► VOCABULARY

1. atrophied
2. exacerbations
3. neuralgia
4. ptosis
5. demyelination
6. plasmapheresis
7. fasciculations
8. acetylcholinesterase

► PERIPHERAL DISORDERS

*Errors are in **boldface**.*

1. Miss Mary Garvey sees her physician because she has been seeing double off and on for several weeks and has been fatigued. Her physician suspects myasthenia gravis and schedules her for a **carotid ultrasound.** He confirms his suspicions with a Tensilon test. He explains to Miss Garvey that she has a disease that is characterized by a decrease in the neurotransmitter **norepinephrine.** He begins her on **Mastadon** and prednisone. Her nurse teaches her the importance of getting regular exercise and recommends **joining a local health and exercise club.**

   Electromyography (EMG), not ultrasound, is likely to be done. Receptor sites for the neurotransmitter acetylcholine are affected. Mestinon, not Mastadon, is an anticholinesterase drug used to reduce symptoms. (A mastadon is a prehistoric elephant.) It seems wise to recommend exercise, but individuals with myasthenia gravis become very fatigued, and rest, not exercise, is the only way to relieve it. Moderate exercise as tolerated is a better recommendation.

2. Mr. Tom Neura has a history of trigeminal neuralgia. He enters the emergency department with severe pain in his **left wrist.** The physician orders a narcotic analgesic because Mr. Neura's **third** cranial nerve is inflamed. Once the acute pain has subsided, Mr. Neura is discharged with instructions to get plenty of **fresh air** and to take his phenytoin (Dilantin) as ordered.

   Pain in the face, not the wrist, characterizes trigeminal neuralgia. The trigeminal nerve is the fifth, not the third, cranial nerve. Fresh air may aggravate pain because even a breeze on the face can cause excruciating pain.

3. Mrs. Mattie Schultz is admitted with exacerbated multiple sclerosis (MS). Her legs are becoming weaker, causing difficult walking, and she has been having difficulty swallowing. You know that **buildup** of myelin on her neurons is responsible for her weakness. You assess her for stressors that might have caused her exacerbation, such as urinary tract infection (UTI) or upper respiratory tract infection (URI). Mattie is started on **thyroid stimulating hormone (TSH) to stimulate her thyroid,** which will help reduce her symptoms. She is also placed on Bactrim for the UTI you identified through your excellent assessment and on **Valium for urinary retention.**

   Patch degeneration, not buildup, of myelin accounts for symptoms of MS. Adrenocorticotropic hormone (ACTH) to stimulate the adrenal cortex to secrete cortisol is given to reduce inflammation and relieve symptoms. Valium might be given for muscle spasms, but bethanechol (Urecholine) or oxybutynin (Ditropan) are given for urinary problems.

► CRITICAL THINKING

1. Amyotrophic lateral sclerosis (ALS) is a nerve disease in which the nerves that stimulate the muscles to make them contract degenerate and form scar tissue. This makes it difficult for muscles to contract.
2. Nerves that control the muscles in his legs are becoming more affected. A referral for physical therapy and a cane or other walking aid might help Reverend Wilson continue to function for as long as possible.
3. He should know that ALS does not affect thinking. Therefore, as long as he can function physically, there is no reason to quit his job.
4. Muscle spasms can be relieved with medications such as baclofen (Lioresal) or diazepam (Valium).
5. Reverend Wilson's muscles that control swallowing are probably affected now. An appropriate nursing diagnosis is impaired swallowing related to muscle weakness. Because his swallowing is unlikely to improve dramatically, a good

344

goal might be that he will not aspirate. The physician might order a swallowing evaluation by a speech therapist, who can recommend interventions to help prevent aspiration. Additional interventions include making sure he is sitting up straight to eat, staying with him during meals in case he has difficulty, having him swallow each bite twice, and having him avoid thin liquids. Eventually he and his wife may need to decide if they want to consider tube feedings.

6. Possible nursing diagnoses include disturbed body image, imbalanced nutrition, impaired oral mucous membranes, impaired mobility, risk for impaired skin integrity, and ineffective coping. Note that these are only possible ideas and would need to be verified with a thorough assessment.

▶ REVIEW QUESTIONS

*The correct answers are in **boldface**.*

1. **(d)** is correct. Guillain-Barré syndrome is most likely caused by an autoimmune process. (a, b, c) are not causes of Guillain-Barré syndrome.
2. **(b)** is correct. Arterial blood gases (ABGs) monitor respiratory function. Deteriorating ABGs signal respiratory failure from weakening respiratory muscles. (a) signals kidney disease, which is not a common problem in Guillain-Barré syndrome. (c) Bleeding and (d) electrolyte imbalances are not associated with Guillain-Barré syndrome.
3. **(d)** is correct. Tensilon is given to determine if it is effective in reducing muscle weakness. (a,b) there is no such thing as a Mestinon test or a Quinine tolerance test. (c) Pulmonary function studies might be done if respiratory muscles are affected, but would not be diagnostic for myasthenia gravis (MG).
4. **(a)** is correct. Anticholinesterase drugs reduce activity of cholinesterase, leaving more acetylcholine available to aid in muscle contraction. (b) Anticholinergic drugs will worsen symptoms. (c, d) Adrenergic or beta blockers will not help.
5. **(d)** is correct. Myelin is damaged in MS. (a, b, c) are not related to MS.
6. **(b)** is correct. ACTH stimulates the adrenal cortex to release cortisol, which reduces inflammation and may induce remission. (a, c, d) are not used to treat MS.
7. **(b)** is correct. Elevating the head of the bed will reduce the workload of the respiratory muscles. (a) Antibiotics given when infection is not present can lead to resistant strains of bacteria. (c) Bed rest can increase risk of respiratory complications, and (d) suction should be done only when necessary.
8. **(d)** is correct. The patient with Bell's palsy may have difficulty closing the affected eye, and eyedrops will keep the eye lubricated. (a, b, c) are not useful for Bell's palsy. Heat, rather than ice, is sometimes used.
9. **(c)** is correct. The only way to know if nutrition is adequate without blood work is to monitor weights. Monitoring (a) meal trays, (b) intake and output (I&O), and (d) swallowing are all good interventions but will not show whether nutrition has been maintained. Serum albumin is also sometimes used to monitor nutrition status.
10. **(a)** is correct. These symptoms describe Navajo neuropathy. (b, c, d) do not have these specific symptoms.
11. **(a)** is correct. Muscle twitchings are called fasciculations. (b) Atrophy is wasted muscles, (c) chorea is movements found in Huntington's disease, and (d) neuropathy is nerve pain.
12. **(b)** is correct. Eating uses muscles innervated by the fifth cranial nerve and is most likely to cause pain. (a, c, d) do not use the facial muscles and are less likely to cause pain. Sleeping usually relieves pain.

48

ANSWERS

▶ STRUCTURES OF THE EYE

Superior rectus muscle

Ciliary body

Suspensory ligaments

Conjunctiva

Cornea

Iris

Pupil

Lens

Canal of Schlemm

Aqueous humor { Anterior chamber
Posterior chamber

Vitreous humor

Fovea

Optic nerve

Retinal artery and vein

Optic disc

Retina

Choroid layer

Sclera

Inferior rectus muscle

► STRUCTURES OF THE EAR

► VISION
1 A, 2 D, 3 F, 4 B, 5 G, 6 C, 7 E

► HEARING
1 A, 2 E, 3 C, 4 H, 5 B, 6 D, 7 F, 8 G, 9 I

► VOCABULARY
Nystagmus
Definition: Constant involuntary cyclical eyeball movement.
Tropia
Definition: Deviation of eye away from visual axis.
Accommodation
Definition: Adjustment of the eye for distance to focus the image on the retina by changing lens curvature.

Ptosis
Definition: Drooping of upper eyelid from paralysis
Arcus senilus
Definition: Opaque white ring around the periphery of the cornea in aged persons from deposits of fat.
Ophthalmologist
Definition: Physician trained to diagnose and treat eye conditions and diseases.
Optometrist
Definition: Doctor of optometry who diagnoses and treats certain eye conditions and diseases.
Optician
Definition: Makes prescribed corrective lenses.

► DIAGNOSTIC TESTS

Assessment Test	Purpose of Test	Normal Test Results
Snellen chart	Visual acuity	Right eye (OD) 20/20, left eye (OS) 20/20, each eye (OU) 20/20
Visual fields	Peripheral vision	Equal to examiner's
Cardinal fields of gaze	Extraocular movement	Follows in all fields without nystagmus
Accommodation	Pupillary response to near and far distances	Eyes turn inward and pupils constrict when focusing on a near object
Rinne	Differentiate between conductive and sensorineural hearing loss	Air conduction > bone conduction
Weber	Hearing acuity	Heard equally
Romberg's	Balance/vestibular function	Able to maintain standing position without loss of balance

► CRITICAL THINKING

1. Eye strain from computer use.
2. The nurse should assess the position of Ms. LittleThunder's computer and the lighting of the office. The nurse should also assess the size of font that Ms. LittleThunder is using.
3. The position of the bottom of the computer monitor should be 20 degrees below the line of sight and should be positioned 13 to 18 inches from the eyes. Glare should be reduced by situating the computer screen away from windows and lights. The font size should be increased if the letters on the screen appear too small.

► REVIEW QUESTIONS

*The correct answers are in **boldface**.*

1. (**b**) The first distance recorded when conducting the Snellen test is the distance from which the patient can clearly read the alphabetical line on the chart. The second distance recorded is the distance from which a person with normal vision can see the same alphabetical line. (a, c) are incorrect. (d) is incorrect because normal vision is 20/20.
2. (**d**) Symmetrical eye muscle strength keeps the eyes in the same position, and the light is reflected in exactly the same place. (a) is incorrect. (b) defines accommodation. (c) defines the pupils' reaction to light.
3. (**c**) P = pupils, E = equal, R = round, R = reactive, L = to light, and A = accommodation. (a, b) are incorrect. (d) is incorrect because PERRLA is the expected finding.
4. (**a**) Visual fields test peripheral vision. (b, c, d) are incorrect because near vision is tested with a handheld chart or by reading a book, distance vision is tested with a Snellen chart, and central vision is tested with an Amsler grid.
5. (**d**) Arcus senilis, though a physical eye finding, does not cause visual problems. (a, b, c) can lead to visual disturbances.
6. (**c**) Air conduction is heard longer than bone conduction. (a) defines bone conduction. (b) is incorrect because air conduction is more efficient. (d) is incorrect.
7. (**d**) Patients with hearing loss sometimes speak unusually loud or soft. (a, b, c) indicate that the patient is hearing well enough to communicate.
8. (**b**) Air conduction is heard longer than bone conduction. (a) indicates the normal findings of a Weber test. (c, d) indicate abnormal findings.
9. (**c**) Ototoxic is ear toxicity. (a) Otoplasty is ear repair. (b) Otalgia is ear pain. (d) Tinnitus is ringing in the ears.
10. (**d**) Seeing halos around lights would be an important visual finding. (a, b, c) are incorrect.
11. (**a**) Darwin tubercle is a normal finding at any age. (b, c, d) are incorrect.
12. (**d**) is correct. (a) is for balance. (b) examines the tympanic membrane. (c) assesses the reflex that controls balance.
13. (**a**) Otorrhea is ear drainage. (b) Otalgia is ear pain. (c) Ototoxic is toxic to ear. (d) Tinnitus is ringing in the ears.
14. (**c**) Presbycusis is loss of high-pitched sounds due to aging. (a) Plasty is ear repair. (b) Otalgia is ear pain. (d) Tinnitus is ringing in the ears.

ANSWERS

VOCABULARY
1. (E)   4. (F)
2. (D)   5. (B)
3. (C)   6. (A)

ERRORS OF REFRACTION

A Hyperopia

B Myopia

PRESBYOPIA

Corrections are in **boldface.**

Presbyopia is a condition in which the lenses **lose** their elasticity resulting in a decrease in ability to focus on **close** objects. The loss of elasticity causes light rays to focus **beyond** the retina, resulting in hyperopia. This condition usually is associated with aging and generally occurs **after** age 40. Because accommodation for close vision is accomplished by lens contraction, people with presbyopia exhibit the **inability** to see objects at close range. They often compensate for blurred close vision by holding objects to be viewed **further away.** Complaints of eye strain and mild **frontal** headache are common.

VISUAL AND HEARING DATA COLLECTION

Macular degeneration. The patient reports slow, progressive loss of central and near vision in one or both eyes. The visual loss is described as blurred vision, distortion of straight lines, and a dark or empty spot in the central area of vision. Examination of visual acuity for near and far vision will reveal loss of vision. Use of the Amsler grid will allow the examiner to detect central vision distortion. The examiner may use intravenous fluorescein angiography to evaluate blood vessel abnormalities.

Cataract. The patient complains of difficulty seeing at night, when reading, and in bright light; increased sensitivity to glare; double vision; and decreased color vision. Visual acuity is tested for near and far vision. The direct ophthalmoscope and slit lamp are used to examine the lens and other internal structures. The lens will appear cloudy on examination, and the visual acuity may be reduced.

Hordeolum. Small, raised, lightly colored area on the palpebral border without pain.

Acute angle-closure glaucoma. The patient complains of unilateral severe pain of rapid onset, blurred vision, halos around lights, sensitivity to light, and tearing. The patient may complain of nausea and vomiting. A tonometry test will reveal increased intraocular pressure (IOP). The visual field examination may demonstrate a loss of peripheral vision.

External otitis. The patient complains of pain and may complain of pruritus. Redness, swelling, and drainage may be observed during otoscopic examination. Rinne and Weber tests may indicate conductive hearing impairment. Laboratory tests such as complete blood count (CBC), white blood cell (WBC) count, and culture may indicate infection.

Impacted cerumen. The patient may experience hearing loss, a feeling of fullness, or blocked ear. Otoscopic examination reveals cerumen blocking the ear canal. Audiometric testing, whisper voice, and Rinne and Weber tests may indicate conductive hearing loss.

Otitis media. The patient may complain of fever, earache, and a feeling of fullness in the affected ear. If purulent drainage has formed, there may be pain and conductive hearing loss. Otoscopic examination will reveal a reddened and bulging tympanic membrane. Audiometric studies and Rinne, Weber, and whisper tests will likely reveal hearing loss. Laboratory studies may indicate an elevated WBC.

Otosclerosis. The patient will have progressive bilateral hearing loss, particularly with soft low tones. The patient may experience tinnitus. Otoscopic examination may reveal a pinkish, orange tympanic membrane. Audiometric testing and the whisper voice test will show decreased hearing. The patient will hear best with bone conduction in the Rinne test, whereas lateralization to the most affected ear will occur with the Weber test. Imaging studies will indicate the location and the extent of the excessive bone growth.

▶ GLAUCOMA

Corrections are in **boldface.**

Glaucoma is characterized by abnormal pressure **within** the eyeball. This pressure causes damage to the cells of the **optic** nerve, the structure responsible for transmitting visual information from the **eye** to the brain. The damage is **silent,** progressive, and **irreversible** until the end stage, when loss of **peripheral** vision occurs and eventually blindness. Once glaucoma occurs, the patient **will always have it and must follow treatment to maintain stable intraocular eye pressures.**

▶ CONDUCTIVE HEARING LOSS

Corrections are in **boldface.**

Conductive hearing loss is interference with conduction of **sound impulses** through the external auditory canal, eardrum, or middle ear. The inner ear is **not** involved in a pure conductive hearing loss. Conductive hearing loss is a **mechanical** problem. Causes of conductive hearing loss include cerumen, foreign bodies, infection, perforation of the tympanic membrane, trauma, fluid in the middle ear, cysts, tumor, and otosclerosis. Many causes of conductive hearing loss such as infection, foreign bodies, or impacted cerumen **can be** corrected. Hearing devices **may improve** hearing for conditions that cannot be corrected. Hearing devices are most effective with conductive hearing loss when **no** inner ear and nerve damage are present.

▶ OTOSCLEROSIS

Corrections are in **boldface.**

Otosclerosis results from the formation of new bone along the **stapes.** With the new bone growth, the **stapes** becomes **immobile** and causes conductive hearing loss. Hearing loss is most apparent after the **fourth** decade. Otosclerosis usually occurs **more** frequently in women than in men. The disease usually affects **both** ears. It is thought to be a hereditary disease. The primary symptom of otosclerosis is **progressive** hearing loss. The patient usually experiences bilateral conductive hearing loss, particularly with soft, **low** tones. **Stapedectomy** is the treatment of choice.

▶ CRITICAL THINKING

1. The key symptom that this older adult is having is visual loss without pain. The nurse's examination reveals opacity of the lens, a primary indicator of cataract formation. The vision is diminished because the light rays are unable to get to the retina through the clouded lens.

2. Cataract formation is diagnosed through the eye examination. Visual acuity is tested for near and far vision. The direct ophthalmoscope and slit lamp are used to examine the lens and other internal structures. Instruct the patient that it is important for him to remain still while the health care practitioner uses the handheld ophthalmoscope. The slit lamp will require the patient to rest his chin and forehead against the machine while the health care provider performs this painless test. Instruct the patient that both tests require shining a bright light into the eye, which may be uncomfortable for a few seconds.

3. Refer to Nursing Process for Patients Having Eye Surgery in Chapter 49. Areas to include in a teaching plan are disease process, surgical intervention, preoperative and postoperative restrictions, use of dark glasses, medication administration, eye protection, and activities to be avoided.

▶ REVIEW QUESTIONS

The correct answers are in **boldface.**

1. **(d)** Loss of central vision occurs with macular degeneration and is tested using the Amsler grid. (a, b, c) are incorrect because the patient with macular degeneration may have decreased distinction of colors, slow loss of vision, and loss of near vision.

2. **(b)** Myotics lower intraocular pressure by stimulating pupillary and ciliary sphincter muscles. (a) is incorrect because osmotics decrease IOP by decreasing vitreous humor production. (c) is incorrect because mydriatics dilate pupils. (d) is incorrect because cycloplegics paralyze the muscles of accommodation and can increase IOP.

3. **(c)** Dilated pupils cannot protect the eye from the sun by constricting. (a, b, d) are incorrect.

4. **(d)** A stapedectomy involves removing or replacing part or all of the stapes with a prosthesis. Otosclerosis is the hardening of the stapes, so a stapedectomy is the treatment of choice. (a) is incorrect because a myringotomy is an incision made in the tympanic membrane to drain out fluid or suction the inner ear. (b) is incorrect because a myringoplasty is reconstructive repair of a perforated tympanic membrane. (c) is incorrect because a mastoidectomy is the excision of mastoid cells.

5. **(a)** There are no specific medicines to relieve dizziness; however, antihistamines are helpful for some patients. (b, c, d) are incorrect.

6. **(a)** Hearing aids amplify sound and are most useful with conductive hearing loss. Hearing aids are less useful when nerve damage is also present. (b, c, d) are incorrect.

7. **(d)** is correct. (a, b, c) are incorrect.

8. **(a)** These three symptoms are known as the triad of symptoms of Meniere's disease. (b, c, d) are incorrect.

9. (**b**) The labyrinth is involved with balance and equilibrium. Avoiding sudden movements can help prevent dizziness. (a, c, d) are incorrect.

10. (**d**) is correct. (a, b, c) are incorrect.

11. (**c**) Blurring of vision is the first symptom of cataracts due to the clouding of the lens. (a, b, d) are incorrect.

12. (**c**) is correct. (a, b, d) are incorrect.

13. (**c**) Sudden onset of acute pain could indicate increased IOP, bleeding, or detachment; all could lead to permanent eye damage. (a, b, d) are important nursing interventions with lesser priority.

14. (**b**) The intraocular pressure increases as the aqueous humor is prevented from flowing from the anterior to the posterior chamber. (a, c, d) are incorrect.

15. (**c**) is correct. (a) occurs in detached retina; (b) lens opacity is usually found with a cataract; and (d) occurs in Meniere's disease.

16. (**b**) Coughing, sneezing, bending over, and vomiting all increase intraocular pressure and put the patient at risk of hemorrhage. (a, c, d) do not directly increase IOP.

50

ANSWERS

► INTEGUMENTARY STRUCTURES

1. (E)	6. (C)
2. (D)	7. (H)
3. (G)	8. (A)
4. (B)	9. (F)
5. (I)	

► VOCABULARY

1. (E)	4. (C)
2. (A)	5. (D)
3. (B)	

► PRIMARY SKIN LESIONS

1. (C)	6. (G)
2. (F)	7. (D)
3. (A)	8. (E)
4. (I)	9. (H)
5. (B)	

► DIAGNOSTIC SKIN TESTS

1. (B)	3. (A)
2. (D)	4. (C)

► CRITICAL THINKING

1. Left-sided paralysis; immobility; confusion; nothing by mouth and lack of adequate nutrients being provided to maintain healthy tissue; diaphoresis causing skin excoriation and breakdown; thin build, which provides less padding and greater pressure on blood vessels, resulting in ischemia and tissue necrosis.

2. Approximately 170 calories per 1000 mL of 5-percent dextrose, which is less than the recommended daily calorie intake.

3. Risk of impaired skin integrity: Assess skin every 4 hours; keep linens and clothing clean and dry; place on turning schedule every 1 to 2 hours; keep skin dry; avoid massaging reddened or bony areas.

Impaired mobility: Place on turning schedule every 1 to 2 hours; perform active or passive range of motion; encourage patient to participate in activities of daily living.

Imbalanced nutrition, less than body requirements: Assess patient's daily fluid, caloric, and nutrient needs; consult dietitian; request referral to speech therapist for swallowing studies; provide fluids and nutrition as ordered (tube feedings, hyperalimentation).

4. He is high risk and needs constant pressure relief below the 25 to 32 mm Hg that closes capillaries and causes ischemia. A pressure-relieving device provides this relief for high-risk patients.

► REVIEW QUESTIONS

*The correct answers are in **boldface**.*

1. (**a**) is correct.
2. (**d**) is correct.
3. (**c**) is correct.
4. (**b**) is correct.
5. (**a**) is correct.
6. (**c**) is correct.
7. (**d**) is correct. (a, b, c) are younger and have more moisture and elasticity.
8. (**a**) is a bluish color resulting from a decrease in tissue oxygen. (b) is a reddish color. (c) is a yellowish color. (d) is a pale color.
9. (**c**) results in the decreased ability to maintain warmth. (a, b, d) do not affect warmth.
10. (**d**) provides protection for a skin tear. (a) is used for a deep or infected wound. (b) is used for deeper pressure ulcers. (c) is used to fill in a deep wound.
11. (**c**) Petechiae indicate a clotting problem, so the physician must be informed immediately. (a, b, d) are not of use because this is a clotting problem.

51

ANSWERS

▶ VOCABULARY

1. **(S)**	11. **(I)**
2. **(R)**	12. **(H)**
3. **(Q)**	13. **(G)**
4. **(P)**	14. **(F)**
5. **(O)**	15. **(E)**
6. **(N)**	16. **(D)**
7. **(M)**	17. **(C)**
8. **(L)**	18. **(B)**
9. **(K)**	19. **(A)**
10. **(J)**	

▶ BENIGN SKIN LESIONS

1. **(C)**	4. **(F)**
2. **(E)**	5. **(A)**
3. **(D)**	6. **(B)**

▶ PLASTIC SURGERY PROCEDURES

1. rhinoplasty
2. face lift
3. blepharoplasty

▶ CRITICAL THINKING

1. Diabetes, immobility, hypotensive period that resulted in ischemia, poor initial circulation indicated by need for femoral-popliteal bypass.
2. Sacrum: stage III. Heel: stage II
3. Turning every 2 hours relieves pressure, but this is not frequent enough to prevent ischemia in the high-risk patient because it begins to develop in 20 minutes. Elevation of the right foot relieves pressure and is very helpful. Sheepskin is used for comfort only; it does not relieve or reduce pressure, so it is not effective in preventing pressure ulcers.
4. The patient is at high risk for pressure ulcers, and sheepskin provides only comfort, not pressure relief, which the patient requires. An order for a pressure relief device should be requested, such as a special air mattress or bed.

▶ REVIEW QUESTIONS

The correct answers are in **boldface.**

1. **(c)** is correct. Shear can result from pulling a patient up in bed, leading to tissue injury and a pressure ulcer. (a, b, d) help prevent pressure ulcers.
2. **(c)** is correct. A stage III ulcer is deep but has not entered the muscle or bone area.
3. **(a)** is correct. A nonocclusive dressing should be used on an infected wound. (b, c, d) are occlusive dressings that are contraindicated for infected wounds.
4. **(b)** is correct because it describes light red (blood-tinged) drainage. (a, d) There is no indication of infection or pus. (c) There is not a large amount.
5. **(b)** is correct. Because the wound is not infected, gentle flushing produced by a needleless syringe is desired. (a, d) are pressure flushing techniques for infected wounds. (c) will cause further tissue damage.
6. **(d)** is correct. This burn has damaged all the skin layers. (a, b, c) are incorrect.
7. **(d)** is correct. These are signs of an infection, which is a common cause of death in burn patients. The physician must be notified immediately. (a) removing the dressing will not help, (b), an occlusive dressing can worsen the infection, and (c) an antibiotic must be ordered by the physician.
8. **(a)** is correct. This describes basal cell carcinoma. (b, c) are incorrect.
9. **(c)** is highly metastatic and requires prompt treatment. (a, b) are not highly metastatic.
10. **(a)** is correct. A fungal infection has most likely developed due to the use of the antibiotics. (b, c, d) do not fit the description.

52

ANSWERS

▶ **STRUCTURES OF THE IMMUNE SYSTEM**

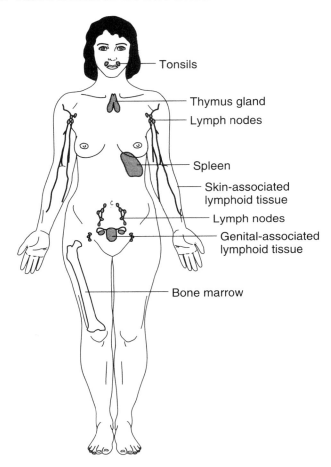

- Tonsils
- Thymus gland
- Lymph nodes
- Spleen
- Skin-associated lymphoid tissue
- Lymph nodes
- Genital-associated lymphoid tissue
- Bone marrow

► IMMUNE SYSTEM CELLS

1. (D)	5. (C)
2. (G)	6. (A)
3. (E)	7. (F)
4. (B)	

► ANTIBODIES

1. IgA
2. IgG
3. IgD
4. IgE
5. IgG
6. IgA
7. IgM

► VOCABULARY

1. Antigens
2. Immunity
3. Natural killer cells, T cells, B cells
4. T cells (or T lymphocytes)
5. Immunoglobulins
6. Cell mediated
7. Naturally acquired active
8. IgG
9. Inflammation
10. Neutrophils

► IMMUNE SYSTEM

1. (G)	5. (B)
2. (D)	6. (H)
3. (E)	7. (C)
4. (A)	8. (F)

► NURSING ASSESSMENT— SUBJECTIVE (HISTORY)

Corrections are in **boldface.**

Demographic Data

The patient's age, gender, race, and ethnic background are important. Systemic lupus erythematosus affects **women** eight times more frequently than **men.** The patient's place of birth gives insight to ethnic ties. Where the patient has lived and does live may shed light on the current illness. The patient's occupation such as that of a coal miner may contribute to **respiratory** symptoms.

Common signs and symptoms found with immune system disorders include fever, fatigue, joint pain, swollen glands, **weight loss,** and skin rash.

History

Food, medication, and environmental allergies should include those that the patient experiences and those present in the family history. With a family history a previous exposure to a substance is **not** required before a severe reaction occurs. Conditions such as systemic lupus erythematosus, ankylosing spondylitis, and asthma are thought to be either familial or have a **genetic** predisposition. If the patient's thymus gland has been removed (thymectomy), **T**-cell production may be altered. Corticosteroids and immunosuppressants **alter** the immune response. The patient's lifestyle may place the patient at **high** risk for contracting the human immunodeficiency virus. The patient's diet and usage of vitamins give insight into the **reserve** of the immune system. Stress (environmental, physical and psychological) can **depress** immune system function.

► CRITICAL THINKING

1. Demographic data (age, gender, race and ethnic background, place of birth, place of residence, occupation [past and present]); patient history (blood transfusions, high-risk behaviors, allergies [drug, food, environmental], surgeries, diagnosed medical conditions [past, present]); physical (general appearance, cardiovascular, skin, mucous membranes, respiratory, gastrointestinal, renal, musculoskeletal, nervous).

2. Normal lymph nodes are not palpable. Nodes that are nontender, hard, fixed, and enlarged are frequently associated with cancer.

3. If cancer is suspected: recent weight loss, occupational exposures, any high-risk lifestyle behaviors such as smoking, sexual patterns, previous medical history, family history.

► REVIEW QUESTIONS

The correct answers are in **boldface.**

1. **(a)**	8. **(c)**
2. **(b)**	9. **(c)**
3. **(d)**	10. **(a)**
4. **(a)**	11. **(b)**
5. **(b)**	12. **(c)**
6. **(b)**	13. **(b)**
7. **(d)**	

53

ANSWERS

VOCABULARY

1. (J)	10. (F)
2. (K)	11. (G)
3. (H)	12. (A)
4. (M)	13. (E)
5. (C)	14. (L)
6. (I)	
7. (N)	
8. (B)	
9. (D)	

IMMUNE DISORDERS

1. type I, type I, type III, type IV
2. hay fever
3. sinusitis, nasal polyps, asthma, chronic bronchitis
4. Infection
5. epinephrine
6. hives
7. is less pruritic, has more diffuse edema, may last longer
8. Coombs' test
9. Shock, renal failure
10. penicillins, sulfonamides
11. MSG, bisulfates
12. Poison ivy (or oak)
13. vitamin B_{12}
14. Erythrocytapheresis
15. sacroiliac, costovertebral, large peripheral

REVIEW QUESTIONS

*The correct answers are in **boldface**.*

1. (**a**) an infection can develop if treatment is not followed. (b, c, d) are incorrect.
2. (**c**) The physician must be informed to determine if the medication should be given. It is not within the nurse's scope of practice to make that decision. (a, b, d) are incorrect.
3. (**d**) the antibiotic, which is the cause of the problem, should be stopped immediately so that no more medication enters patient. (a, b) would be done next or as the antibiotic is stopped if assistance is available. (c) is incorrect.
4. (**d**) respiratory distress with wheezing occurs in anaphylaxis. (a, b, c) are incorrect.
5. (**a**) Epinephrine is the initial treatment for anaphylaxis. (b, c, d) are incorrect.
6. (**a**) Red blood cells are destroyed by this condition, so red cell fragments would be present. (b, c, d) are incorrect.
7. (**b**) When a portion of the stomach is removed, intrinsic factor, which is necessary for the absorption of vitamin B_{12}, is reduced. Patients must have lifelong vitamin B_{12} injections to prevent pernicious anemia from developing.
8. (**b**) is correct. (a, c, d) are incorrect.
9. (**d**) is correct. (a, b, c) are incorrect.
10. (**c**) Respiratory distress occurs in anaphylaxis. (a, b, d) are incorrect.
11. (**b**) Opening windows will allow pollen to enter the car. (a, c, d) will control the allergy.
12. (**d**) is correct. (a, b, c) are incorrect.
13. (**a**) is correct. (b, c, d) are incorrect.
14. (**b**) is correct. (a, c, d) are incorrect.

54

ANSWERS

► VOCABULARY
1. Acquired immune deficiency syndrome (AIDS)
2. CD4$^+$ cell
3. Viral load
4. Opportunistic infections
5. Human immunodeficiency virus (HIV) wasting syndrome
6. Enzyme-linked immunosorbent assay (ELISA) test

► DIAGNOSTIC TESTS
1. ELISA test. The typical HIV diagnostic tests and testing pattern include the following:
   A. ELISA test is done to detect antibodies to HIV antigen on test plates.
   B. If positive, the ELISA test is repeated.
   C. If the ELISA test is again positive, another test, often the Western blot, is done for confirmation.
   D. If all test results are positive, the patient is HIV-antibody positive.
   E. Other tests can be used, especially if initial test results are not conclusive. It is important that the patient be counseled before and after the ELISA test is done. Patients need to be instructed on safe-sex practices, resources, and support systems.
2. Viral load: Measures the amount of HIV RNA in plasma and is extremely important for determining prognosis and monitoring the response to antiretroviral therapy. Viral loads should be preformed 1 month after initiation of new treatments and at 4-month intervals thereafter.
3. CD4$^+$ cell count: Is essential for evaluating the status of the immune system. In healthy adults, levels average approximately 600 to 1400/mm^3. It is recommended that CD4$^+$ cell counts be preformed at 4-month intervals for most patients.

► HIV
1. Blood, semen, vaginal secretions
2. Many
3. Early
4. Women

► HIV AND AIDS
1. True
2. False—end stage of HIV infection is AIDS
3. False—anyone may contract HIV if exposure occurs
4. True
5. False—an incubation period occurs following exposure, so testing 1 to 2 days later would be inconclusive; antigens are detectable 2 weeks after infection with the virus
6. False—standard precautions are used with all patients, so isolation is not routinely necessary for patients with AIDS unless ordered for special reasons

► CRITICAL THINKING
1. The patient is told that he is HIV positive but does not have AIDS at this time. With treatment, HIV is considered a chronic condition that may not develop into AIDS for many years. If AIDS develops, there is currently no cure.
2. CD4$^+$ T-cell count of less than 200/mL and the presence of 1 of 25 clinical conditions. These conditions are often opportunistic infections or cancers.
3. To prevent opportunistic infections from developing.
4. (a) Candidiasis, medications, and peripheral and central nervous system disease tend to decrease the senses of taste and smell. This, along with discomfort, anorexia, and fatigue, predisposes the patient with AIDS to nutritional deficiencies. (b) Medicated swish and swallows, topical anesthetic sprays, and flavor enhancers may promote an increased food intake.
5. It occurs from encephalopathy caused by direct infection of brain tissue by HIV.
6. Bodily secretions of infected person coming in contact with recipient's blood through a break in the skin.
7. The recommended disinfectant is household bleach in a 1:10 dilution mixture. Use it to (a) clean toilet seats and bathroom fixtures; (b) clean inside the refrigerator to avoid growth of mold; and (c) wash clothing separately that is soiled with blood, urine, feces, or semen. Dishes are washed normally in hot soapy water and rinsed thoroughly after use.

▶ REVIEW QUESTIONS

The correct answers are in **boldface.**

1. (**d**) is correct. (a, b, c) are incorrect.
2. (**d**) is correct. (a, b, c) are incorrect.
3. (**a**) is correct. (b, c, d) are incorrect.
4. (**d**) is correct. (a, b, c) are incorrect.
5. (**c**) is correct. (a, b, d) are incorrect.
6. (**b**) is correct. Fruits and vegetables increase bowel function. (a, c, d) are incorrect.
7. (**a**) is correct. (b, c, d) are incorrect.
8. (**d**) is correct. (a, b, c) are incorrect.
9. (**b**) is correct. Cooked vegetables are safer. (a, c, d) are incorrect because they contain raw foods, which are riskier for infection.
10. (**b**) is correct. Standard precautions are used for all patients. (a, c, d) are incorrect.

55

ANSWERS

VOCABULARY

1. Coping
2. cognitive
3. Psychopharmacology
4. biofeedback
5. phobia
6. obsession
7. bipolar
8. psychosomatic or somatoform
9. schizophrenia
10. delirium tremens

DEFENSE MECHANISMS

1. Denial
2. Rationalization
3. Reaction formation
4. Compensation
5. Repression
6. Displacement or transference
7. Projection
8. Restitution
9. Avoidance
10. Conversion reaction

CRITICAL THINKING

1. Dirty hair, clothing, and personal hygiene are not normal. Neither is morbid obesity. A good way to open up communication related to the subject is to ask if she would like you or an assistant to help her with a bath. If her state of cleanliness is bothersome to her, she will most likely welcome the help and maybe even share information as to why she has been unable to bathe. On the other hand, if she refuses help or says she doesn't need a bath, further assessment of her ability to care for herself is warranted.

2. It should become fairly obvious whether Mrs. Jewel knows where she is and whether she is oriented to person and time during routine data collection. If you have any doubts, ask specific questions such as "Where are you? Why are you here? Who is this sitting over here?" (Point to a family member if one is in room.) "What year is it?

Who is the president of the United States?" (Or other questions most people should know.)

3. During routine data collection, listen carefully to Mrs. Jewel's responses. Document any irrational or inconsistent responses.

4. For recent memory, ask questions such as what she ate for breakfast, or ask about a news event in the last week that everyone should have heard about. For remote memory, ask questions about her younger years, such as where she lived, the name of her grade school, or the year she got married.

5. There is no special questioning needed to assess communication ability. Simply pay attention to her responses to routine questions. Document unusually fast or slow speech, stuttering, inappropriate volume, or difficulty getting ideas across.

6. *Affect* is the outward expression of emotion. If this expression does not match what Mrs. Jewel is telling you, or if it is inconsistent with her situation, her affect is inappropriate. For example, it would be unusual to be laughing about being in the hospital.

7. Asking her to explain a proverb (such as "a stitch in time saves nine") will help determine if she has good judgment. In addition, you might ask her what she would do under certain circumstances, such as if her blood sugar was low. Keep in mind that her response might reflect both judgment and knowledge.

8. *Perception* is the way a person experiences reality. Pay attention to her responses to your questions. For example, if she stopped taking medication for her diabetes because some little voices told her to do so, her perception is faulty. Normal responses are based on reality.

REVIEW QUESTIONS

*The correct answers are in **boldface**.*

1. (**b**) is correct. Appropriate behavior is a sign of mental health. (a, c, d) may or may not correlate with mental health.

2. (**b**) is correct. Blaming is a type of projection. (a, c, d) do not necessarily involve blaming others.

3. (**c**) is correct. It is important to establish a therapeutic relationship for psychotherapy to be effective. (a, b, d) are not helpful for the patient with mental health problems.

4. (**a**) is correct. This amount of sleepiness is unusual. (b) may be true, but this is not a decision you should make independently; (c, d) are not independent nursing actions.

5. (**c**) is correct. Drinking alcohol before flying could impair judgment and cause harm to the pilot and others. (a, b, d) are all reasonable and safe responses to anxiety.

6. (**b**) is correct. The patient may be disoriented following electroconvulsive therapy (ECT). Maintaining safety is a primary goal during this time. (a) restraints are inappropriate, (b) the patient should not be discharged until he or she is oriented and safety is ensured, and (d) oxygen is not standard treatment following ECT.

7. (**d**) is correct. A stressor must be defined by the patient. (a, b, c) although surgery, divorce, and loss of a job would seem stressful to most people, it is important to allow the patient to identify for herself or himself what is stressful.

8. (**c**) is correct. This response lets the patient know what is real, then distracts with a walk. (a, d) do not correct her misperception, and (b) is not speaking respectfully.

9. (**b**) is correct. Fluctuations in sodium affect metabolism of lithium. (a, c, d) are not known to affect lithium.

10. (**c**) is correct. Pill counts, although unreliable at times, are the most reliable source of data of the responses given. (a) The patient or (b) significant other may not provide accurate or truthful data, and (c) refills may or may not have been taken.

11. (**a**) is correct. Group support is one of the most effective treatments for alcoholism. (b) Drugs may be used during acute withdrawal but are not ideal for long-term therapy, (b) ECT is not a treatment for alcoholism, and (d) reducing alcohol consumption is not successful for most people.

12. (**d**) is correct. Speaking to other staff so that the patient cannot hear may be interpreted personally by the patient. (a, b, c) are therapeutic for the patient with schizophrenia.